PICTURING MEDICAL PROGRESS

FROM PASTEUR TO POLIO

A HISTORY OF MASS MEDIA IMAGES AND POPULAR ATTITUDES IN AMERICA

BERT HANSEN

RUTGERS UNIVERSITY PRESS

NEW BRUNSWICK, NEW JERSEY, AND LONDON

Library of Congress Cataloging-in-Publication Data
Hansen, Bert, 1944–
Picturing medical progress from Pasteur to polio : a history of mass media images and popular attitudes in America / Bert Hansen.
   p. ; cm.
Includes bibliographical references and index.
ISBN 978-0-8135-4526-4 (hardcover : alk. paper)
ISBN 978-0-8135-4576-9 (pbk. : alk. paper)
1. Medicine—United States—History. 2. Medical innovations—United States—History. 3. Medical illustration—United States—History. 4. Health in mass media—United States—History. 5. Popular culture—United States—History. I. Title.
[DNLM: 1. History of Medicine—United States. 2. History, 19th Century—United States. 3. History, 20th Century—United States. 4. Mass Media—history—United States. 5. Public Opinion—United States. WZ 70 AA1 H25p 2009]
R151.H25 2009
610—dc22   2008038707

A British Cataloging-in-Publication record for this book is available from the British Library.

Visit our Web site: http://rutgerspress.rutgers.edu

Manufactured in the United States of America

CONTENTS

ACKNOWLEDGMENTS

Early assistance in exploring popular images of medical discovery came from undergraduate students at SUNY-Binghamton and from medical students at New York University who undertook research on the news coverage of one or another medical discovery, including Eleanor Langer, David Leibowitz, Thomas Moffe, Theresa Pagliuca, and John Rescigno. David's research paper won the Osler Medal of the American Association for the History of Medicine and was eventually published. Research by New York University graduate students Ersi Demetriadou, Jean Howson, and Mark C. Young further expanded my knowledge. A course paper by Richard E. Weisberg at NYU grew into a dissertation demonstrating important changes in the portrayal of physicians in nineteenth-century French painting. Ronald J. Fasano, a graduate student at Baruch College and my research assistant for two years, created the initial database for my collection of medical history images.

Fellow historians and friends have been generous with informal advice, encouragement, insights, and research assistance on matters large and small over many years. I am indebted to Susan Abrams, Vincent DiGirolamo, Ann Downer-Hazell, David Gaudette, Normand Gauthier, the late Gerald L. Geison, Victoria A. Harden, Jon Harkness, Paul Jackson, Craig Long, Howard Markel, Barbara Melosh, Harvey Mendelsohn, the late Dorothy Nelkin, Gregory Robinson, Michael Sappol, Darwin H. Stapleton, Alexandra Stern, Elizabeth A. Toon, Linda Ehrsam Voigts, Judy Tzu-Chun Wu, and Masha Zakheim. Strangers, too, have pitched in, often by means of the Internet. I thank the following individuals, whose specific assistance is acknowledged in the book's notes: Leslie Bailey, Ron Goulart, Richard F. Krentz, Janet K. Mock, the late Gerard Piel, Cecilia Rasmussen, Roger K. Smith, and Maggie Thompson.

The contributions of librarians, archivists, and curators to historical scholarship are always vital and often invisible. Several colleagues have helped me repeatedly: Adele A. Lerner of New York Hospital/Cornell Medical Center, Miriam

Mandelbaum of the Rare Book Collection at the New York Academy of Medicine, Stephen E. Novak of the Health Sciences Library of Columbia University, Michael Rhode of the National Museum of Health and Medicine of the Armed Forces Institute of Pathology, Randall W. Scott of the Popular Culture Collection of the Michigan State University Libraries, Arlene Shaner of the Rare Book Collection at the New York Academy of Medicine, Micaela Sullivan-Fowler of Historical Services at the Ebling Library for the Health Sciences at the University of Wisconsin–Madison, and George A. Thompson, Jr., of the Bobst Library at New York University. For help with specific inquires, I also thank Carol Bodas of the Library of the Salk Institute, Jack Eckert of the Countway Library of Medicine, Michele Lyons of the Stetten Museum at the National Institutes of Health, Jeffrey A. Mifflin of the Archives of the Massachusetts General Hospital, Karen Nickeson of the Billy Rose Theatre Division of the New York Public Library, Sarita B. Oertling of the Moody Medical Library of the University of Texas Medical Branch at Galveston, and Annick Perrot of the Musée Pasteur in Paris. This project would have been impossible without the steadfast professionalism of Baruch College's Interlibrary Loan Service, especially the energetic assistance of Louisa Moy and Eric Neubacher.

The George and Mildred Weissman School of Arts and Sciences of Baruch College has supported my research generously over the years with time released from teaching. The History Department's strong commitment to scholarly research has been essential. At Baruch and the City University of New York, I owe special thanks for the steadfast encouragement of Myrna Chase, Matthew Goldstein, James McCarthy, Kathleen Waldron, and Cynthia Whittaker. Through the kindness of Dean Chase, the Weissman School provided a subvention for this book's color plates. Over many years, research expenses were supported in part by grants from the City University of New York's PSC-CUNY Research Award Program. I am also honored to acknowledge a Eugene M. Lang Junior-Faculty Research Fellowship at Baruch in the summer of 1998. Second only to the continuing research support from my own university, a major contribution to my scholarship was made by the Institute for Advanced Study, where I was in residence for the academic year 1984–85 and the fall of 1997. The institute provides a most congenial environment for scholarship, and I am grateful for its support of my research.

Several colleagues and friends have provided constant encouragement and enthusiasm over the time I worked on this book. That they also read drafts and suggested cuts has been immeasurably helpful. Roslyn Bernstein has been a wonderful colleague, a critical sounding board, and an engaged reader. Jacalyn Duffin and I have been talking, arguing, and laughing together about images in the history of medicine for more than a decade; her good sense and her encouragement have been crucially important. Janet Golden expressed enthusiasm for the project at a critical turning point; she also gave a much longer version of this book a critical reading to help sharpen its focus and arguments. Caitlin Hawke and I have been sharing an interest in things Pasteurian for more than a decade, and it has always been a pleasure to work with her on common projects. William H. Helfand is well known for his generosity in sharing both his profound knowledge of medical history images and access to his rich personal collection of graphic art. I am indebted to him for many kinds of help, and he has long been an enthusiastic friend of this project. Doreen Valentine has been a great collaborator, and she is an editor par excellence. The talents of Andrew Katz sharpened the work during copyediting, and I am especially gratified by his design and layout for the book. I thank them all for their contributions to making this a better book, while acknowledging that its errors and infelicities are my responsibility alone.

Material from three articles of mine is used with permission of the journals.

"America's First Medical Breakthrough: How Popular Excitement about a French Rabies Cure in 1885 Raised New Expectations of Medical Progress," *American Historical Review* 103:2 (April 1998), 373–418.

"New Images of a New Medicine: Visual Evidence for Widespread Popularity of Therapeutic Discoveries in America after 1885," *Bulletin of the History of Medicine* 73:4 (December 1999), 629–678.

"Medical History for the Masses: How American Comic Books Celebrated Heroes of Medicine in the 1940s," *Bulletin of the History of Medicine* 78:1 (Spring 2004), 148–191.

Permission to reprint copyrighted images is acknowledged in the individual captions. I extend a special note of thanks to Regina Feiler at Time Inc. and to Julie Grahame, the Karsh Representative for North America. The original illustrations reproduced here are all in my personal collection except for color plate 22 and figures 2, 17, 23, 25, 27, 29, 38, 40, 44–50, 55, 66, and 108. An extended passage from *Microbe Hunters* by Paul de Kruif is quoted with the permission of Houghton Mifflin Harcourt Publishing.

PART I

THE SETTING

CHAPTER 1

MEDICINE IN THE PUBLIC EYE, THEN AND NOW

F OR AMERICANS OF THE 1950s, the single most important newspaper and magazine story was the successful field trial of Jonas Salk's new vaccine to prevent infantile paralysis. Fear of polio had been pervasive in the lives of ordinary people, heightened by the uncertainty of when, how, and where it would strike. Although polio cases were measured in the thousands, not millions, infantile paralysis was every parent's fear. With the vaccine breakthrough, feelings of hope and relief overwhelmed the more than twenty million U.S. households with children.

The publicity surrounding this triumph was unprecedented in magnitude, as was the enormous number of people involved in the clinical trial and the rapid mass distribution of the new vaccine. The press and the public of the 1950s had been somewhat prepared for such medical advances, with penicillin and "blue baby" surgery in the 1940s, but no one could have foreseen the tidal wave of enthusiasm and appreciation for the new polio shots. Typical of many such front pages in the evening papers on April 12, 1955, was this two-line banner headline above the masthead of the *Chicago Daily News*: "Victory against Polio! Salk's Vaccine Works." Secondary headlines explained, "Salk's Vaccine Does the Job against Polio: 80 to 90 Per Cent Effective, Medical Jury Tells the World."[1] Use of the new shots began immediately. Less than twenty-four hours after the announcement, children in Los Angeles were receiving the vaccine. A photograph of the first child ran the following morning in the *Los Angeles Times,* along with an article reporting that President Dwight D. Eisenhower had decided to share vaccine data even with "red countries."[2]

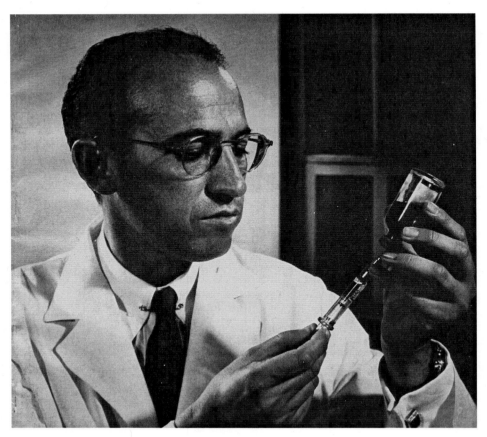

FIG. 1. "Dr. Jonas E. Salk: Portrait by Karsh of Ottawa," © Yousuf Karsh, used with permission of the Karsh estate. All rights reserved. This image appeared as the cover of *Wisdom: The Magazine of Knowledge for All America* 1:8 (August 1956); magazine dimensions: 10.5 by 13 inches. Author's collection.

Although a number of scientists and doctors received credit for the years of work leading to this triumph, physician Jonas Salk gained the lion's share. He was often photographed as a contemplative medical research worker, emblematic of the entire enterprise, in an iconic pose that originated in a famous painting of Louis Pasteur from the late nineteenth century. For example, in a portrait by Canadian photographer Yousuf Karsh (fig. 1), Salk's eyes focus intently on the bottle of vaccine, almost as if it were a holy object. *Wisdom* magazine put this photograph on its cover for August 1956.[3] *Life* magazine employed the same iconography, opening a major article with a photograph by Alfred Eisenstaedt in which Salk holds a large culture bottle of polio virus over his head toward the light and stares intently at the liquid.[4]

But even as such images idolized the triumphant doctor's mysterious genius, they included recognizable tools of medical work such as the vaccine bottle and the syringe. These features made him immediately recognizable as a medical hero, even if a viewer might not find the face familiar. This style of heroic medical portraiture employing symbols of laboratory activity or clinical care—though quite familiar today—was not an age-old tradition in pictures of doctors. During the eighteenth and nineteenth centuries, such accoutrements had been absent from honorific portraits and news drawings of physicians. They made their initial appearance in the 1880s with popular images of Louis Pasteur. The seventy years from Pasteur's rabies shots to Salk's polio shots thus constitute a single era of medical imagery, marked off from a prior era that had its own quite different image of the successful physician. This iconography continued beyond Salk's era, but it lost dominance in the later decades of the twentieth century, when medical discovery became less personalized and when doubts arose about medical progress. This book explores that seventy-year era between Pasteur and Salk but looks first at images of the prior era to establish a clear contrast with the innovations of the 1880s.

A second image of the 1950s concisely embodies both the sequence of changes from Pasteur to polio and a popular notion of the twentieth century. "Slow but Sure," an editorial-page cartoon by Bruce Shanks, appeared in the *Buffalo Evening News* during the first week's excitement about the polio vaccine (fig. 2). "Father Time" enters the Salk vaccine into the great book of medical history, adding polio to a list of diseases that medicine has conquered: smallpox, diphtheria, and pneumonia. Cancer and heart disease still await solutions, but the overall picture celebrates progress in medicine. This drawing not only elevated the vaccine's debut as an event on the world-historical stage but also confirmed the mass-culture view that saw medicine as steadily making progress with a series of giant steps. Shanks himself won a Pulitzer Prize for editorial cartooning just a few years after this drawing was published.[5]

Through such graphic documents of popular culture, this book analyzes the general public's image of medical advance from the mid-nineteenth century to the mid-twentieth. It describes the static picture of doctoring in the era when medical advances were neither expected nor greeted with public enthusiasm. It demonstrates that only in the 1880s did a new iconography emerge through the media coverage of the work of Louis Pasteur's rabies shots. And unlike many other transitions from a traditional to a modern outlook, this change was not gradual but sudden and swift. This study documents the new imagery, claiming also that the social history of the popular images can provide historians with access to the thoughts and feelings of people at the time. It argues that key features of the Pasteur episode served as a template shaping the perception of succeeding breakthroughs. This transformation added the promise of cure to the older expectation of care as a characteristic of medicine's public image. Most prominent among the features of the new consciousness that arose in the 1880s were popular curiosity about medical discovery, enthusiasm for medical advance, a belief that novelty in medical treatment is desirable, and expectations that scientists will produce ever-more-powerful and ever-more-numerous practical innovations.

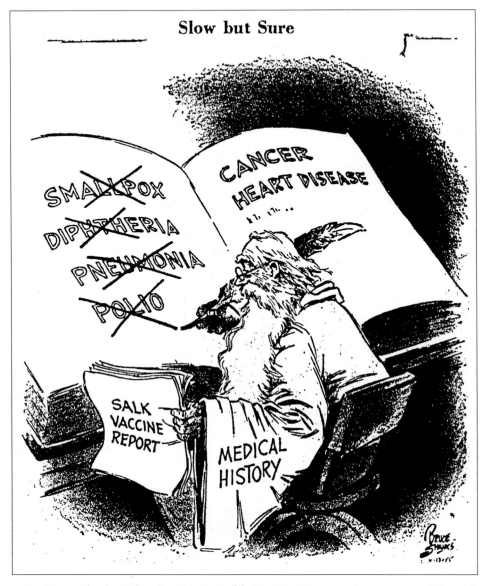

FIG. 2. Bruce Shanks, "Slow but Sure," *Buffalo Evening News,* April 13, 1955, 44. Editorial-page cartoon. © 1955. Used with permission of The Buffalo News. All rights reserved.

This book also illustrates how institutional developments well beyond science and medicine facilitated these innovations. For example, the timing of the first breakthroughs resulted from a convergence of scientific change with new technologies and new business structures in the mass media. Among the consequences of the public enthusiasm for laboratory medicine engendered by the first breakthrough was the unprecedented emergence of institutes to undertake substantial scientific research. The popular picture of those new institutions was shaped by structural innovations in the media, namely, a new economic base for magazine distribution and new technologies to reproduce graphic images, including photographs. Entirely new media were invented, and for the generation after World War I, radio, motion pictures, photojournalism, and comic books became the vehicles through which images of medical progress were disseminated. In the 1920s, the history of medicine made its debut in mass culture, taking a place alongside ongoing reports of new medical advances. As the pictorial record in these media makes clear, the initial Pasteur episode had been iconographically so powerful that it continued to shape people's ideas and emotions about medicine through the middle of the twentieth century.

A comprehensive collection of images has been tapped for examples, and they have been interpreted with a strict focus on their meaning to ordinary people at the time they were published. The effort has been to see those images as people saw them then, to discern what contemporaries found in them, and to recognize which images were deeply assimilated into the general public's outlook.

Graphic images are historically significant because they often convey more specific meanings, prompt more intense feelings, and engender more lasting effects than discursive communications. Popular pictures provide access to ordinary people's thinking, but they are often ephemeral, appearing in less prestigious media. The imagery in editorial cartoons, magazine stories, magazine advertising, health education pamphlets, radio shows, Hollywood movies, or children's comic books has been largely ignored by historians of art and underutilized by historians in general. More typically, historians of science and medicine have written about oil paintings, precious objects, pages from illustrated books and professional journals, and rare photographs. But such visual materials did not circulate widely and cannot offer much information about the thoughts and feelings of ordinary people. In trying to re-create something of the feelings among ordinary Americans in the past, this study restricts itself to images and documents that were reproduced in large numbers for wide general consumption.

In pursuing a history of popular ideas and culture, this study intentionally makes little use of the insider reports that are so valuable for recovering the history of scientific and medical discovery: articles in professional journals, papers delivered at scientific conferences, diaries and laboratory notebooks, personal letters, unpublished photographs. Further, this quest directs its attention to the effects of public images and does not usually go behind the media stories to consider why the artists created their images, how the editors made their decisions, or what social forces impinged on them both. Instead, the most important primary sources for this study are documents from the regular life of the ordinary citizen: daily newspapers, popular magazines, radio shows, and movies. Even though these sources may well be less than accurate for revealing the making of an advance, they are the best key to documenting the public awareness of what was changing in science and medicine. These verbal and visual productions preserve the imagery that was in wide circulation. Additionally, they make it possible to track a continued engagement with discoveries, as certain stories are retold and commemorated repeatedly in a range of popular media.

It would be risky simply to presume that publications, even those printed in large numbers and widely distributed, were always read closely or that their contents were fully absorbed. Hence, the challenge for a historian is to find as often as possible some additional evidence confirming how ordinary people responded to the published imagery. Sometimes this additional evidence means letters to the editor. Sometimes it means people flocking to see a display or event. Sometimes it means work by writers and artists that presumed that ordinary folks were already familiar with a phenomenon, an idea, an image, a point of view. Special evidentiary value is thus found in jokes and editorial cartoons that would not have "worked" unless the audience already had certain images in their heads. A popular song sheet about Brown-Séquard's Elixir, an electioneering cartoon that adapted medical scenes to its own purposes, a milk-bottle cap honoring Dr. Salk, or commercial advertising that invoked a discoverer's name can provide the best indication —other than a contemporary opinion poll might offer—of what people knew and felt about medicine.

One little scene from pictorial newspapers in 1886 illustrates these general points. Though this particular engraving was printed in France and then in Denmark and was perhaps not published in the United States until the twentieth century, its place of origin is less significant than the questions it prompts.[6] The subject of the engraving is Louis Pasteur watching a boy being injected with the rabies vaccine in a medical clinic swarming with onlookers (fig. 3). These injections were brand new in late 1885 and, hence, a good subject for popular news magazines such as *Le Journal Illustré* and *Nutiden* in early 1886.[7]

This image, which I found in the mid-1970s in a picture book on modern biology, first prompted for me the question of why rabies shots had caught the attention of the general public. That busy crowd, together with the fact that the media were recording the public's curiosity and excitement about the procedure (and in the process inducing further curiosity in others), gave unambiguous evidence that this particular medical innovation was a public event, not just a scientific one, that it was something being widely talked about at the time, and that it was regarded as something exciting enough to go out of your way to see—even though there was little to see besides a fine needle injecting a small amount of fluid under the skin of a patient's belly. I also began to wonder which other medical advances might have been accorded this level of mass popular interest. What I did not know as I began my exploration of these questions was that no one had examined the history of medical breakthroughs or established how they first arose. Nor could I confirm before completing several years of research that the rabies breakthrough, on which I had accidentally stumbled, was clearly the very first medical breakthrough that played out on the public stage in the United States. Nor did I realize then how powerful some of the Pasteur images had been in establishing an entirely new and enduring iconography of the medical scientist at work.

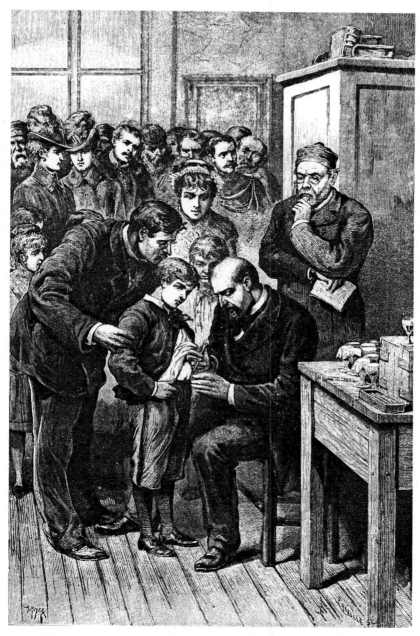

FIG. 3. "Vakcination hos Pasteur," *Nutiden* 507 (June 6, 1886), 359. This weekly Danish newspaper reprinted the image found in a French magazine, *Le Journal Illustré* of March 28, 1886. In translation, the French caption reads, "Rabies vaccination session at the laboratory of the Ecole Supérieure in the presence of Louis Pasteur, Dr. Grancher, and [their assistant] Eugene Viala, drawn from life by Meyer, engraved by Meaulle." Author's collection.

Novelties that enamored the public were not always the same as those that garnered the medical profession's approval at the time. Nor were they the ones that dispassionate scholarship has judged most significant over the long term. This book's narrative, focusing on popular enthusiasms, includes episodes that have seemed unimportant to historians, if they have been noticed by them at all. Conversely, it pays little attention to advances, even objectively important ones, if they made no splash at the time in the public consciousness, such as the introduction of ether anesthesia in 1846. In popular culture, in contrast to the history of medical discovery per se, each country or culture will have a different series of medical breakthrough enthusiasms. This is the U.S. story, even though the medical heroes that thrilled Americans were sometimes French or German, Italian or Canadian.

Americans still have a passion for medicine and a romantic view of medical discovery, although tragedies, failures, and scandals starting in the late 1950s prompted occasional disillusion with medical research and introduced cracks of hesitation and skepticism in the prior era's overwhelming enthusiasm for medical progress. Those challenges to credibility and confidence did not, however, completely halt the romance with medical research that first blossomed in 1885 and bloomed steadily for seventy years.

CHAPTER 2

BEFORE THERE WERE MEDICAL BREAKTHROUGHS

DISEASES AND DOCTORS IN THE PICTORIAL PRESS, 1860–1890

[*The* Daily Graphic] *is a marvelous paper. . . . I hope you will be able to keep it going all the time, for I don't care much about reading . . . but I do like to look at pictures, and the illustrated weeklies do not come to me as often as I need them.*

—Mark Twain, letter in the *New York Daily Graphic*, March 14, 1873

S INCE MEDICAL BREAKTHROUGHS as far-reaching media events were entirely unknown in the United States before 1885, what pictures of health care did ordinary people have in mind before this change? How did the graphic media portray medicine? If change was not paramount, what were the enduring commonplaces? Between 1860 and 1885, the imagery changed little, and popular sentiment retained the centuries-old understanding, shared by physicians and patients alike, that little ever changed in medicine. Even by the early 1880s—with important new scientific discoveries being made in anatomy, physiology, cell biology, and bacteriology—medicine had seen few successful advances in therapy and none that made a sensation in the press.[1]

Evidence of negative feelings about doctors and doctoring in this era of transition is widely available. Two brief jokes that appeared in *Judge,* a national weekly paper of political and social satire, neatly illustrate how longstanding cynicism was repackaged in the 1880s. In late 1885, readers were told, "A doctor in Chicago became crazy by dosing himself with cocaine. The case is a rare one. It is to the credit of the intelligence of the medical profession that they do not often make the mistake of taking their own medicines."[2] A few weeks later, *Judge* targeted the profession again, leavening this assault with antifeminist sentiments: "Five times as many ambitious women take to medicine as to law. This contradicts that generally-received idea of the sex that they delight in scandals and quarrels, but abhor cruelty and killing."[3]

Still, the widespread pessimism about the quality of medicine did not entirely inhibit people's seeking out professional medical help when they were seriously ill. Nor did it keep them and their doctors from having confidence that the treatments often "worked."[4] Popular culture is never entirely consistent.

Images in daily newspapers before the 1890s were generally small enough to fit within a single column of type. Large woodcuts and lithographs appeared in weekly publications. Around midcentury, photographs became useful as a supplement to artists' sketches as the source of images that were drawn onto blocks or stones for reproduction, but photographs could not be effectively printed in large press runs before the 1890s. The wood engravings and lithographs (including chromolithographs) that appear in this book fall into roughly three types: direct copies of a painting, drawing, or photograph; cartoons and caricatures drawn by artists; and pictures based on an artist's sketch (sometimes imagined and sometimes recorded on the spot). The last might be "action shots" of newsworthy activities or portraits of worthy or interesting people or buildings.

Pictorial news reporting came into its own in the United States with the establishment of *Frank Leslie's Illustrated Newspaper* in late 1855.[5] The specific story that first gave critical momentum to the use of on-the-spot illustrations was *Frank Leslie's* exposé of the so-called swill milk problem in New York City dairies where cows were fed on brewery waste.[6] Pictures not only enlivened the reporting but made it seem accurate and true; frequent drawings showing the paper's artist at the scene were intended to confirm the authenticity of the images and, hence, of the articles themselves. *Harper's Weekly: A Journal of Civilization,* founded in early 1857, did not start out to emulate *Frank Leslie's* but soon adopted its model.[7] Like *Frank Leslie's, Harper's Weekly* had been including some graphics from the start, but in the pre–Civil War years the text remained paramount. The success of *Frank Leslie's* persuaded *Harper's Weekly* of the public's strong interest in seeing what was happening in the field during the war, forcing *Harper's Weekly* to abandon the primacy of text and make pictures central to its character.[8]

Graphic images of health and medicine also frequently appeared in two nationally circulated magazines of political commentary and social satire: *Puck* (German-language edition founded in 1876, English-language edition in 1877) and *Judge* (founded in 1881).[9] Both these weeklies were slightly smaller in format than the news weeklies, but their circulation was enhanced and their identity established by the full-page color images on the front and back covers and on a double-page center spread. *Puck* usually inclined toward supporting Democratic Party figures, but it could be quite independent. *Judge* was more usually Republican but liked the reforming tendencies of the Democratic Party's candidate, Grover Cleveland, in 1884. *Frank Leslie's, Harper's Weekly, Judge,* and *Puck* could all be found in middle-class homes, as well as in libraries, men's clubs, barbershops, taverns, and railroad waiting rooms.

Aggressively appealing to lower levels of taste and income across the country was the *National Police Gazette.* This pictorial weekly purveyed "sporting news" for the barbershop and racetrack crowd, focusing its attacks more typically on personal and sexual scandals than on politics and policy. But occasionally its lurid images and its sensationalized text included physicians and scientists, including the French chemist Louis Pasteur. Founded in 1847, the *Gazette* became a financial success and a cultural force only in 1878.[10] It was printed on notorious pink paper; its woodcuts were crude compared to those in *Harper's Weekly* and *Frank Leslie's,* but they were large, lively, and splashy.

Another newspaper important for its use of graphics at this time is the *New York Daily Graphic.* It was established in 1873 and lasted only until 1889. Although it did not have as full a national presence as the other papers had, it is remarkable for producing five times a week an eight-page issue filled with timely and generally well-crafted wood engravings. It had an impressive broadsheet size, with a single large picture on the front every day. Its graphics included news sketches, joke cartoons, and social and political satire.[11] These six periodicals were by no means the only newspapers and magazines carrying pictures, but they are the ones that provided the richest presentation of medicine before the 1890s.[12] Circulation numbers varied considerably, but approximate numbers are still useful. The circulations of *Judge* and *Puck* rose over time to roughly ninety thousand copies a week. For *Frank Leslie's* and *Harper's Weekly,* the numbers approached two hundred thousand by the 1890s.[13]

PHYSICIANS

By the mid-nineteenth century, doctors had long been a socially recognized group, but most people most of the time avoided them even when injured or sick. Further, only a few doctors in this era, quite unlike their twentieth-century descendants, were well-off, of high social status, or intellectually supported by a demanding education. In the 1860s, many doctors lacked a medical diploma and had been trained only through an apprenticeship. Furthermore, formal medical schools did not expect a baccalaureate degree of their applicants, or even a high school diploma.[14]

Still, a doctor was recognizable in life and in newspaper graphics, cartoons, and caricatures as a man (almost always) wearing a dark suit, what one weekly referred to as "his professional broadcloth and fine linen," and often holding or wearing a top hat.[15] The high hat was as characteristic of doctoring then as the stethoscope and the lab coat are in the present day. Beards were a common style for doctors in this era, and in time they came to be an expected part of a physician's appearance. For example, in an 1889 cartoon satire, "The Importance of the Beard" by Frederick Opper, a serious young doctor without a beard lacks for patients, while his slack but bearded colleague has a crowded practice.[16] A St. Louis doctor's personal statement in a newspaper made the same point: twenty-six-year-old Dr. Chapman V. Dean remarked, "Don't you know that if I could raise a beard my practice would be twice, and possibly three times, as large as it is?"[17]

That doctors were not visually differentiated from other men of a similar social or professional class is clearly evident, for example, in the numerous news drawings of the bedside of President James A. Garfield in the several weeks between his being shot by assassin Charles Guiteau on July 2, 1881, and his death on September 19. The male doctors were largely indistinguishable by attire, posture, and activity from politicians and male relatives.[18] The medical attendance on President Garfield was somewhat unusual in including a woman doctor, "Mrs. Dr. Susan Edson," who can be seen fanning the president to provide relief from the oppressive summer heat and humidity of Washington, D.C. (fig. 4). The engraving reproduced here was on the cover of a pictorial newspaper published in London, England, but it is a close copy of the main section of a double-page engraving appearing in *Harper's Weekly* three weeks earlier.[19] Readers of *Harper's Weekly* learned from the text associated with this image that Mrs. Garfield and Dr. D. Willard Bliss were standing at the head of the bed and that General David G. Swaim, an old friend, was seated. But without such verbal assistance, a viewer would be unable to recognize simply from appearance which persons in the picture were the doctors.[20]

A contemporary political satire (fig. 5) presents a strong contrast in tone and artistic style to the news drawing of President Garfield's sickbed, while portraying the appearance of doctors in much the same way. These "doctors" are consulting on the case of a sick political party, the Democratic Party, in bed with "softening of the brain." From left to right, the physician caricatures are recognizable as Samuel J. Tilden, a leading Democratic politician from New York and the defeated presidential candidate in 1876; Charles Dana, editor of the *New York Sun*; and Henry Watterson, editor of the *Louisville Courier-Journal*. In the caption, Dr. Dana says, "It's almost too good to hope for, Gentlemen; but I think the 'Bad-Republican-Nomination Cordial' may pull the old fellow through yet!"

Clearly the medical activity of these consultants is verbal, not manual, though someone may have written prescriptions for the tonics and pills piled up on the bedside table. No medical instruments and no characteristic garments are in evidence. In fact, a viewer recognizes these figures as physicians only from the setting and the caption, as their gentlemanly dress would not by itself signify their profession.

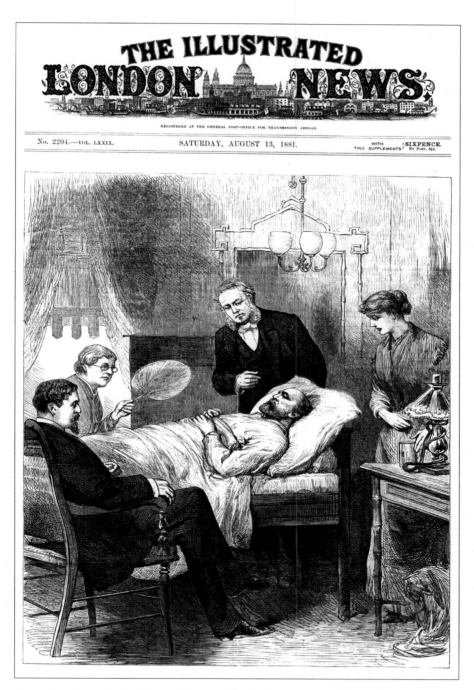

FIG. 4. "President Garfield Lying Wounded in His Room at the White House, Washington," *Illustrated London News* 79:2204 (August 13, 1881), cover (141). Unsigned wood engraving. This image was not credited to another magazine, but it is clearly based on a center spread, "The President's Room," *Harper's Weekly* 25:1283 (July 23, 1881), 504–505. Author's collection.

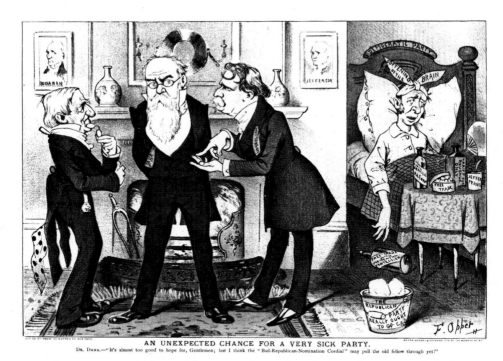

AN UNEXPECTED CHANCE FOR A VERY SICK PARTY.

Dr. Dana.—"It's almost too good to hope for, Gentlemen; but I think the "Bad-Republican-Nomination Cordial" may pull the old fellow through yet!"

FIG. 5. "An Unexpected Chance for a Very Sick Party," *Puck* 15:379 (June 11, 1884), back cover (240). Chromolithograph by F. Opper. Author's collection.

Before 1890, it was rare for newspapers and magazines to picture physicians as physically active in the work of healing; they were most commonly sitting or standing in the patient's bedroom, often consulting with other physicians. Timing the pulse with a pocket watch was the most common patient-care activity depicted. From time to time, doctors were portrayed giving a minimal health examination to immigrants or performing vaccinations. When in the 1880s New York City provided a "summer corps" of physicians to visit the poor in their homes as a step toward reducing contagious diseases, especially among children, one of these young doctors was illustrated on the cover of *Harper's Weekly*.[21] The wood engraving by William A. Rogers shows the young doctor standing with a woman in her living room. She is holding a child, and the doctor has his ear against the baby, listening for heart or bowel sounds without a stethoscope. Except for a "doctor's bag," no medical accoutrements are evident, and he wears normal business attire. Even when a doctor's medical career was celebrated, as in magazine stories about a prominent physician or in obituaries, his accompanying portrait would have been indistinguishable from that of a politician or a banker. A typical example of such a portrait is the engraving of Dr. J. Marion Sims in a June 1876 *Harper's Weekly*.[22]

A cartoon that emblematically paired a doctor with a lawyer makes the same point and highlights the longstanding conventions often used to indicate these professions. Although comic in style, this 1873 cover of the *New York Daily Graphic* (fig. 6) was merely illustrating the story of a professional convention, not mocking the participants. A local celebrity, Clark Bell, the chairman of the medico-legal dinner, is caricatured sympathetically for his role in bringing doctors and lawyers together. Two figures represent these learned professions, and each bears symbols

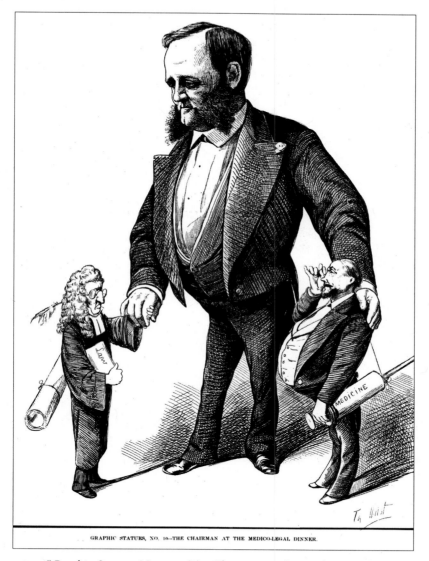

GRAPHIC STATUES, NO. 10—THE CHAIRMAN AT THE MEDICO-LEGAL DINNER.

FIG. 6. "Graphic Statues, No. 10 — The Chairman at the Medico-Legal Dinner [Clark Bell]," *Daily Graphic* 1:40 (April 18, 1873), cover (1). Wood engraving from drawing by Theodore Wust, full page of a daily newspaper in a larger format than the weeklies: this page is 14 by 20.5 inches; for comparison, *Harper's Weekly* and *Frank Leslie's Illustrated Newspaper* were usually about 11.5 by 16 inches. Author's collection.

identifying him to viewers, much like saints in a religious painting. The attorney is recognized by his wig, a scroll, and a book labeled "Law." The physician is known by a large clyster, a centuries-old sign of doctors' role in stimulating the evacuation of the bowels. But note that without the clyster, his attire and posture would offer no clue, as the dinner chairman, a lawyer, wears the same suit and vest as the doctor. Before the 1890s, doctors looked largely the same across a range of news drawings, joke cartoons, and political caricatures, whether they were being honored or mocked.

And mocked they often were—for failure to cure, for ignorance, for venality. Physicians were a natural target for negative feelings because they earned their living from other people's misfortune and because they were associated with pain and death, even when they were not the cause of it. Pessimistic, cynical, and disrespectful cartoons and verbal jokes about doctors were common in newspapers and magazines of the era. When covering the trial of a pharmacist for making a fatal error in preparing a remedy, for example, the *New York World* reported with no apparent sense of exaggeration, "There were so many doctors present that District Attorney Winfield said that all the patients in Hoboken would get well if the trial lasted a week."[23] Since prosecutor Winfield needed physicians as witnesses, he could not have been expressing personal hostility but only joking about a common view of doctors. Similar skepticism about the benefits of a doctor's care appears in a cartoon entitled "A Wise Precaution," in which an old man is speaking with his wife at home. The man remarks, "I really must get my life insured; I am not feeling very well. I think I will call in on Dr. Gilbert and get some medicine, and to-morrow I will get insured." His wife replies, "Don't you think, Tommy dear, it would be safer to get insured first?"[24]

More antagonistic than the sarcasm of such humor were portrayals of doctors as recklessly self-serving, especially when linked with commercial enterprises or public agencies that failed to protect the public from danger. In "The Streets of New York" (fig. 7), cartoonist T. Bernhard Gillam shows an undertaker expressing gratitude on behalf of his friend, the doctor, for the city's failure to clean the streets. In "Our Mutual Friend," the doctor and the cemetery manager congratulate each other on the presence of poisonous colorings used in candy as redounding to their benefit (see color plate 1). Here, as elsewhere, verbal captions are needed for a viewer to know which man in a suit is the doctor.

HOSPITALS AND MEDICAL CHARITY

That very few images before the turn of the twentieth century showed doctors in hospital settings might seem odd to modern observers, given the huge presence that our hospitals have as the site of complex medical care. But during the nineteenth century, hospitals were few in number, and hospital care was avoided except by the

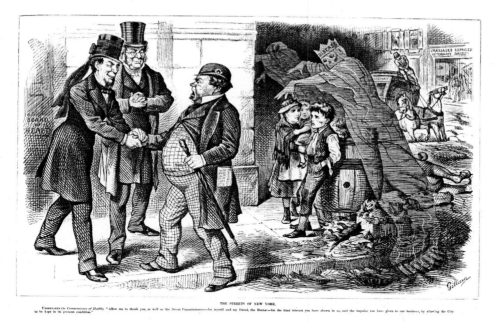

THE STREETS OF NEW YORK.

FIG. 7. "The Streets of New York," *Harper's Weekly* 25:1261 (February 26, 1881), 135. Full-page cartoon by T. Bernhard Gillam. Author's collection.

most desperate patients. Most doctors did not receive any of their training inside hospitals. Only a tiny number of American doctors chose to serve a term as a resident physician or, once well established in a career, contributed to medical care for the poor by serving in the role of attending physician. Hospitals were managed by laypersons as charitable, not medical, institutions.[25]

Hospitals' buildings, however, did appear frequently in the illustrated newspapers (fig. 8). The papers rarely showed interiors or any medical activity. Hospitals were routinely portrayed as architectural achievements, monuments to civic pride, or important changes to the landscape or cityscape.[26] Notably, they were not celebrated as sites of therapeutic interventions or lives saved.

Even bedside scenes in hospitals seldom showed physicians or nurses at work. Occasionally, hospital wards could be glimpsed in images soliciting donations in support of hospitals, showing charity work by laywomen in hospitals, or providing exposés of hospital management failures. These images, both positive and negative, were especially influential in shaping many people's notions of hospitals, since most Americans never entered their doors. Only the very poor stayed in hospitals before the 1890s, and visiting hours were so restricted that even family members of patients had limited opportunity to enter their precincts.

Apart from municipal hospitals in a few larger cities and federally funded care for out-of-town merchant seamen, nineteenth-century U.S. hospitals were generally established and maintained by Protestant denominations, Jewish congregations, and

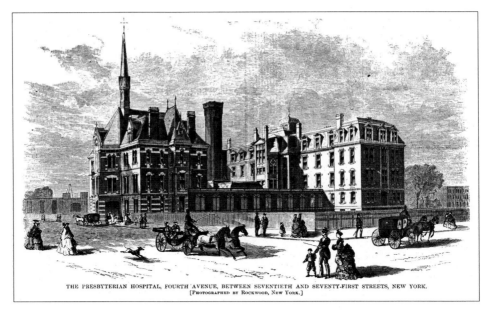

THE PRESBYTERIAN HOSPITAL, FOURTH AVENUE, BETWEEN SEVENTIETH AND SEVENTY-FIRST STREETS, NEW YORK.
[Photographed by Rockwood, New York.]

FIG. 8. "The Presbyterian Hospital," *Harper's Weekly* 16:829 (November 16, 1872), 901. One-third-page wood engraving. Author's collection.

Roman Catholic dioceses and orders. A special offering to support the local hospital was commonly collected once a year, often in the week between Christmas and New Year's Day. As this pattern coalesced, organizations such as the Hospital Saturday and Sunday Association evolved to coordinate a cooperative pooling of the donations from individual congregations and to redistribute it among the hospitals according to need.[27]

Puck magazine's routine support for the Hospital Saturday and Sunday Association with cover and center-spread images illustrates just what was and what was not salient about hospitals. In "Puck's Hint for Hospital Sunday" in December 1884 (color plate 2), the spirits of an injured boy on crutches are raised by the charitable help he has received in the hospital, symbolized by a bouquet of flowers. The verses on the collection canister read, "Here Christian, Jew, and Pagan meet / All meaner thought above, / To lay at Charity's dear feet / The offerings of love." In the background, a large hospital ward is visible, with attendants at work. One of the nurses appears to be a nun, perhaps a member of the Sisters of Charity, who staffed hospitals in many cities.[28] In a similar promotional image on *Puck's* cover two years later, an injured workingman is shown being helped through these donations; and in the background, large edifices carry these hospital names: Presbyterian, St. Luke's, German, Skin and Cancer, and Mount Sinai.[29]

None of these promotional images featured a physician, medical devices, or any stronger symbol of cure than centuries-old crutches and bandages. In 1889, another

Puck cartoon, this time a huge, colorful center-spread image, presented the Hospital Association as more worthy than several other charities; but, here too, there was no symbolism showing medical care as the main purpose of hospitals.[30] To the public, as to the weeklies' artists, hospitals were still primarily charity-funded custodial enterprises, not curative ones.

Whereas middle- and upper-class husbands were expected to make cash donations to hospital work, their wives and daughters gave of themselves by organizing visits to hospital patients and by collecting donations of cut flowers for delivery to hospitals and shut-ins. In the illustrated newspapers, sketches of these activities open the sick rooms to our view, just as a century ago they opened a view for the great number of people who never entered a hospital themselves or observed it firsthand. Although the artists' subject matter was charity, the images also helped readers envision the hospitals' space and furnishings, the appearance of patients, and the absence of medical equipment. Such generic images cannot, of course, be read as records of a particular patient or hospital, but they must have been generally true to reality at that time or they would not have served their purpose. In November 1868, *Harper's Weekly* offered a scene of two ladies visiting a sick woman in a ward at the hospital for incurables on Blackwell's Island, New York (fig. 9). Since many hospitals did not accept cases of chronic illnesses, we may take this image as being of a patient in a particularly desperate situation.[31]

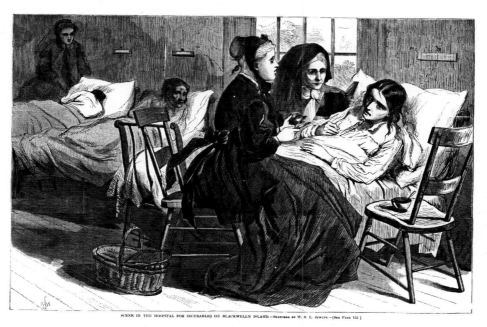

SCENE IN THE HOSPITAL FOR INCURABLES ON BLACKWELL'S ISLAND.—Sketched by W. S. L. Jewett.—[See Page 135.]

FIG. 9. "Scene in the Hospital for Incurables on Blackwell's Island," *Harper's Weekly* 12:583 (February 29, 1868), 136. Full-page wood engraving from sketch by W.S.L. Jewett. Author's collection.

During the nineteenth century, when hospitals served only the poor and their functions remained more custodial than medical, the public seems to have had kindly feelings toward them, sympathetic both to the misfortunes of the patients and the tribulations of the managers. There were few scandals or attempts at systematic reorganization or reform despite frequent deficiencies in staffing, visiting hours, food quality, and general upkeep. But at least once, editorial outrage sketched a disturbing scene that has been often reprinted and has thus become quite familiar today. This unsigned drawing of a scene in New York's Bellevue Hospital (fig. 10) appeared on the cover of *Harper's Weekly,* and its story, "Rats in the Hospitals," opened on the cover and continued on the second page. The report indicated that, a few weeks earlier, the stillborn child of Mary Connor had been eaten by rats. The report acknowledged that "the artist has peopled the scene to bring its horrors vividly before the public mind," while maintaining that "published evidence" proves "it is no exaggeration."

Despite the naturalistic style of this image, it was not like a "spot news" image in the modern sense; it was more akin to an editorial cartoon, endeavoring to motivate outrage about a general problem rather than to capture a specific situation. In the context of the entire page, with its masthead, border, and a benign unrelated image above it, the sketch's impact was probably not nearly so stark at the time as when cropped and isolated in modern reproductions.[32] Furthermore, the everyday familiarity with household vermin in the nineteenth century probably made this image less horrifying to people in the 1860s than to those of us looking back from our day. In both rural and urban settings, rats and mice were present always and everywhere. They scurried through school rooms and churches, storerooms and shops, kitchens and bedrooms. Even the richest in the fanciest homes would not have found it unimaginable to hear in the dark the sounds of rodent feet—however successful their household help might have been in preventing this intrusion most of the time. The everyday presence of rats and mice, even in middle-class homes, is confirmed by a line from the famous Christmas poem "A Visit from St. Nicholas," traditionally attributed to Clement Clarke Moore: "Not a creature was stirring, not even a mouse." That *Harper's Weekly* attributed the sanitation problems more to corruption than to vermin per se was confirmed in the following week's issue with a far less familiar cartoon, "The Night Superintendent of Bellevue Hospital" (fig. 11). The contented, large-bellied rat in a vest bears the same repulsive smugness of successful politicians often seen in political cartoons by Thomas Nast in *Harper's Weekly.* An editorial in this issue, "The Alms-House Rat," condemned the rat, asserting that he "personifies the corruption and waste and gross profligacy which corrode the public charities of New York."

If hospitals were places to be avoided as much as possible, even by the desperate poor, public dispensaries and charitable clinics were heavily used by a wide segment of the poor, the working class, and (if physicians' complaints are to be believed) by some middle-class patients who were able to afford private doctors.[33] Even more than hospitals, dispensaries were illustrated in the papers sympathetically, as calm

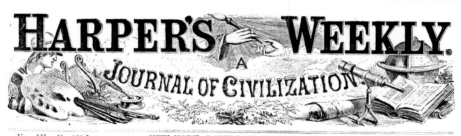

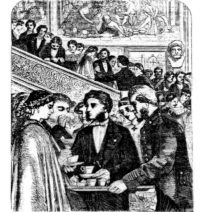

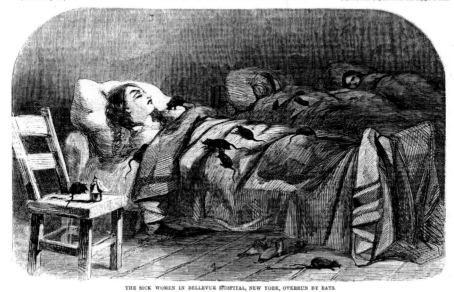

FIG. 10. *Harper's Weekly* 4:175 (May 5, 1860), cover (273). Two unsigned wood engravings: "Hearts May Be Broken by Light Words Spoken" and "The Sick Women in Bellevue Hospital, New York, Overrun by Rats." Full page. Author's collection.

yet crowded places where devoted caregivers served patients (fig. 12). It was reported that the New York Eye and Ear Infirmary served about 150 "sufferers" each day, over 10,500 in the prior year, and a grand total of 186,000 since it opened in 1820.[34] Although the doctors in this 1875 scene are better dressed than their patients and most of them wear full beards, all are in dark suits with a vest, without any evidence of a medical or surgical garment, apron, or even a cloth for wiping one's hands. A few metal tools are shown, but no antiseptic bath is yet visible.

Nurses—at least in their familiar modern incarnation as alert but gentle females in starched uniforms, often at a doctor's side—did not have a significant presence in U.S. graphic media prior to coverage of the Spanish-American War in 1898. This absence might seem surprising given that volunteer nurses served in military hospitals during the Civil War. But the actual numbers were low: only about three thousand nurses served on each side.[35] Starting in 1873, formal nursing schools were opened at a handful of U.S. hospitals. But the number of trained nurses in the United States was very low until the 1890s. Their presence was actually as

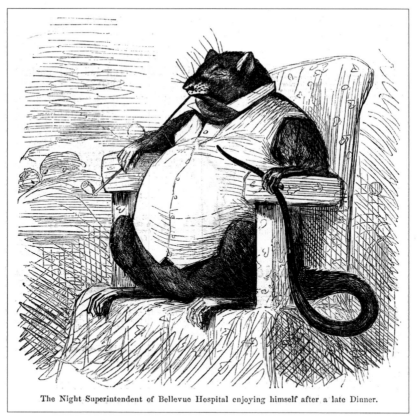

The Night Superintendent of Bellevue Hospital enjoying himself after a late Dinner.

FIG. 11. *Harper's Weekly* 4:176 (May 12, 1860), 304, "The Night Superintendent of Bellevue Hospital enjoying himself after a late Dinner." One-sixth-page anonymous wood engraving. Author's collection.

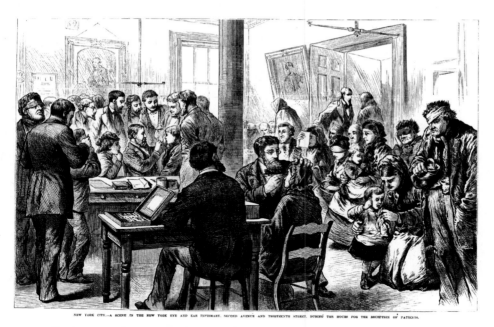

NEW YORK CITY.—A SCENE IN THE NEW YORK EYE AND EAR INFIRMARY, SECOND AVENUE AND THIRTEENTH STREET, DURING THE HOURS FOR THE RECEPTION OF PATIENTS.

FIG. 12. "A Scene in the New York Eye and Ear Infirmary, Second Avenue and Thirteenth Street, during the Hours for the Reception of Patients." *Frank Leslie's Illustrated Weekly* 40:1019 (April 10, 1875), 73. Anonymous wood engraving, full page. Author's collection.

sparse in the society as it was in the pictorial newspapers of the era. On occasion, a nurse might be illustrated as part of a military or hospital scene. The limited public consciousness of trained nurses before the end of the century is also evident in that only around 1900 did the medical sense of the word "nurse" begin to replace the older, common usage indicating a caretaker of young children. In the 1880s and 1890s, for example, there were many political cartoons that placed male politicians, or Uncle Sam himself, in the role of "nurse," with long skirt, full bosom, apron, and bonnet. But these were all children's nurses.[36] Nor did nurses gain any visibility during the flood of media images connected with the first decade of medical breakthroughs that began in 1885.[37]

FEMALE PHYSICIANS

Just as women in the domestic sphere (and men in the hospital setting) had been performing nursing functions long before the mid-nineteenth-century invention of formal nursing training and the beginnings of professionalism, some women without degrees had been providing medical care as "lady doctors" long before medical schools started admitting women at midcentury. But when women started earning the M.D. degree around 1850, it was the beginning of a significant if gradual transformation of the character of the medical profession, despite the small numbers of women medical students through the 1890s.

In January 1849, Elizabeth Blackwell, a young woman born in England who had lived in the United States since childhood, earned the first medical degree awarded to a woman in the United States. There were brief news reports on the event, largely as a curiosity, but evidently no pictorial coverage. The popular press did not treat Blackwell's early career either as a scandal or as a major change for the medical profession. Like some other midcentury events that were later to be celebrated by historians as medical firsts (such as Dr. William Beaumont's experiments on the physiology of digestion or the introduction of ether anesthesia for surgery), women's securing credentialed entry into the profession passed largely unnoticed at the time. From time to time over the next few decades, however, the public found female physicians pictured in their newspapers and magazines and could read about the new institutions they opened to serve female patients.

The most substantial illustrated account appeared in an April 1870 issue of *Frank Leslie's Illustrated Newspaper,* and it offered remarkable portrayals of activities at the Women's Medical College of the New York Infirmary, which had opened in 1868.[38] This infirmary and its medical school had been founded by Elizabeth Blackwell, and in 1870 it was under the direction of her sister, Dr. Emily Blackwell. The bulk of the newspaper's front cover was given over to a close-up view of a female medical student dissecting a cadaver's right leg (fig. 13). The student, with a metal instrument in each hand, seems to be lifting flesh with a forceps and measuring an interior part with calipers. She works alone, as calmly as if she had been doing embroidery, seemingly oblivious to the ghoulish setting. She may not be looking at the corpse as a whole, but we are, standing at the foot of the slab, forced to look first at the cadaver's bare feet and legs, its torso and arms covered (except for the hands) by a sheet, with another sheet covering the head, which is distinctly visible.[39] That this is not butchery but a science lesson is conveyed not only by the student's dignified focus on the work but also by the open box of anatomy tools and by the diagram of leg muscles visible in the open textbook at her elbow.

Inside the paper, this story included three more large images: "The Anatomic Lecture-Room," where about twenty seated students watch a female demonstrator point to parts of a partially draped cadaver; "The General Lecture Room," where seated students listen to a bearded man who reads from a book while standing near a microscope and a hanging skeleton; and "Dissecting Room—Students at Work" (fig. 14), where the women work in pairs on separate cadavers, each woman with an open book nearby, and an instructor walks around to help. This unusual set of images demonstrates that the new women doctors had been quietly assimilated into the public's notion of what constitutes a doctor, symbolized by their participation in the traditional rituals of the gross anatomy course and their entitlement to traffic in dead bodies, even defacing them in the course of learning to heal.[40] But in the 1870s, women doctors were still being inducted into the "old medicine." A "new medicine"—in which anatomy would be displaced by the study of microbes,

FRANK LESLIE'S ILLUSTRATED NEWSPAPER

Entered according to the Act of Congress in the year 1870, by FRANK LESLIE, in the Clerk's Office of the District Court for the Southern District of New York.

No. 759—VOL. XXX.]   NEW YORK APRIL 16, 1870.   [PRICE, 10 CENTS. $4 00 YEARLY. 13 WEEKS, $1 00.

MAJOR-GENERAL THOMAS.

HISTORY has not yet pronounced on the question, Which of the great military leaders of our late war is entitled to rank first as a soldier? If consummate military knowledge and skill, with the capacity to devise and the power to execute, and not the mere *prestige* resulting from a favorable conjunction of circumstances, are to determine the question, then the late Major-General George H. Thomas will stand on the record as the greatest captain our country has yet produced.

But General Thomas was more than a sol-

dier. His noble unselfishness, his proud modesty, and severe simplicity, were among the qualities that distinguished him, at a time when they were not conspicuous among the men accepted by a grateful country as among its heroes.

The military reputation of General Thomas, and the loftiness and dignity of his character as a man, had pointed him out as the probable, we had almost said undoubted, successor of the distinguished general now at the head of the nation. Had he lived, he would have been the almost unanimous choice of his countrymen, to whom his military career

would have been a great, but by no means his first, recommendation. As described by a daily contemporary:

"It is as the best type of the American soldier and patriot that his grateful countrymen will mainly choose hereafter to point to George H. Thomas. But since the close of the war, he has exhibited qualities of statesmanship of no ordinary kind. It would be unjust to forget the admirable, and, in some respects, unmatched, services which he has rendered to the political reconstruction of that Union which his sword helped to save. He came out of the war with a vast popular prestige, and he gave it all to the country. His very name was a tower of strength, and he lent it, unhesitatingly and utterly, to the policy of reconstruction settled on by Congress. He took the part of

the freedmen, and helped them to protect themselves. He was the terror of the Kuklux cut-throats, and the shield of order and society against anarchy and chaos at the South. The service he so rendered to the Union was hardly surpassed by the Mill Springs, the Chickamaugas and the Nashvilles, which his skill and valor had won, because his simplicity, his sincerity, his utter freedom from political bias, and his disgust of partisan tricks, were as well known as his masculine judgment, his strong common sense, and his incapacity to be deceived in what he saw, or to report it other than as he saw it. Hence his denunciations of anarchical elements at the South, and his bold advocacy of stringent means to remedy them, produced a wide-spread effect among impartial men of all parties, and words which might have been scouted as fanatical from others, came from him, as those of truth and soberness."

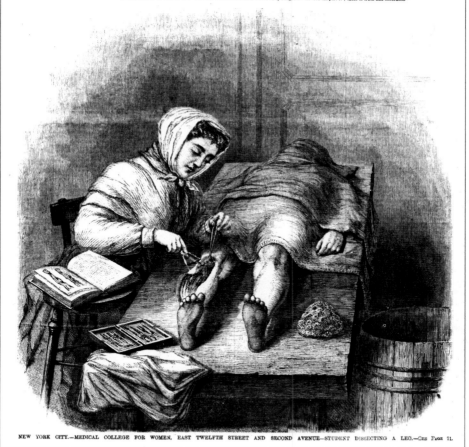

NEW YORK CITY.—MEDICAL COLLEGE FOR WOMEN, EAST TWELFTH STREET AND SECOND AVENUE—STUDENT DISSECTING A LEG.—SEE PAGE 71.

FIG. 13. "Medical College for Women. East Twelfth Street and Second Avenue—Student Dissecting a Leg," *Frank Leslie's Illustrated Newspaper* 30:759 (April 16, 1870), cover (65). Author's collection.

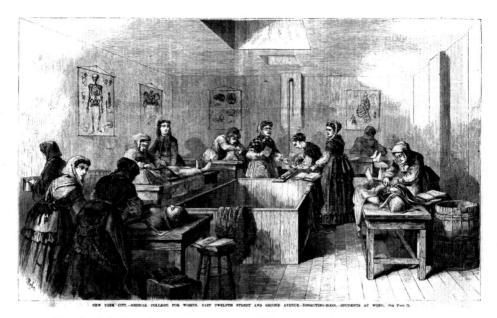

NEW YORK CITY.—MEDICAL COLLEGE FOR WOMEN, EAST TWELFTH STREET AND SECOND AVENUE—DISSECTING-ROOM.—STUDENTS AT WORK.   See Page 73.

FIG. 14. "Medical College for Women. East Twelfth Street and Second Avenue—Dissecting Room—Students at Work," *Frank Leslie's Illustrated Newspaper* 30:759 (April 16, 1870), 73. Full page. Author's collection.

and heroic chemical medicaments would face competition from "biologic" remedies originating in the research laboratory—lay in the future, far beyond anyone's imagination.[41]

THE TRANSFUSION OF BLOOD

An unusual and risky medical novelty made an appearance in the pictorial press of the 1870s and 1880s, showing up first in news drawings of a European experiment and then in several political cartoons: the transfusion of blood from a healthy human donor (or sometimes from a sheep) directly to a patient. In the summer of 1874, a news drawing of a crowded hospital bedside where a blood transfusion was taking place covered a full page in the Supplement section of *Harper's Weekly* for July 4; the same image reappeared a few weeks later in *Scientific American*.[42] In the procedure shown in these periodicals (fig. 15), the donor's blood spurted like a fountain, falling into a funnel connected to the patient with flexible tubing. When the funnel and tube had filled with blood, the funnel could be raised up to aid its flow by gravity into the patient's vein.

Transfusion was then a far from common medical practice, and it did not become a common one until an understanding of blood types was developed, clotting could be prevented, and other technical problems solved after about 1900. But the basic idea was simple enough that it could serve as the vehicle for a political metaphor even though the procedure would not have been part of the reader's experience, or even the experience of most physicians.[43]

In the political cartoons, the fountain-to-funnel apparatus was replaced with tubing interrupted by stop-cocks and a squeeze-bulb pumping device. Pictures of such devices were probably available to artists in medical instrument catalogues or medical textbooks. Both types of transfusion apparatus were fully illustrated, for example, in the huge *American Armamentarium Chirurgicum* published by George Tiemann and Co. in 1889.[44]

During the election campaign in October 1880, *Harper's Weekly* used an almost-full-page drawing by artist W. A. Rogers, "Transfusion of Blood—Is It Too Late?" (fig. 16), to characterize the Democrats' candidacy of Winfield Scott Hancock, a Civil War general, as an attempt to revive a completely debilitated Democratic Party. The physician figure, here as in so many other popular images of this period, has no characteristic attire and does not perform the operation in a recognizably medical setting. The election of the Republican candidate James A. Garfield a few weeks later confirmed that any such transfusion had indeed been too late to save the party. Rogers's interest in this metaphor may well have been prompted just a few months earlier by two long and detailed articles in the *New York Times*, one about

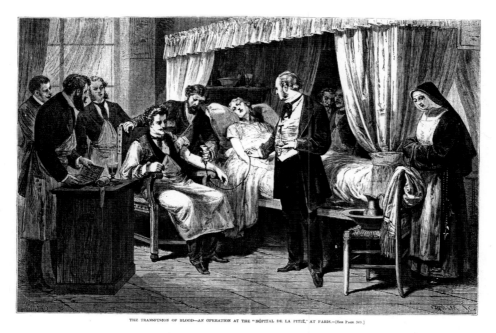

THE TRANSFUSION OF BLOOD—AN OPERATION AT THE "HÔPITAL DE LA PITIÉ," AT PARIS.—[See Page 569.]

FIG. 15. "The Transfusion of Blood—An Operation at the 'Hôpital de la Pitié,'" *Harper's Weekly* 18:914 (July 4, 1874), 570. Anonymous wood engraving, full page. Author's collection.

transfusion apparatus on public display in New York City and the other about successful operations.[45] The political metaphor did not originate with this artist, however, and it may have been commonplace. For example, three years earlier an untitled editorial in the *New York Times* included this remark: "The experiment of trying to rejuvenate the moribund organism [i.e., the Democratic Party] by a transfusion of Republican blood has been found a failure."[46]

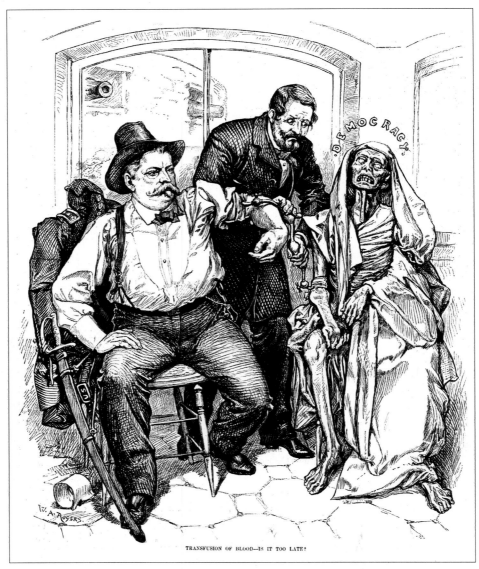

TRANSFUSION OF BLOOD—IS IT TOO LATE?

FIG. 16. "Transfusion of Blood—Is It Too Late?" *Harper's Weekly* 24:1240 (October 2, 1880), 637. Nearly-full-page wood engraving from drawing by W. A. Rogers. Author's collection.

In late 1884, after the election of Democrat Grover Cleveland as president on a "clean government" platform that drew reform votes from across party lines, a large, color center spread in *Puck* magazine by artist Joseph Keppler pictured the result in a cartoon using this metaphor again: "The Transfusion of Blood—May the Operation Prove a Success."[47] In this case, the donor of blood for the tired old Democratic Party is not the candidate himself but the strong, young "Independent Citizen." The character of Puck himself acts as the physician, timing the procedure with a pocket watch. The doctors in attendance are recognizable as caricatures of various Cleveland supporters. The point for my purpose in this book is not the political message but the public's access to imagery of an unusual medical procedure and of physicians as gentlemen in dark suits who gather to consult on cases, not yet as white-coated knights of the laboratory. Again, the procedure is portrayed simply as a dire expedient, not as an advance or a breakthrough. Progress was not yet a hallmark of medicine.

Four years later, the metaphor reappeared, this time in *Judge* magazine. In a full-page cartoon signed by "Hamilton M.D." (for artist Grant Hamilton), "Doctor Mills" (Roger Quarles Mills, congressman and later senator from Texas, who sponsored a "free trade" bill) proposes to the "American Workingman" that he risk donating his blood by giving up protectionism in order to save the languishing English industries (color plate 3). John Bull, the symbol for England, sobs in the background, and the hearty workingman is watched carefully by President Grover Cleveland while being warned against the procedure by "Doc Watterson" (Henry Watterson, editor of the *Louisville Courier-Journal*).[48] This cartoon provides less detail of the apparatus for blood transfusion than earlier ones, but it does include political versions of typical old-fashioned medications such as "free trade tonic," "free trade pills," and a tank of "free trade gas," to which is attached either a funnel-shaped ether mask or a mistakenly connected transfusion funnel.

In all the graphic renderings of blood transfusion, the procedure was shown as a desperate experiment of uncertain outcome, not as a successful innovation that might bring major changes to medical practice.

MEDICINE MEMORIALIZED AND MOCKED

Most of this chapter has explored medicine's imagery indirectly from pictures created for other purposes such as illustrating news or feature articles, praising or maligning political figures, satirizing social mores, and raising money for charity. Equally important are the less common artifacts of popular culture in which the primary visual message is a direct statement about the character of medicine or the medical profession, such as a medical exhibition in the nation's centennial year and editorial cartoons criticizing the medical profession per se.

National anniversary celebrations and especially the exhibitions that came to be known as "world's fairs" routinely offered the public at large an elaborate vision of notable achievements, past and present. Characteristically, these venues celebrated past advances and promised more in the future. At the world's fairs of 1904 in St. Louis, 1933 in Chicago, and 1939 in New York, medical achievements were prominent. But they were not so prominent at Philadelphia in 1876 or Chicago in 1893. For 1876, one looks in vain through *Frank Leslie's Illustrated Historical Register of the Centennial Exposition,* an oversize volume of 320 pages detailing the exhibits of the U.S. centennial exhibition, for any hint that medical science or medical care had changed over the preceding hundred years. Medicine was not even listed as a focus of interest in the official classifications of the exhibition's materials.[49]

There was, to be sure, a pavilion for health and medicine at Philadelphia's Centennial Exposition. But what did the organizers choose to feature there? Not the world's first successful ovariotomy by Dr. Ephraim McDowell in 1809, not the unprecedented experiments on the physiology of digestion by Dr. William Beaumont, published in 1833, that gained him international recognition within the medical world, not the introduction of ether anesthesia for surgery in Boston in 1846, not the successful repair of vesico-vaginal fistula by Dr. James Marion Sims performed in the 1840s and published in 1852—all of these advances appear prominently on later lists of the country's special contributions to the advancement of medicine. Rather, the exhibition's medical materials were all contained within the model post hospital of the U.S. Army. And in *Leslie's Register of the Centennial Exposition,* there is not even a mention, let alone an image, of the reconstructed army hospital.

The model hospital exhibit consisted of the hospital itself with twenty-four beds, showing the "arrangement of the beds and the conveniences provided in the army hospital for attending to the wants of the sick and wounded" (fig. 17). Mannequins in the beds indicated the proper treatment of injuries. Walls carried "photographs of difficult and successful amputations." Also on display were models of Civil War hospitals, models of hospital steamers, a display case of medical curiosities from the Army Medical Museum, a dispensary room with supplies, an office with instruments, books, and forms for medical records, a dining room and its furnishings, and a kitchen with its equipment and utensils. Additional items in the exhibit included medicine chests, litters, trusses, artificial limbs, hospital tents, ambulances, and wagons.[50] Though these items may have been up-to-date, they were all examples of traditional medical and surgical practice. There seems not to have been anything representing the new Listerian antisepsis. Tellingly, there was no laboratory, apparently no sterilization apparatus, no gallery of great doctors, and no list of medical advances—all of which the public regularly found at world's fairs after the turn of the twentieth century.

One physician did have a modest presence at the Centennial Exposition, though this was only by accident. The Philadelphia surgeon Samuel Gross was the subject of a new painting submitted by Thomas Eakins for exhibition in the fair's Art Gallery. But after this canvas was rejected by the fine-arts exhibit committee for being

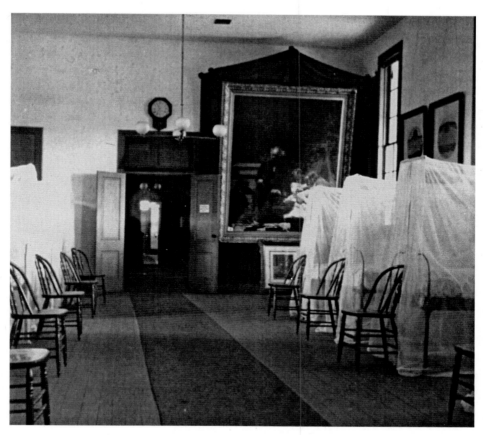

FIG. 17. Photograph of ward of the model Post Hospital, Medical Department, Philadelphia Centennial Exposition, 1876, with Thomas Eakins's painting of the Gross Clinic on the rear wall. Photograph Expo1876-05 of the National Museum of Health and Medicine, Armed Forces Institute of Pathology, Washington, D.C. Used with permission.

indelicate, it found itself hanging incongruously on a wall of the army hospital.[51] Significantly, it was the politics of art and decency—to be sure, it is a rather bloody picture—that brought Dr. Gross's portrait into the medical exhibit, not some plan to feature leading lights of U.S. medicine there.

While few doctors were being memorialized in the press for medical advances, many were being mocked for their foolishness in joke cartoons and editorial caricatures. Some images satirized them for personal faults; others berated the profession as a whole for its inability to effect cures. If most of these graphics were relatively gentle, editorial cartoons sometimes blasted systematic failings in the profession with a hostility that can be shocking to modern viewers in a time of enthusiasm for the benefits of advanced medicine. These cartoons—comic and critical at the same time—round out a picture of the public's mind-set prior to the advent of medical breakthroughs.

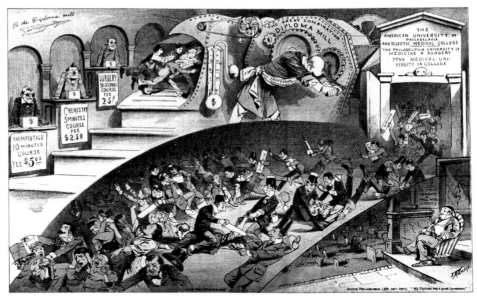

THE PHILADELPHIA PHYSICIAN-FACTORY.

FIG. 18. "The Philadelphia Physician-Factory," *Puck* 7:162 (April 14, 1880), 94–95. Double-page chromolithograph by J. A. Wales. Author's collection.

In early 1880, for example, *Puck* artist J. A. Wales created "The Philadelphia Physician Factory" (fig. 18), a center-spread cartoon in full color with the industrial imagery of a "diploma mill" that pulled boys into a hopper and cranked crowds of them out an exit chute as top-hatted doctors brandishing surgical saws and other instruments ready to assault unwilling patients. According to the editorial, this cartoon was definitely not attacking "the old-fashioned practitioner" or the profession at large but was attacking a Dr. Buchanan of Philadelphia, who had become a controversial figure for the way his proprietary school was pumping out graduates, essentially selling diplomas by mail order.

> Nothing is necessary [in the Philadelphia institutions]—no study, no love for the profession, no intellect—nothing but a face and a pocket full of brass. . . . But where is the old-fashioned practitioner by the side of the Philadelphia physician? The "Eclectic" College man can kill ten patients while the old fogy is curing one; he can spread disease like a pestilence incarnate; he can maim more men, if his taste happens to run to surgery, than a first-class civil war. Why, at the end of a long and busy life, the Philadelphia physician, sitting at the door of his noble mansion, and looking proudly over the well-filled aisles of his own private graveyard, can say to himself, with sweet complacency: "It's just as well that I never took the trouble to study—always got along just the same."[52]

Yet because this image was separated from the editorial text by six pages, it might not have been read as applying its aggressively negative image of doctors only to

those of a small number of disreputable schools. All medical schools in Philadelphia were loosely implicated in the broad sweep of the condemnation, and a reader
—knowing that caricatures often use one example to stand for a whole category—
might well have seen the diploma mill as standing in for all medical colleges. After
all, in this period, almost all medical schools were still proprietary, even those with
a formal connection to a general college or university. Moreover, similar surgery-
happy doctors appeared in other cartoons with no reference to fake diplomas, and
the link between doctors, undertakers, and cemeteries was a well-established trope
in cartoons of the era.

A cover image from *Puck* about three years later is less frantic but even more
vitriolic.[53] Its target is not the more common ones (quackery or venality) but rather
the inhumanity of the mainstream doctor, "the old-fashioned practitioner" who had
been treated so favorably in the words of *Puck's* 1880 editorial.[54] In the image, a
desperate mother's plea for help from a regular, or allopathic, physician is denied
because of his refusal to consult with a sectarian physician whom she had called first
(fig. 19). Dr. All. O'Path's gold-headed cane bears a death's head on the handle. As
Puck explained itself in its editorial,

> Professional etiquette is a very pretty thing. So is a discriminating wisdom in the choice
> of associates. So is the courage of one's opinions. But there are times when a too rigid
> adherence to these pretty things is, to say the least, undesirable. . . . Perhaps it is well that
> Dr. Oldschool should keep his professional broadcloth and fine linen free from all con-
> tamination. But the etiquette of the world prescribes limitations to the etiquette of the
> profession.[55]

As with the "diploma mill" image a few years earlier, *Puck's* editorial text was gen-
tler than the artwork, and the words made clear that not all physicians were being
criticized. But once again, the power of the graphic imagery probably overwhelmed
such distinctions.

In a striking image one year later, no distinction among doctors is made at all,
and thus there is no ambiguity in or limit to *Puck's* cynicism about the value of doctoring. In this image, all doctors are portrayed as worthless or dangerous and in ca-
hoots with the undertakers. Medical colleges are to be regarded as an unredeemable
source of human misery.[56] *Puck* ran "Our Merciless Millionaire" on its cover (see
color plate 4). The event that had occasioned this outburst of hostility was the proposed gift to the College of Physicians and Surgeons at Columbia College of half
a million dollars from William H. Vanderbilt.[57] Over a caption of "The Public Be
—Doctored!" Puck himself tries to protect the public by holding Vanderbilt back
from presenting the gift. In 1882, it had been widely circulated that Vanderbilt said,
"The public be damned" when a Chicago reporter asked whether he was running
his railroads for the benefit of the public or for his shareholders.[58] Although the formal focus in the drawing is *Puck's* challenge to Vanderbilt's planned donation, the
background figures reinforce opposition to this generous charitable gift: on the left,

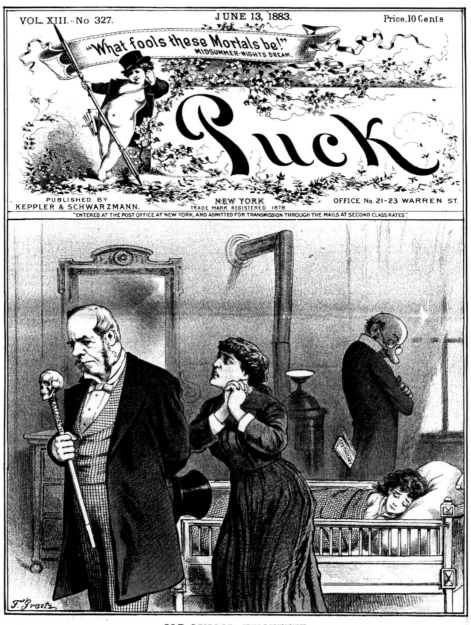

OLD–SCHOOL ETIQUETTE.

Dr. All. O'Path:—"Very sorry, madam, if your child must die; but you ought not to have called in a Homœopath first."

FIG. 19. "Old School Etiquette. Dr. All. O'Path—'Very Sorry, madam, if your child must die; but you ought not to have called in a Homoeopath first,'" *Puck* 13:327 (June 13, 1883), cover (225). Full-page chromolithograph by F. Graetz. Author's collection.

awkward-looking medical students wave their scalpels and surgical saws; in the center is a cemetery; and on the right is the delighted and grateful proprietor of "Crape & Planten Undertakers," with a sign announcing the establishment's references: "Dr. Give-em-up, Dr. Killem, and Dr. Skinner." This is a very dreary view of what doctors do, unrelieved by humor or irony, with even the puns making resolutely negative reference to the sorry effects of having to see a doctor.

The historical importance of an image such as this one—on the cover of a popular weekly paper of political and general humor with liberal leanings and a national readership in a German-language edition as well as in English—is found not in the artist's and editor's goal in printing it or in what specific and local effects it had on Mr. Vanderbilt or the Columbia medical school but in its upholding attitudes common as late as 1884 that medicine should be avoided and not promoted, that medical progress was not an element in medical care, and that medical education was not a deserving charity. A different kind of medical charity—custodial care for the poor in hospitals through the Hospital Saturday and Sunday Association—was highly laudatory. And, as seen earlier, *Puck* was for it.

In 1884, there was yet no public image in U.S. culture of medical research as an interesting or commendable activity. Medicine had nothing at all comparable to the radical innovations seen in science and technology, a cumulative series of discoveries celebrated under the rubric of progress. This was the era of the phonograph, the telephone, the electric light bulb, and the lightweight cables of the Brooklyn Bridge —all of them popular subjects of newspaper stories and images.[59] *Puck* cheerfully supported science, if not medicine, conspicuously honoring Charles Darwin and mocking his detractors in many cartoons. At Darwin's death in 1882, for example, he was illustrated in *Puck* as the sun shining high in the heavens and scattering the clouds of ignorance. He was acclaimed as "A Sun of the Nineteenth Century" in a pun on traditional accolades that celebrated great achievers as sons of their century.[60] But there were no similar accolades for medical innovators.

GENERAL IMPRESSIONS

Stepping back from *Puck* and its mockery of doctors to look at the images in this chapter as a group highlights a few general features. In popular media prior to the 1890s, doctors were attired as gentlemen, as members of a learned profession in "broadcloth and fine linen." The identifying symbols of their profession were not the stethoscope or the fever thermometer (though both had come into use), not the microscope (which, though widely known, was not yet seen as a medical tool), not the injection syringe with hollow needle; they were primarily a confident manner, a top hat, and a watch to time the pulse. Serious portraits and news drawings rarely illustrated doctors with scalpels and surgical saws, but humorous and satirical prints did.[61] Talking was their most commonly observed medical activity, consulting more often with one another than with the patient. When they were portrayed attending a patient in bed, they were seen taking a person's pulse, giving pills and spoons of liquid medicine, and charging for services whether or not the patient survived. In the pictorial media of this era, doctors appeared to have only a minor place in public health reform or in campaigns against poisons and adulterants in food. More frequently they were portrayed as conspirators in the corruption perpetrating these abuses. Although a few elderly doctors and medical professors garnered respectful obituaries in the national press, sometimes with portraits that looked just like those of bankers or politicians, none was celebrated for a life-saving discovery. None was a household name.

Considering this long-term stasis, in which medical practice seemed to change little and certainly seemed not to be growing in strength, might an acute observer still have discerned changes on the horizon? Were there hints of the developments that were to burst onto the scene in 1885? Were the sounds of experimental animals scurrying in cages and of glassware clinking on lab benches even faintly audible behind the everyday din of illness, accident, birth and death, crisis and recovery, fear of epidemics, and neglect of routine hygiene and food safety that made most people fatalistic about disease and about doctoring? The hints were few and unconnected; only in hindsight might an emerging trend be recognized. Even within the profession, there was no consensus that the novelties encountered by the recent American medical graduates who studied in Europe were more than curiosities.

In the mid-1880s, anesthesia for surgery and childbirth had been around for about forty years and was becoming more common, but it was still not universally applied, nor was it seen as the revolution that historians and patients later deemed it.[62] Listerian antiseptic procedures, introduced in the mid-1860s, gained some ground in a hit-or-miss fashion, especially with publicity they received when Joseph Lister toured the United States demonstrating his surgical techniques in the centennial year. Yet still, in 1881, when President Garfield was wounded by an assassin's bullet, the nation's best doctors casually probed his wound with dirty fingers and no anesthetic. If those initial examinations were not sketched for publication in the press, later efforts, when his condition stabilized, were illustrated in popular papers. In a large image of "The Discovery of the Location of the Bullet" (fig. 20), the public saw how Alexander Graham Bell, the telephone's inventor, was brought in to help the doctors determine the bullet's location with a new piece of apparatus he designed for this purpose.[63]

Ideas about distinct types of germs as causes of specific diseases had not yet coalesced into a coherent theory of infection. Discoveries being made in animal physiology through vivisection were, likewise, not yet changing much of medical practice, and they were seldom illustrated in the U.S. press, even by the opponents of such experiments. One large graphic of an electrical experiment on dogs did fill the front page of *Frank Leslie's Illustrated Newspaper* in August 1888. Four serious gentlemen are shown observing on a lab bench the reaction of a dog fitted with wires when the current is turned on. But the image does not depict a medical experiment;

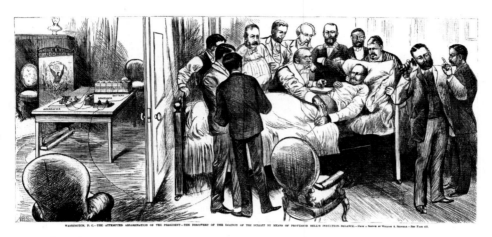

FIG. 20. "Washington D.C.—The Attempted Assassination of the President—The Discovery of the Location of the Bullet by Means of Professor Bell's Induction Balance," *Frank Leslie's Illustrated Newspaper* 52:1351 (August 20, 1881), 412–413. Upper portion of center-spread wood engraving "from a sketch by William A. Skinkle." Author's collection.

the experiment was engineering research to establish guidelines for the use of electrocution to replace hanging in capital punishment.[64] Still, it is noteworthy that a family paper could print a potentially disturbing image without fear of heavy criticism. Similarly, these family magazines repeatedly published illustrations of just how unclaimed, stray dogs in city dog pounds were dispatched by lowering a huge cage packed with animals into the river to drown them.

In the same year that *Puck* skewered medical education with "Our Merciless Millionaire," the *New York Daily Graphic, Harper's Weekly,* and *Frank Leslie's* all ran a few modest drawings of some of Louis Pasteur's experiments with rabbits, dogs, and monkeys. On June 16, 1884, the *Daily Graphic* ran a group of three sketches (a caged dog, an inoculated monkey in a cage, and Pasteur standing between two rows of rabbit cages), credited to *L'Illustration*. *Leslie's* ran Pasteur among the rabbit cages in its regular feature "The Pictorial Spirit of the Illustrated Foreign Press." Neither paper had any accompanying text. *Harper's* ran a short article with its page of naturalistic sketches entitled "Hydrophobia—M. Pasteur's Experiments" (fig. 21).[65]

This engraving of Louis Pasteur among his caged rabbits seems immediately accessible and intelligible, and it has thus become a popular choice for reproduction in the twentieth century. It seems to take us directly into his laboratory, and as historians, we are delighted to be offered such access. Yet, for all its seeming transparency as a document of its time, we must read it cautiously to discern just what the readers at the time it was published knew or thought about Pasteur's work. The *Harper's* piece was not a news story about a breakthrough for human medicine; it was a low-key report of interesting work in "experimental pathology." As explained in the *Harper's* text, the goal of the experiments was to find a way to prevent dogs from getting rabies and thereby to protect people from exposure to the disease. Medical

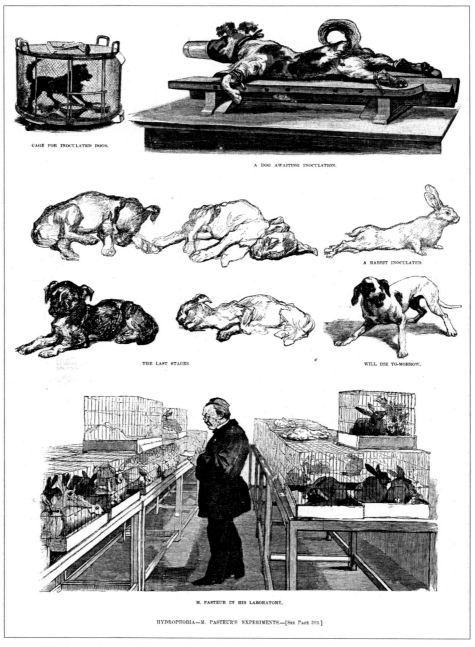

CAGE FOR INOCULATED DOGS.

A DOG AWAITING INOCULATION.

A RABBIT INOCULATED.

THE LAST STAGES.

WILL DIE TO-MORROW.

M. PASTEUR IN HIS LABORATORY.

HYDROPHOBIA—M. PASTEUR'S EXPERIMENTS.—[See Page 395.]

FIG. 21. "Hydrophobia—M. Pasteur's Experiments," *Harper's Weekly* 28:1435 (June 21, 1884), 392. Unsigned wood engraving. Author's collection.

treatment for people bitten by a rabid dog was not mentioned as an element of this work. Furthermore, Pasteur was a chemist, not a physician, and his was not yet a household name. He was known to a limited number of Americans for work on silkworm diseases and for procedures to improve the keeping quality of beer and wine. Pasteurization of milk did not become familiar for another two decades or more. In the 1884 image, Pasteur stands contemplatively among the animal cages —heavy ones of iron for angry dogs and lightweight wire cages for innumerable, placid rabbits. It is a slightly exotic scene, almost like exhibits at a country fair, except for distressing images of dogs showing the stages of paralysis leading to death. As with the electrocution experiments on dogs, this family publication, though often sentimental in style, had no qualms in the 1880s about explicit pictures of such material.

In less than two years' time, however, the results of Pasteur's hydrophobia experiments were to feed a new frenzy of enthusiasm for laboratory discoveries with the immediate power to save human lives. This unprecedented excitement was to create new popular expectations about the value of doctoring, about medical advance, and about medical philanthropy.

PART II

A NEW REGIME OF MEDICAL PROGRESS

CHAPTER 3

HOW MEDICINE BECAME HOT NEWS, 1885

Of late M. Pasteur's name has become a house-hold word in every country.
— exhibition catalog, Eden Musée, 1886

WHEN LOUIS PASTEUR announced the successful inoculation of a person with his experimental rabies vaccine in 1885, he was already well known to the French public. The chemist had been celebrated in France for such intellectual and practical achievements as preventing spoilage of wine and beer, saving the silk industry from a silkworm disease, and inventing a vaccine to protect cattle and sheep from anthrax. Across the Atlantic, however, his science and his name were familiar to only a small number of Americans, largely careful readers of *Scientific American* and younger physicians who had recently completed medical training in Europe.[1] The survival of the first rabies victim to be treated by Pasteur's method (Joseph Meister, who had been badly bitten by a dog and rushed from Alsace to Paris in hopes of a miracle cure) seemed likely to be quickly forgotten in the United States with no lasting effect on popular consciousness. Initial news coverage of Pasteur's discovery was hardly remarkable. The *Chicago Tribune,* for example, announced it as part of a cable dispatch from Paris on October 29, and the *New York Herald* reported it on the thirtieth, adding some reactions of New York doctors and the American Society for the Prevention of Cruelty to Animals. The *St. Louis Globe-Democrat* of

November 1 carried a report on Pasteur's first two patients. Routine articles in the *New York Times* and other papers gave it no greater attention. Then nothing significant appeared in the press until an accident made Pasteur's discovery newsworthy again in North America.[2]

In early December, a dog ran through the early morning streets of Newark, New Jersey, biting seven other dogs and six children. This event made the afternoon papers. Such occurrences were common and were commonly reported in the daily press, but this time the situation was different. Pasteur was quickly cabled for advice, and he agreed to receive and treat the young Americans. Their Paris journey to secure life-saving treatment created a sustained media sensation across the United States and Canada. This small incident abruptly transformed a trickle of modest news reports about a scientific announcement into a torrent of news articles, features, illustrations, editorials, jokes, published letters, cartoons, and even political satire. The excitement lasted several months, and it catapulted Louis Pasteur and medical research to celebrity—and to everyday familiarity—across North America.

THE SETTING FOR A MEDICAL SENSATION

The trip by four Newark boys to Paris is a story worth telling in its own right, but its significance lies in the ways the adventure prompted so much sustained attention by the press and the public that it changed popular expectations about medicine more generally. When U.S. newspapers and magazines devoted extravagant attention to the first Americans treated with Pasteur's brand-new rabies cure, they were not simply reporting an event with engaging human-interest elements. They were also elaborating a story of medical discovery as something useful and exciting to ordinary people. In the process, they were cultivating a thrill about medicine's being newly powerful and about scientific knowledge making a difference beyond the walls of the medical school and the laboratory. As a result, Pasteur's rabies treatment, though far from the most significant discovery of the age and not connected with the United States except by accident, stimulated a series of events and expectations that set a pattern through which later discoveries would be experienced.

Compared to cholera, tuberculosis, and the other major infections of the nineteenth century, the incidence of rabies (usually called hydrophobia in human cases) was very low.[3] Furthermore, its treatment was not based, as were several others, on the positive identification of the infecting microorganism. The introduction of diphtheria antitoxin in late 1894 has commonly been considered the pivotal episode for scientific medicine, when the honor is not assigned to ether anesthesia, aseptic surgery, or the germ theory. Though historians have largely ignored the rabies treatment and its effects on society and culture, the hydrophobia cure of 1885 may justly be called the first medical breakthrough for the way it galvanized the American public.[4]

Today we use the word *breakthrough* to designate the phenomenon of a *publicly recognized* major advance in science or technology. Not all advances are experienced as breakthroughs in this sense; some significant changes are not widely recognized, either because they are not useful (or not seen as such) or because they develop by gradual steps without having a concentrated impact. A new idea or invention is, in general, more likely to become a breakthrough to the extent the advance is seen as large, sudden, useful, already practicable rather than just potentially of use, and relevant to a wide public. These five possible attributes of a discovery are often mutually interdependent, but each is analytically important. Taken together, they highlight the most important general feature of a breakthrough: it is a social phenomenon, it exists only if it is something widely noticed at the time. And the very notice it receives often creates further effects.

Indeed, although the rabies-cure phenomenon was not called a breakthrough in its day, it exhibited these five attributes. Several months of incessant attention to the workings of laboratory science prompted by the cure helped to create new iconography and even new institutions. In the process, popular consciousness gained an entirely new idea that medical research could provide widespread benefits. This new expectation about progress helped to displace a centuries-old understanding (shared by physicians and patients alike) that little ever changed in medicine. Although mechanical inventions by Thomas Edison and others had generated grand enthusiasms at times, a medical development had never before captured the headlines in the United States with sustained popular attention. One important feature of the rabies vaccine that distinguished it from the typical benefits of germ theory was that it was used for therapy, not just diagnosis or prevention. Technically it was a preventive, as the injections were given after a dog bite to still-healthy people before any symptoms had appeared. Yet because people feared bites from a suspicious dog as tantamount to getting hydrophobia, the procedure was universally, if not accurately, viewed as a cure. This common misconception is important because, in the emotional ranking of popular enthusiasms, knowledge about disease without immediate application is hardly worth noting, preventives are mildly interesting, therapies are far more appealing, and successful cures (whether real or apparent) are at the top.

The phenomenon of the rabies breakthrough was also made possible by several changes in the newspaper business that converged in the 1880s. Although the image of American newspapermen rushing to get the latest news off the press and into the hands of waiting readers goes back to James and Benjamin Franklin and to Paul Revere, industrial innovations of the mid- and late nineteenth century first made it possible to bring the same news at the same time to large masses of people. High-speed, rotary presses powered by steam replaced the hand-cranked, flat-bed mechanism of the Franklins. By the mid-nineteenth century, newspapers could roll off the presses at the rate of tens of thousands per hour. The introduction of the land telegraph, followed by the laying of a transatlantic cable, improved remote access to the latest happenings. As the country became united by a network of railroads, editors everywhere could readily read—and often reprint for a local audience—other editors' long stories about faraway events. Additionally, when newspapers departed from their origins as organs of political parties and aggressively sought unaffiliated readers, especially new immigrants, they used both hot news and human-interest stories to attract them. Joseph Pulitzer successfully exploited these developments and helped reshape an entire industry. Though Pulitzer was hardly alone and though his paper was to play a smaller role in the Pasteur/hydrophobia mania than was the *Herald* of James Gordon Bennett Jr., Pulitzer's move to New York from St. Louis in 1883 to purchase the *World* was a major step in escalating the pursuit and creation of newsworthy thrills.[5]

THE EVER-PRESENT THREAT OF RABIES

When popular enthusiasm for a new kind of medicine did appear in the United States, it did not spring from Pasteur's pioneering 1882 vaccine for anthrax or Robert Koch's identification of the cholera bacillus that same year or Koch's discovery of the tubercle bacillus in 1883—all major landmarks in scientific medicine.[6] However much these advances appear momentous from our vantage point, they simply did not receive substantial treatment as news. The transformation in expectations about medicine's power to cure came rather from Pasteur's triumph over a quite minor disease. Rabies was a malady that killed people by mere dozens each year, in contrast with such major slayers as tuberculosis, pneumonia, smallpox, diphtheria, and infant diarrhea, which slew hundreds of thousands annually.[7] Hydrophobia in the United States, as in Europe and elsewhere—though well-known and widely feared—was a quite infrequent illness.[8] It was, however, invariably fatal. And since there was no sure way to determine whether an animal that inflicted a bite was rabid or not, fear of a horrible death followed every dog bite for weeks or months before one could be confident that the incubation time had been safely passed. A small wound or its quick healing did not mean one was out of danger, as people learned from frequent stories in the press.

In cities of that era, stray and feral dogs were remarkably numerous—if impossible to count. But an indication of the magnitude of the problem in New York City can be found in an official report in the 1880s tabulating the dead animals received at the docks for disposal; it records some eight thousand horses and twenty-three thousand dogs in one twelve-month period (with countless others incinerated, buried, tossed in sewers, and so on).[9] Contemporary estimates of the city's dog population, including both the strays and those with owners, ranged from 225,000 to 300,000. When Brooklyn, Newark, and other suburbs were added in, there were perhaps more than half a million dogs within forty miles of New York City.[10] In most cities, controlling a large dog population was nearly impossible. The sight of a policeman shooting at a dog was not uncommon, both on the street and in the pictorial press. On one magazine's cover in the summer of 1874, for example, a policeman aims his revolver at a saliva-drooling dog (fig. 22). Nearby, a fashionably

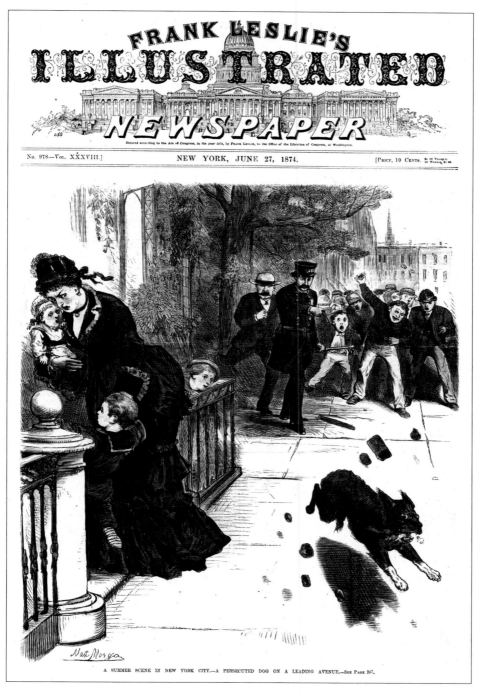

FRANK LESLIE'S ILLUSTRATED NEWSPAPER

No. 978—Vol. XXXVIII.]   NEW YORK, JUNE 27, 1874.   [Price, 10 Cents.

A SUMMER SCENE IN NEW YORK CITY.—A PERSECUTED DOG ON A LEADING AVENUE.—See Page 247.

FIG. 22. "A Summer Scene in New York City.—A Persecuted Dog on a Leading Avenue," *Frank Leslie's Illustrated Newspaper* 38:978 (June 27, 1874), cover (241). Wood engraving by Matt Morgan. Hand coloring was added later to the copy reproduced here; the original was not colored. Author's collection.

dressed lady is trying to protect three small children. Behind the policeman is a crowd of men and boys hurling rocks and cans as they chase after the dog.[11] Equally visible to the public was the official practice of drowning the impounded strays after a brief holding period; in a less squeamish era than ours, this procedure was graphically portrayed in the pictorial press.[12]

Although cases of hydrophobia were numerically infrequent (seldom running to ten a year even in a large city), newspaper editors believed their readers to be interested in the fascinatingly gruesome details. One typical account may stand in for hundreds of similar articles; it is quoted in full to illustrate the brief, but detailed, narrative into which ordinary newspaper readers of the era could imaginatively place themselves (and their children). This article ran in the *New York Times* on June 9, 1881. In addition to reporting local cases, U.S. dailies and weeklies regularly reported numerous rabies deaths even in far distant cities and towns.

DYING OF HYDROPHOBIA—TERRIBLE STRUGGLES OF A BOY WHO WAS BITTEN BY A VICIOUS DOG
A vicious dog was shot in the area of the residence of Mr. F. Gilbert, No. 208 Fifth-avenue, on the 2d of April. Several boys had been attacked and bitten by the animal, which was a half-bred Newfoundland bitch, on the West Side of the City, whence it had been chased. One of the boys, Frederick Herrman Kruger, aged 11½ years, died yesterday morning of hydrophobia, at No. 380 West Forty-second-street.

On the day that he was bitten, he had just returned from the Fortieth-street public school, and was playing with another boy in front of his home when the animal came along from Eleventh avenue pursued by men and boys. It jumped at Frederick, threw him in the gutter, and tried to seize him by the throat. The boy held his chin down, and the brute caught him by the nose and nearly bit off the end of it. The animal then escaped, and was seen later in the day at Thirty-first-street and Tenth avenue. It was again chased and was killed by Officer Link, of the Twenty-ninth Precinct.

Mrs. Kruger sent for Dr. Alfred W. Maynard, of No. 353 West Forty-second-street, who cauterized the wound and stitched the end of the nose in place. The injuries healed, leaving an ugly scar, and the incident was almost forgotten.

On Saturday, Frederick, who had been playing in the street, went home and asked his mother for a drink of water. She gave him some in a glass from a hydrant in the yard, but when he attempted to raise it to his lips the muscles of his throat contracted spasmodically and his features became distorted. Handing the glass back to his mother, he said that he was ill and asked for water that was not cold. Mrs. Kruger gave him a glass of tepid water, but he was unable to swallow this and was seized with convulsions.

Dr. Maynard at once detected unmistakable symptoms of hydrophobia. He administered hydrate of chloral and bromide of potassium until the convulsions were allayed, but they returned whenever water was offered to the patient.

Up to Tuesday the boy's condition changed little, but in the afternoon of that day he imagined that dogs were under the bed trying to bite him, and that some one was in his room ready to shoot or cut him. He kept his hand over his nose as if to shield it, and screamed so loudly at times that he could be heard a block away. Violent convulsions set in during the evening and three persons were required to hold him. Large quantities of morphine were administered hypodermically every half-hour.

In spite of this, the convulsions returned with increased force, and his cries, while they lasted, were agonizing. At 5:30 o'clock yesterday morning, when he died, his struggle was so great that three strong men, who were holding him down in bed, were exhausted. It is said that another boy who was bitten in the cheek by the same dog lives in the neighborhood.[13]

In this newspaper story, one is confronted not only with the pain of rabies but also with the terror of facing such a death, whether for one's children or for oneself. This article is typical in providing names, addresses, the biting encounter, the medical care, the healed wound, the helpless doctors, and the last agonies, including the ferocious, almost inhuman strength manifested by the victim near the end.

LOUIS PASTEUR'S RESEARCH

With a profound appreciation for the power of the fear and fascination of rabies, Louis Pasteur proclaimed in October 1885 that such tragedies were henceforth preventable. Pasteur was hardly alone in seeking to identify the microbial causes of human diseases. The 1870s and 1880s saw a flurry of such work, largely stimulated by Pasteur's discoveries in fermentation and the complex of tentative theories and procedures that came to be called "the germ theory of disease." In addition to seeking the etiological agents, Pasteur and his collaborators pioneered experiments to attenuate, or weaken, an infectious agent so as to reduce its capacity for causing serious illness, while preserving its ability to provoke in an inoculated animal a natural protective response and thereby prevent a subsequent infection by that same agent. Only one such protective sequence was known when Pasteur began his work, the prevention of smallpox in persons by inoculating them with smallpox matter or, more safely, with cowpox matter. (Since cowpox was also known as vaccinia, the process was called vaccination. After Pasteur achieved successful prevention of chicken cholera and anthrax, he applied the word vaccination to this process in general, no longer restricting it to inoculation with cowpox virus.)

Several characteristics of rabies made it an attractive subject for research: it was a well-recognized specific disease, easily distinguishable from other ailments; it was transmitted by a known route of contagion (unlike tuberculosis, plague, typhus, yellow fever, and many other common diseases at that time); and it had a determinable and relatively long incubation period. Pasteur's search for the causative microbe was unsuccessful, as was that of other researchers.[14] Rabies' characteristic fury and paralysis drew investigators to the nervous system as the site of the unseen microbe, and Pasteur's laboratory developed clever techniques of transmitting the disease from one animal to another by removing pieces of the brain or spinal cord and applying them directly to the exposed brain of a new subject. Opening the skull (trephination) was a surgical technique dating to ancient times in both the Old World and the New. Pasteur's assistants did it well, carefully using the newly discovered anesthetics of his era to keep the dogs and rabbits asleep for the surgery.[15]

By passing the undetectable rabitic agent through several generations of experimental animals, Pasteur was able to achieve a highly virulent infective matter of standardized potency (as measured by a consistent incubation time when new animals were inoculated). Once he had produced infective matter of known potency, he experimented with means of attenuating it and eventually established that air drying of infected marrow from a rabbit's spinal cord reduced its potency from maximum to minimum in about fourteen days.

According to Pasteur's reports in the 1880s and the widely disseminated biography by his son-in-law, René Vallery-Radot, he was successful using a remarkably simple procedure to create a natural resistance. Pasteur gave healthy dogs a series of inoculations with pieces of marrow that had been dried for a decreasing number of days, ending up on the final day with highly virulent marrow that was known to kill an animal after a short incubation period. This weakest-to-strongest system appeared successful in creating a refractory, or resistant, state in his experimental dogs.[16] Pasteur tested this state, his reports implied, by exposing treated dogs not only to virulent injections but also to natural rabies from bites by a rabid dog, and he announced a preventive vaccine for canine rabies in August 1884 at an international scientific congress at Copenhagen. During 1884, this work on canine rabies received an illustrated article in *Harper's Weekly* and a few brief notices in the daily press (see figure 21).[17]

Given the long incubation period of natural cases of rabies, Pasteur wondered if it would be possible to start the process of artificially creating resistance *after* an animal (or a person) had been bitten, with the hope that it might take hold before the "street infection" could do its lethal work. According to Pasteur's published accounts, he worked in the winter of 1884–1885 on vaccinating dogs after they had received rabid bites, and in March 1885 he began to consider the possibility of human trials, first on himself.[18] In the summer of 1885, fate intervened when Joseph Meister, a badly bitten nine-year-old boy from Alsace, showed up with his mother at Pasteur's laboratory. The tense scene was described in the biography written years later by Pasteur's son-in-law:

> Pasteur's emotion was great at the sight of the fourteen wounds of the little boy, who suffered so much that he could hardly walk. What should he do for this child? Could he risk the preventive treatment which had been constantly successful on his dogs? Pasteur was divided between his hopes and his scruples, painful in their acuteness.[19]

After consultations with physicians, Joseph Meister was given, under Pasteur's supervision, the first full human rabies treatment of twelve injections beginning on July 6, 1885, in a least-to-most-virulent series.

Although Pasteur valued press coverage, often cooperating with reporters to the point of co-opting them, he intentionally held back when it came to this human experiment and allowed no press coverage for fear of the public's misinterpretation of any failure. Keeping awareness of this experiment within a small circle, Pasteur worried privately through July and much of August that Meister might die and that blame would fall on Pasteur's efforts, whether or not his inoculations were at fault. As August progressed and young Joseph remained well, Pasteur regained his usual self-confidence, but he still made no public announcement. In mid-September, however, word of Meister's survival (and possible cure) started to become public even prior to Pasteur's making an official report to the Académie des Sciences. The first news reports were favorable but short and little noticed.

In mid-October, a second child was brought to Pasteur for treatment. Jean Baptiste Jupille, a fourteen-year-old shepherd, had courageously turned to face a rabid dog chasing five younger boys. He wrestled the dog to its death while suffering severe bites on both hands. Pasteur confidently invited the boy to Paris and began treatment about October 20.

On October 26, Pasteur presented a triumphant account of the Meister treatment at the Académie des Sciences, ending with the story of young Jupille's heroism. Leaders of the academy, medical and scientific, praised Pasteur effusively and applauded the youth's bravery. The press reported at modest length on the address and the meaning of the achievement, but time was needed to change a transient curiosity into a rampant enthusiasm. Reports in the U.S. press were dutiful and encouraging but lacked any human-interest angle. Through November, the articles resembled the brief items on other scientific and medical news in the 1870s and early 1880s, and most were shorter than the typical report about a death from hydrophobia or about cases of trichinosis after eating ham at a picnic.[20] But then everything changed radically in early December.

FROM LOCAL INCIDENT TO INTERNATIONAL EVENT

On December 2, 1885, in Newark, New Jersey, as on many other days in large cities and small towns, schoolchildren were bitten by a stray dog that also bit other dogs and was then chased and killed. As was common, the accident was duly reported in the newspapers. On the very same day, a hydrophobia death in Milwaukee, that city's second in six months, was reported as a news item in the *St. Louis Globe-Democrat* hundreds of miles away.

On December 3, a day after the Newark children were bitten, a powerful new element emerged when a local physician's letter on the front page of the *Newark Daily Journal* urged that the children be sent immediately to Paris for the new treatment and asked the public to contribute to their expenses if the children's families could not afford it. Within hours, workingmen had collected donations and brought them to the office of the doctor who had written the letter, William O'Gorman. Pasteur was asked by cable if he would receive the children; the papers printed his swift reply: "Si croyez danger envoyez enfants immediatement" (If you believe they are in danger, send the children immediately) (*Newark Daily Journal,* December 4; *St. Louis Globe-Democrat,* December 5). Arrangements were made for passage a few days later on a French steamer; more donations were accepted, with contributors' names printed in the newspapers. As interest in the boys' story grew, the press expanded its attention to include their families, the donation of warm clothing for their winter voyage across the North Atlantic, Pasteur's other discoveries, supposed remedies for hydrophobia, the problem of stray dogs in U.S. cities, methods of dog control, the variety of opinions among local physicians and medical professors on hydrophobia, the mechanism of the inoculation process, Pasteur's experiments, the germ theory in general, and the outfitting of a hospital room in the steamer. Over the following four months, newspapers all across the United States also reported at length on such topics as other countries' rabies patients being treated in Paris, several attempts to produce the vaccine in the United States, the death of a young girl in Paris after she had received the new treatment, and the start of an international campaign to raise funds to create the independent research and treatment center in Paris that ultimately opened in November 1888 as the Pasteur Institute.

Already by December 4, a cluster of several interlocking stories was running not only in most New York City and Newark papers but as far west at St. Louis, where the *Post-Dispatch* carried this report: "Six children were bitten by a supposed mad dog in Newark, N.J. yesterday. Twelve dogs were also bitten, of which eight were killed. It is probable that the children will be sent to Dr. Pasteur in Paris for treatment." Four of the six bitten children were judged by local physicians to be hurt seriously enough to need the trip: Eddie Ryan (age five), Patrick Joseph Reynolds (age seven), Austin Fitzgerald (age ten), and Willie Lane, a messenger boy (age thirteen).[21]

On December 8, the *New York Sun* ran the first pictures of the four new celebrities. On the ninth, Joseph Pulitzer's *New York World* offered a picture of Dr. O'Gorman. Also on the ninth, the *New York Times* took the opportunity to acknowledge news of a girl in Pasteur's care who had died after being inoculated, but it carefully reported Pasteur's explanation that "the period of incubation had expired and the treatment was therefore too late." The paper also quoted the chemist's firm assurance, "I am confident my treatment will be successful if commenced at any time before actual hydrophobia sets in, even if a year or more elapses between the bite and the commencement of treatment."

In Chicago on the ninth, the *Tribune* ran a small portrait of Pasteur in an article that registered the general public's engagement with the story. "The name of Pasteur is on every lip, and the confidence that the medical fraternity have in his skill is exemplified in the case of the Newark children who were bitten by a rabid dog. Although the expense of sending these children to Paris will be $2,000, they are to be sent to Pasteur for treatment. The result will be watched with unusual interest by our countrymen." The same portrait appeared by itself in the *Nashville Daily American* on December 11 and among the small pictures of the steamer party in the *New York World* of December 10, "The Children's Farewell" (fig. 23). Newspapers ran postage-stamp-sized images like these because they had not yet adequately solved the technical problem of holding together a page of type in which anything broke the rigid boundaries of the column rules. Despite the images' minute size and generalized character, they convey what was offered to satisfy the public's curiosity: the children boarding the ship, the stateroom converted into a dormitory (labeled "The Steamer's Hospital," despite the fact that all four were in good health), portraits of the four boys, a head-shot of Dr. Pasteur, and a full-length figure of Dr. Frank Billings in top hat with cane (an expert in animal diseases who was to accompany the children and introduce them to Pasteur's laboratory, where, it was said, he had studied).[22] The boys' pictures in the *World* were probably copied from the *Sun*'s four portraits printed two days earlier, and the image of Pasteur is not a good likeness. The *New York Evening Post* caustically suggested that the image was simply the face of a local politician relabeled to fill a sudden need. My interest is not in judging the accuracy of the images or in settling the priority disputes but in noticing how images and comments about them added momentum to the tidal wave of this sensation.[23] The unpictured members of the party were Mrs. Ryan, the mother of one of the bitten boys, and her youngest son, Willie, not bitten but too young to be left home without his mother.

FIG. 23. "The Children's Farewell. Dr. Pasteur's Little Patients Sail on the Steamer Canada," *New York World*, December 10, 1885, 5.

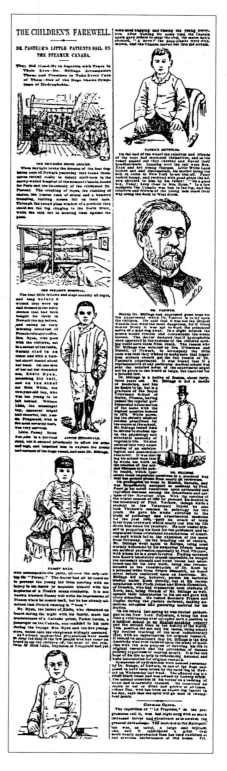

For the days that the boys were at sea, there could be no news of them in an era before the development of radio, so the papers kept the public engaged with stories about the dog pound and strays, about a new rabies victim (with articles showing pictures not only of one Charles Kaufmann, who had been bitten, but also of the dogs involved), about Pasteur's earlier work, and even about the history of applied science in France more generally. For example, on December 14, the *New York Times* ran a substantial article of nearly two full columns on the longstanding rivalry between the École Polytechnique and the École Normal Supérieure. A long, illustrated article gracing the Sunday morning edition of the *St. Louis Globe-Democrat* set the Newark cases into a wider context of medical science, citing remarks by a local physician of French origin, Dr. M. E. Chartier.[24] Another type of rabies news during the Newark boys' time at sea was the reporting of new victims around the world, such as Herr Gegner, proprietor of Prague's largest hotel, and his son, who were bitten and going to Paris for treatment (*Boston Evening Transcript, St. Louis Globe-Democrat,* and *St. Louis Post-Dispatch* of December 15).

In the week or so since the Newark boys had been bitten, readers in the New York area—and throughout the United States—had been treated to such extensive coverage that the enthusiasm became a target for satire. The *Puck* issue with a cover date of December 16 ran a cartoon entitled "The New Scheme," showing two hoboes in conversation. The first proclaims, "Congratulate me, old man—I'm going to Paris." The second inquires, "How'd yer work it?" The first explains, "Said I was bitten by a mad dog—pop'lar subscription gettin' up to send me to Pastoor."[25] This mocking of the popular commotion actually appeared far earlier than it might seem from the magazine's date. These weekly magazines were usually distributed six or seven days prior to the publication date on the cover, although in practice there was considerable variation. But the disparity in dates means that satirists had already seized on the phenomenon within one week (not two) of when the Newark boys were bitten.[26] Another indication that the story was on everyone's mind is given by the *Boston Evening Transcript*'s reprinting on December 19 of two hydrophobia jokes taken from small-town papers, the *Lowell Citizen* in Massachusetts and the *Norristown Republican* in Pennsylvania.

But in addition to humorous items such as these, which made fun of the popular enthusiasm, there also appeared satirical caricatures such as the *Puck* cover for December 16, 1885, "Another Patient for Pasteur," in which the intent was political commentary and the rabies-cure sensation was simply a vehicle for other messages (see color plate 5).[27] "Blainiac rabies" in the cartoon's caption refers to James G. Blaine, Grover Cleveland's unsuccessful opponent in the 1884 presidential campaign and a politician infamous for several scandalous indiscretions.[28] The "patient" in this cartoon is Whitelaw Reid, editor of the *Tribune,* who supported Blaine. Reid is being carried aboard by two other New York editors, Carl Schurz of the *Evening Post* and George William Curtis of *Harper's,* both of whom, though Republicans, had nonetheless refrained from backing Blaine in the 1884 election. They were thus free of the (hydrophobic) madness suffered by their colleague. "Blainiac" rabies is, of course, also a pun on "maniac." Scandals involving James G. Blaine and the support he received from Reid had no inherent connection with medical history, yet the image makes clear that the public must already have been quite familiar with the new Parisian treatment.

At least four publications with a cover date of December 19 ran illustrated versions of the Pasteur story (fig. 24). Pasteur watching the injection of Jupille, his second rabies patient, was the graphic centerpiece of a *Harper's Weekly* story.[29] The same image was also published that day in *Scientific American*.[30] This sketch had already appeared on the cover of a French magazine, *L'Illustration,* on November 7, 1885, and had also been reproduced in New York's *Daily Graphic* on November 19, weeks prior to its use by *Harper's Weekly* and *Scientific American.* Even the *National Police Gazette* ran a half-column story and a small portrait on the nineteenth.[31] Two other "action shots" of Pasteur at work circulated widely in the popular media of France, England, and the United States: Pasteur standing between two rows of rabbit cages and Pasteur peering through a microscope.[32] Also during 1885, an

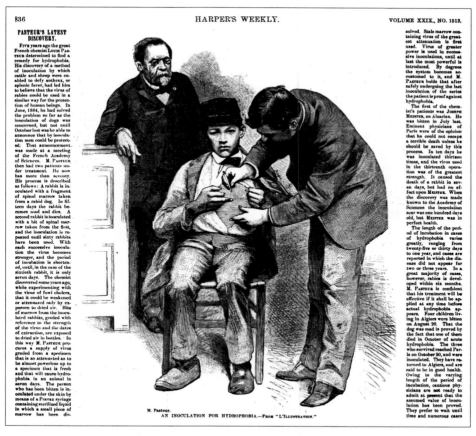

FIG. 24. "An Inoculation for Hydrophobia—From *L'Illustration,*" *Harper's Weekly* 29:1513 (December 19, 1885), 836. Author's collection.

important painting of Pasteur in his laboratory by Albert Edelfelt was completed and shortly thereafter exhibited at the Paris Salon, but copies of this image seem not to have appeared in a U.S. publication until 1890.

Frank Leslie's Illustrated Newspaper took a different approach, calling its story "M. Pasteur and His Patients" and running four small drawings of the Newark boys (based it seems on those published in the *World* and/or the *Sun*), along with a large, uncredited reproduction of an engraving showing the scientist at work, "experimenting on a chloroformed rabbit" (see figure 31 in chapter 4). A small version of the *Frank Leslie's* engraving was reprinted without acknowledgment two days later in the *Evening News* of Danbury, Connecticut, and perhaps in other dailies as well. The *Frank Leslie's* article opened with a prescient forecast, calling this "an international episode of peculiar interest . . . which will occupy public attention in both France and America for some weeks to come."[33] Although the French newspapers did not sustain their curiosity about "les quatre petits Américains" for long, the Americans did so with a vengeance.

While the news sketches in the illustrated papers were becoming repetitive, the *Daily Graphic* showed originality on that same December 19 by covering its entire front page with nine drawings and cartoons about dogs, rabies, and the fashion of seeking cures in Paris—all surrounding the powerful image of a revolver aimed at a cowering dog. One of the cartoons, showing a young girl in a pharmacy, predicted vaccines as a commonplace of the future. In a parody of the traditional scene of a daughter buying her father's beer (fig. 25), the girl's request to the clerk behind the counter is "Fifteen Cents Worth of Hydrophobia Virus, Please, for Pa."[34] Another vignette on this page, entitled "The Rush to Paris," showed a long queue of people waiting to board a ship bearing the sign "Line Direct to Pasteur."

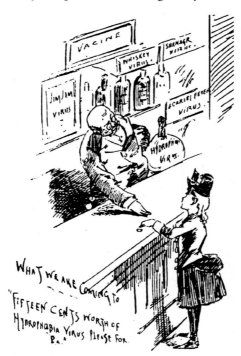

FIG. 25. "What We Are Coming To: Fifteen Cents Worth of Hydrophobia Virus for Pa," *New York Daily Graphic* 39:3976 (December 19, 1885), cover (1). Detail from full-page spread of ten cartoons, "Hydrophobia!" by H. C. Coultaus.

By December 21, Mrs. Ryan, Dr. Billings, and the boys had arrived in France, and the transatlantic telegraph cable could transmit dispatches to New York in about six hours, with reports coming daily and sometimes even more frequently. The next day, the *New York Times* carried these headlines over column one on the front page: "In Pasteur's

Laboratory. The Newark Children Inoculated Last Evening. They Reach Paris All Right, Undergo the Operation Bravely, and Then Go to Bed and to Sleep. By Commercial Cable from Our Own Correspondent."

The *New York Herald* was more dramatic, with two huge articles the next day (December 22), each opened by a high stack of headlines. Local news was mostly tragic: "Dogs Making Havoc. Two Men, a Lad and a Girl Torn by Rabid Brutes in Jersey. The End of a Day's Hunting. Alarm at Mattawan, Keyport, Orange, and Englewood. Fido Attacks His Little Mistress. Forty Dogs Killed and a Great Sunday Dog Hunt." The *Herald's* news from abroad ran the gamut: "Pasteur's Patients. Arrival of the Newark Children in Paris. Incidents on the Journey. Patsey Reynolds Attempts to Throw Himself Overboard. The Boys Inoculated. Surprised to Find the Operation Does Not Hurt. Horrible Death in the Laboratory." On the same day, the *Chicago Tribune* told its readers about the Fitzgerald boy's getting hungry en route from Le Havre to Paris and demanding food at Rouen.

For the actual treatment in Pasteur's laboratory, the cable report's exaggerated style used fine-grained precision and mock seriousness to record the historic moment, juxtaposing childish antics with the reality of a mortal threat. The simple headline read, "Willie Lane, the First American Inoculated for the Rabies."

> Dr. Grancher, who performs all the inoculations for M. Pasteur, told Lane to unbutton his jacket. At exactly 7:12 o'clock the Doctor inserted the point of a silver needle beneath the skin of Lane's abdomen and injected the virus. Lane has thus the honor of being the first American ever inoculated for rabies. As the needle was withdrawn he gave a slight squirm and burst out into a boisterous laugh, exclaiming, "Why, it's like the bite of a big mosquito. It don't hurt a bit." Fitzgerald's turn came next. He watched the silver needle intently. . . . Reynolds was next taken in hand. . . . The children then scampered off as cheerful as jay birds and not a bit homesick. The inoculation took place in the same room of the laboratory where a man on Saturday died of rabies.[35]

The mania of all this coverage grabbed the attention of social satirists. But, notably, their work did not puncture the balloon of excitement. Instead they helped to inflate it further. One *Puck* cartoon trumpeted, "The Pasteur Boom—High Times for Hydrophobists. Now Is the Time to Get Bitten by a Rabid Dog and Take a Trip to Paris" (fig. 26). It made light of the masses' enthusiasm for the trip, without challenging its importance to the four little boys and without taking a stand on the value of Pasteur's new therapy. It also mocked both the fashion for ladies' lap dogs and the policeman's traditional role as urban dog killer. Indicative of how the press was feeding on itself in the creation of news is the fact that, when this cartoon arrived in Europe by steamer, it was shown to Pasteur on January 7 by the *New York Herald's* correspondent, who then cabled a report of Pasteur's comments across the Atlantic in time to make the next morning's papers (*New York Herald,* January 8).

Besides the daily reports of the boys' injections, the approach of Christmas occasioned further stories about their Parisian escapades. Then, after the holiday, events

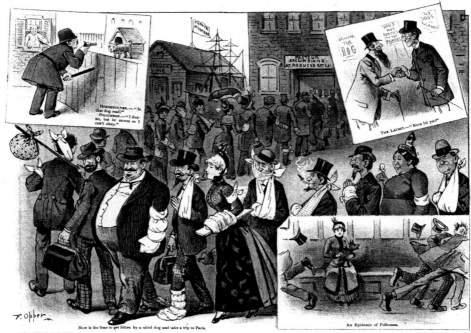

THE PASTEUR BOOM—HIGH TIMES FOR HYDROPHOBISTS.

FIG. 26. "The Pasteur Boom: High Times for Hydrophobists. Now Is the Time to Get Bitten by a Rabid Dog and Take a Trip to Paris," *Puck* 18:459 (December 23, 1885), back cover (272). Full-page chromolithograph by Frederick Opper. Interior captions read, "Householder: 'Is that dog mad?' Policeman: 'I dunno, but he snores so I can't sleep.' The Latest: 'Been bit yet?' An Epidemic of Politeness." Author's collection.

took a more dramatic turn, with complaints from some members of the party. Like other papers, the *New York Times* gave front-page coverage to the party's personal squabbles on December 29 with this stack of headlines: "Mrs. Ryan and Patsy Reynolds Making Trouble. Two Members of the Party Proving Unruly. The Inoculations Becoming Painful. Arrival of Kaufmann." Charles Kaufmann (also "Kauffman" and "Kaufman" in various papers) was the first American dog-bite victim to follow the boys to Paris, having been sent over by Dr. O'Gorman with excess funds contributed for the Newark children. His adventures were usually intertwined in the press with those of the Newark boys.[36]

AMERICAN ENTHUSIASM FOR PASTEUR'S SCIENCE

At the turn of the year, new players were coming onstage. On December 29, the *Boston Morning Journal* commented on the media coverage itself and made a novel proposal:

The popular joke of the day is based upon the Pasteur experiments and the tendency for American dogs to become mad in order that their American owners may take a trip abroad for inoculation against rabies. Going to Paris may be amusing, but it would be interesting to effect a cure at home, if possible. Why could not branches of the Pasteur establishment be opened in this country? We have mad dogs and rabbits and the patients. We have also scientists who might become followers of Pasteur and successful operators of his method.[37]

At just this moment, unknown to the Boston editorial writer, independent groups of physicians in three different cities were all working on initiatives to prepare rabies vaccine that would offer American victims of dog bites better access to the new lifesaving technique. And the news spread quickly.

On December 31, the *St. Louis Globe-Democrat* reported on a local effort: "Inoculation in St. Louis. Physicians of St. Mary's Hospital Following in Pasteur's Footsteps. The Theory of Inoculation for the Cure of Rabies to Be Applied in This City. Mad Dogs for Experiments." The doctors involved were Charles Garcia, M. E. Chartier, and A. Rouif, the last a French veterinary surgeon. On the same day, another St. Louis newspaper, the *Post-Dispatch,* reported on the local activity and also carried news of the New York City effort: "A Good Institution. The Incorporation of the American Institute of Hydrophobia. The First Steps Taken for the [Introduction] in America of Pasteur's Famous Methods. What the Incorporators Have to Say. The Institute to Be Supported by Subscriptions." The American Pasteur Institute was incorporated by eight eminent physicians led by Dr. Valentine Mott (son of Dr. Alexander Mott, who collaborated in this venture, and grandson of the famous surgeon Valentine Mott).

Also on the same day, the Newark doctors' attempt to culture rabies virus in their rabbits was reported, among other places, in the *Chicago Tribune*: "Will Try Dr. Pasteur's Remedy. Veterinary-Surgeon Runge has received from New York the body of a dog which was killed while suffering from rabies, also four cats which were bitten by the dog. He will endeavor to start a laboratory here [in Newark]. A rabbit was inoculated with the virus. This operation is said to be the first of the kind ever performed in this country." On January 1, the *New York Times* and the *Boston Evening Transcript* carried reports about the new "virus farm" in St. Louis, and the *St. Louis Globe-Democrat* called the Newark doctors "American Pasteurs."

All these American initiatives preceded Pasteur's own call for such an institute by over two months, and they were not sanctioned by him. The preliminary (not to say premature) character of these ventures is indicated by the fact that Pasteur had not yet published a full scientific report of his methods, although the general account of the Joseph Meister case, which Pasteur read at the Académie des Sciences of Paris on October 26, had been printed in a French scientific journal and an English translation of it appeared in the January 1886 issue of *Popular Science Monthly*. Widespread interest in the report is indicated by this issue's contents being advertised in daily newspapers (in the *Boston Evening Transcript* of December 22, for example).

A slightly abridged version of the translation even appeared in the *St. Louis Globe-Democrat* on Christmas Day.

In addition to these disinterested groups of physicians, an American with commercial intentions had approached Pasteur, much to his chagrin, with a proposal for a commercial vaccine enterprise, even offering Pasteur two-thirds of the profits. Not surprisingly, Pasteur rejected the offer with a sneer about the United States' famed commercialism, and he told an American reporter, "Vos compatriotes vont trop vite" (Your countrymen are going too fast) (*St. Louis Globe-Democrat,* January 5; and *New York Herald,* January 8).

When American physicians attempted to replicate Pasteur's miracle-making experiments, their imitation was sincere, if clumsy. But because their laboratory efforts had substantial visibility in the daily press, even more people became familiar with this new—and hitherto alien—enterprise. St. Louis readers of the *Globe-Democrat* on January 3 were offered a long and very detailed report entitled "Pasteur's Experiments," even though it was about local work. The article opened this way:

> The First Attempt at Actual Treatment in St. Louis. The brain of the dog that bit George Hudson in Brockman's livery stable on Friday afternoon passed into the possession of Dr. Chartier yesterday, and last night a healthy Newfoundland and Collie dog was inoculated with virus obtained from the cerebral tissue. . . . The operation, which was performed in the basement of a Locust street dwelling, was completed at 9:30 o'clock. The brain of the dead dog, after being scientifically prepared, was subjected to considerable pressure in the hands of Dr. Rouif. A serous fluid with a red tinge oozed from the muslin and was collected in a glass dish.[38]

On that same day in New York, the *Daily Graphic* ran large illustrations of Newark physicians (fig. 27). It labeled them "scientists" and showed them inoculating a rabbit with nerve tissue dissected from a rabbit that had been inoculated with tissue from a rabid dog.[39]

On January 3, many papers also announced the children's departure from Paris; on page 1, the *New York Times* ran this stack of headlines: "Returning from Pasteur. Dr. Billings and His Boys Sail for Home. They Have a Christmas Tree in Their Hotel and Leave Paris Well and Happy. The Farewell Courtesies." During the children's voyage home, the papers again filled the lull in events with reports of other American patients arriving in Paris (*Chicago Tribune,* January 5 and 6) and with retrospective accounts such as a three-and-a-half-column article in the *New York Times* on January 10: "Pasteur and Mad Dogs. His Methods, His Laboratory, and His Patients. Some Facts from His Past Life. The Newark Boys Treated. Scenes in His Workshop—Talks with Him." Other papers provided more details of the rabies work in the United States (*St. Louis Post-Dispatch,* January 12, for example). On January 14, the *Boston Evening Transcript* firmly defended the abundant media coverage: "When the Paris letter writer can think of no other subject to send across the Atlantic, he falls back on Pasteur's laboratory and his manner of concocting virus. It

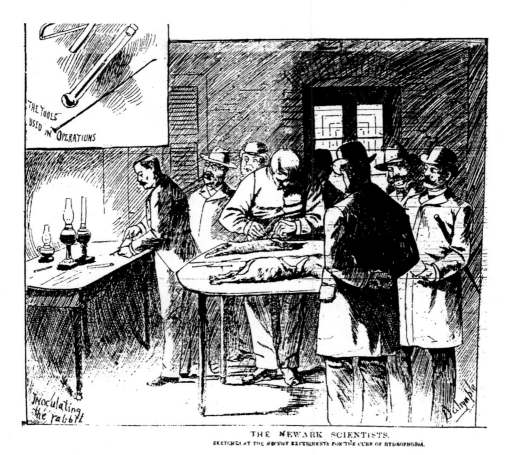

THE NEWARK SCIENTISTS.
SKETCHES AT THE RECENT EXPERIMENTS FOR THE CURE OF HYDROPHOBIA.

FIG. 27. "Inoculating the Rabbit," *New York Daily Graphic* 39:3989 (January 3, 1886), 4. Detail of a page with four drawings entitled "The Newark Scientists. Sketches of the Recent Experiments for the Cure of Hydrophobia."

is a very interesting subject, notwithstanding [that] some carping critics may think it has been slightly overworked." This same paper picked up that issue again on the sixteenth with a long editorial challenging stylistic aspects of the reports on rabies, though not the topic per se, by claiming that they included excessive description and needless human-interest details.

Even before the boys arrived home, American commercialism saw profits to be made from the new folk heroes. The Eden Musée, a popular New York wax museum, defined the boys as the latest sensation by advertising "The Topic of the Day, M. Pasteur Operating on One of the Newark Children."[40] The Pasteur scene was illustrated only very sketchily in the monthly catalogues, but fortunately a full-color advertising card has survived and allows us to see exactly how New Yorkers and tourists envisioned the rabies shots (fig. 28). The museum's printed catalogue confirmed how profoundly Pasteur's work was changing ordinary people's expectations about

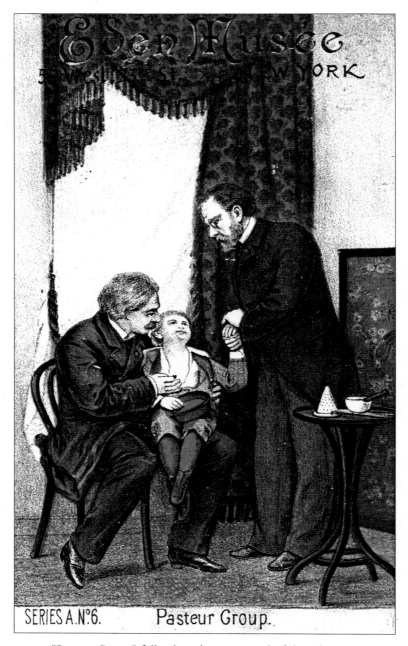

FIG. 28. "Pasteur Group," full-color advertising card of the Eden Musée, undated but almost certainly 1886, 3.0 by 4.9 inches. Text on the back has general information such as hours, exhibit categories, and admission prices (fifty cents, but only twenty-five cents for children and on Sundays), with nothing about this particular exhibit. Author's collection.

medical progress: "Of late M. Pasteur's name has become a household word in every country on account of his experiments in trying to prevent the dreadful effects of the bite of mad dogs, by inoculating the victims with the virus of the rabid animal. ... Patients from all parts of the world have flocked to his laboratory to undergo the new treatment."[41]

A large political caricature from mid-February 1886 documents in concise form just how completely the public consciousness had been saturated with Pasteur's achievement. Pasteur's protective inoculation for rabies reached the pinnacle of visibility for U.S. graphic imagery when one of the United States' leading artists, T. Bernhard Gillam, turned the U.S. president into Louis Pasteur within a satirical setting that placed him in the very center of an oversize color cartoon. In this densely populated center-spread chromolithograph from *Judge,* Gillam employed the device of fashioning about twenty-five of his political targets into wax-museum figures in an elaborate display, "Judge's Wax Works—The Political Eden Musée" (see color plate 6). At the center of the drawing—just above the tiger representing New York's famous Tammany Hall and below the brand-new Statue of Liberty—Grover Cleveland, then president of the United States, is depicted in the posture of Louis Pasteur performing an inoculation of civil-service reform to prevent corruption.[42]

THE UNITED STATES' NEW MEDICAL CELEBRITIES

To satisfy the public's curiosity about the new miracle cure, more elaborate practices materialized—including even performances. In many large cities, dime museums provided exhibits and live entertainment to lower-middle- and working-class visitors, with as many as twenty shows a day. The dime museums in New York City were clustered along the Bowery. More sensationalist than Barnum's American Museum or the Eden Musée, these small establishments, often in storefronts, charged the low admission price conveyed by their name; by contrast, the higher-toned Eden Musée was charging fifty cents admission in 1886. The 1880s were the heyday of dime museums, yet many survived well into the twentieth century.[43] The idea of putting the little Newark boys themselves on exhibit appeared on the front page of the *Newark Daily Journal* on January 13, just before their scheduled return. An article about the parents' anxious wait for the steamer's arrival explained the possibility: "The proprietor of a Bowery dime museum has been working assiduously for several days to secure the children for two weeks to place on exhibition. He offered the parents $15 a week. It is not likely that the proposition will be accepted." The boys' working-class families eventually acceded to this proposition, although they acted with ambivalence and embarrassment, facing condemnation from some middle-class newspapers and an investigation threatened by the Society for the Prevention of Cruelty to Children. But this was, after all, a very attractive offer, given that twelve to fifteen dollars a week were the wages of a skilled workman.[44]

A lengthy article in the *Newark Daily Advertiser* of January 19 that captured the bizarre scene also reveals how medical information was a key part of the spectacle:

> Three of the dog-bitten Newark children, little "Patsy" Reynolds, Austin Fitzgerald, and Willie Lane, were yesterday placed on exhibition at the Globe Museum in the Bowery. They were perched upon a pedestal, with the champion fat woman on one side and a white silk-haired man on the other. Crowds came to see them all day, and at night the museum was packed so full that the spectators could hardly get out.
>
> Prof. Hickey gave the sightseers a complete history of the children from the time they were bitten by the dogs until they were brought to the city for exhibition. He also gave a scientific explanation of Pasteur's method of treatment, and said that hereafter the boys might be bitten by any number of dogs and that it would have no dangerous effects. . . . [Patsy] honored one party of children by shooting orange seeds at them, and an old lady carefully gathered these up to preserve as relics. . . . The managers of the museum had the audacity to ask Dr. Billings to exhibit with the children, and made a similar proposition to M. Pasteur.

When the *New York World* reported on this exhibit a week later, on January 27, the point of its story was not the proceedings themselves but their magnitude: "Three of the Newark boys draw crowds to a Bowery show-house. . . . Three hundred thousand persons have paid 10 cents apiece to get a look at them, and their popularity is increasing daily. Twenty times a day they stand on stage while the manager recites their story. The managers expect to exhibit them in all the large Eastern cities." Three hundred thousand persons represented over 20 percent of New York City's inhabitants at the time, so this figure is surely exaggerated, but perhaps not excessively so, as one historian has reported that attendance at a dime museum could sometimes run as high as ten thousand people each day.[45] Although only three boys were on exhibit for much of the New York run, because of the absence of five-year-old Eddie, the *Newark Daily Advertiser* reported on January 29 that Eddie was due in the New York show "next Monday," shortly before the group was expected to move to Philadelphia. I have not documented any appearance in Philadelphia or other eastern cities, but the children were popular in the West. On February 14, they opened in St. Louis, Missouri, at Broadway and Treyser's Palace Museum. A pictorial flyer that heralded this show has luckily been preserved in a Paris archive (fig. 29): "Palace Museum . . . One Week Only . . . The Newark Children . . . Pasteur's Patients from Paris! Whom we have induced to exhibit, for one week only, at the enormous salary of One Thousand Dollars."[46]

A week later, on February 21, the children began a week-long run in Chicago at Stanhope and Epstean's New Dime Museum, which advertised them along with "the genuine Fiji Cannibals" and "Four Mastodon Halls of Curiosities" in these words: "Of Interest to Everybody! First Appearance in the West of Pasteur's Patients! The World Famous Newark Children! For the past month the Leading New York Sensation! Accompanied by a brief instructive Lecture Illustrating Pasteur's Treatment

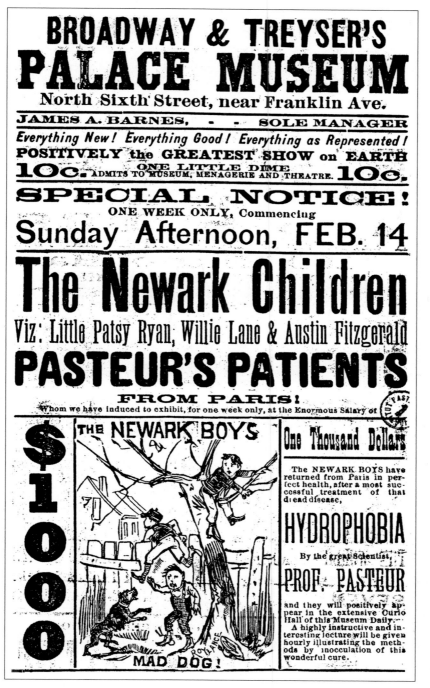

FIG. 29. Handbill promoting the appearance of the Newark boys in a dime museum, February 1886. Reproduction courtesy of the Musée Pasteur, Paris. Although no city is indicated, Broadway and Treyser's Palace Museum was located in St. Louis, Missouri.

and Cure of Hydrophobia. Greatest Scientific Discovery of the Day" (*Chicago Tribune*). A news item in the *Chicago Tribune* on February 23 informed readers that the boys were accompanied for this trip by one of the fathers and one of the mothers and also that—thanks to the art of taxidermy—the exhibit included the very Newark dog that had bitten them. Reports of such appearances flowed back across the Atlantic, prompting at least some hostile reactions. A report from Paris appearing in the *Boston Evening Transcript* on March 13 observed that the exhibition of the children "has been denounced in energetic terms by the Paris press. Much more importance has been given to this matter than it merits, and the accounts of the exhibition which have appeared in the French papers have apparently been greatly exaggerated."

Whatever the attendance figures and however many the cities where they appeared, the reports demonstrate that a large share of the American public experienced a direct and personal engagement with Pasteur's miracle cure. The boys who received their shots in Paris became folk heroes, celebrities toasted across the nation for a few months at least.

However strange it may seem to us to have patients up on a theater stage, the Newark boys' experience was not unique, even if it was rare. Only three other examples of patients on public display in entertainment venues have come to my attention. As medical marvels, Alexis St. Martin and Phineas Gage were exhibited around the country on several occasions in the 1850s, and the incubator babies of Dr. Martin A. Couney were a spectacle for a paying public at Coney Island for much of the first half of the twentieth century.[47] The showman's role in pulling in an audience to pay for expensive medical care for premature infants did have an essential analogue in the 1880s, though the agent was neither Pasteur nor the opportunistic freak-show managers. The key fund-raisers were the editors of the *New York Herald,* the *New York World,* and all the other newspapers, those enterprising men whose articles attracted the money to carry the Newark boys to Paris in the first place.

KEEPING THE STORY ALIVE

In March 1886, the Newark boys returned home from their time on the freak-show circuit, and they apparently remained out of the spotlight except for a striking revival of interest in the 1920s. But as the excitement over the Newark boys began to fade during March, a new and quite different element entered the story, one with far-reaching potential. Louis Pasteur announced plans to establish a large new institute to provide inoculations, and an international subscription campaign was begun.[48] Such campaigns were prominent in the 1880s. Not only had newspapers solicited funds to send the Newark boys to Paris, but a U.S. subscription campaign sponsored by Pulitzer's *New York World* to build the pedestal for Bartoldi's Statue of Liberty (itself a gift from France to the American people for the country's centenary) had reached its goal of one hundred thousand dollars only a few months earlier, in August 1885.[49] A successful fund-raising campaign promoted by newspapers around the world made possible the Institut Pasteur, which opened in Paris in November 1888. Over those two and a half years, U.S. papers reported regularly on the patients of varied nationalities being treated in Paris and on the many donations from around the world.

Many U.S. newspapers kept the rabies-cure excitement going for several more months with a miscellany of stories. They gave much attention to Pasteur's reports that he had lost only one patient in the first 350 cases treated. Then they reported his statement that he intended to try to apply this method to patients of diphtheria (for example, *St. Louis Post-Dispatch,* March 3; and *Boston Evening Transcript,* March 16). And just when excitement might have waned, nineteen Russian peasants who had been severely injured by wolf bites arrived in Paris for treatment (March 16, many papers). On the same day as that sad news, Americans also learned from their papers that the U.S. minister in Paris was shortly to preside at a banquet in Pasteur's honor given by American residents of Paris. The following week, it was reported with some embarrassment that U.S. subscriptions for the Parisian rabies institute were lagging behind those from Portugal and Switzerland (*Chicago Tribune,* March 25). Then there were reports that the Russians had completed their series of injections, although two or three of them could not be helped and had died of their wounds (*Chicago Tribune,* March 25 and April 11). Soon there were reports of four ladies from Athens, Greece, making their way to Paris for treatment (*Boston Evening Transcript,* March 29). In Baltimore, a physician, Dr. Brinton H. Warner, who had been bitten on Christmas, died in the usual excruciating circumstances a few months later (*Chicago Tribune, New York Times,* and *St. Louis Globe-Democrat,* April 7). April saw more American victims of dog bites heading to Paris, including the beautiful and wealthy Amelia Morosini, a daughter of Giovanni P. Morosini, the well-known Wall Street broker and former partner of Jay Gould (*New York Times,* April 20; *St. Louis Post-Dispatch,* April 23). Among Pasteur's patients, Miss Morosini was inscribed in May as number 953 and the first American lady (*St. Louis Post-Dispatch,* May 10). Near the end of May, newspapers carried the encouraging news that the British commission investigating Pasteur's method was tentatively confirming the new method's success (*St. Louis Globe-Democrat* and *St. Louis Post-Dispatch,* May 28). By June 5, the papers could report that Pasteur's treated patients now numbered over eleven hundred (*Chicago Tribune*).

In July, the first patient treated by Pasteur's method in the United States also generated headlines. The treatment was administered by Dr. Valentine Mott, who had gone to Paris for training. He returned to New York with a rabid rabbit infected with Pasteur's fixed strain of virus and began a campaign to raise money that would allow his institute continuously to produce the virus needed for treatments in the United States (*St. Louis Globe-Democrat,* May 24; *New York Tribune,* June 4). Dr. Mott was known to the public, even outside New York, through many articles about his trip to Paris the previous winter. His portrait had even appeared in one of the *Chicago Tribune* articles (February 4).

Quite publicly at 10:55 A.M. on the morning of July 5, 1886, Harold Newton Newell, the young son of a New Jersey physician, Dr. William H. Newell, received the first injection for rabies in the United States in the American Pasteur Institute rooms in the Carnegie Laboratory in New York City (*Boston Evening Transcript, St. Louis Post-Dispatch,* and the *Columbus (Ohio) Evening Dispatch,* July 6). Exactly one year earlier, Pasteur had watched Meister privately receive the world's first successful treatment. Because of the novelty of the procedure, Newell's father signed a detailed consent form, accepting responsibility for any effects on his son and releasing the American Pasteur Institute of liability for the outcome of the injections. The agreement itself was published in at least one newspaper (*St. Louis Post-Dispatch,* July 6).

The following day's *Boston Evening Transcript* complained that the institute had received very little support from the American public, and that it would probably close soon without an increase in donations (*Boston Evening Transcript* and *New York Times,* July 7). Newell's series of injections was ended early "owing to the father's alarm at the illness of his son which followed each inoculation" (*Chicago Tribune,* July 13). Several days later, the boy was reported to be doing well (*New York Times,* July 17). Two days later, it was reported in the *Brooklyn Eagle* that the boy's condition was "growing worse and his relatives fear a fatal result" (July 19). But the story seemed to end there in the press, and I have been unable to find any later reports, favorable or unfavorable. Without a visible success, the American Pasteur Institute in New York, like the one in St. Louis, quickly failed for insufficient public support. The Pasteur treatment was not available in the United States until institutes were established in New York and Chicago in 1890 by physicians who solved the funding problem.

THE MASS MEDIA AND A NEW KIND OF MEDICINE

In just a few weeks in December 1885, the general public assimilated the announcement of a new life-saving discovery, learned that it was made in the bodies of rabbits, faced the puzzling idea that the same virus that killed so brutally could be modified to have fabulous healing power, and became excited with the prospect that these new ideas and techniques could transform the routines of medicine and medical education.[50] This heady moment of rapid change was captured by *Puck* in a cartoon of six frames under the double entendre "The Profession Gone Mad" (fig. 30). The title's pun on "mad dogs" and "mad doctors" suggested that the public's raging enthusiasm for the latest fad was shared by physicians. Six simple vignettes illustrated a major revolution in several dimensions of medical education, research, and practice. Although intended as humor, the cartoon captured in a sophisticated

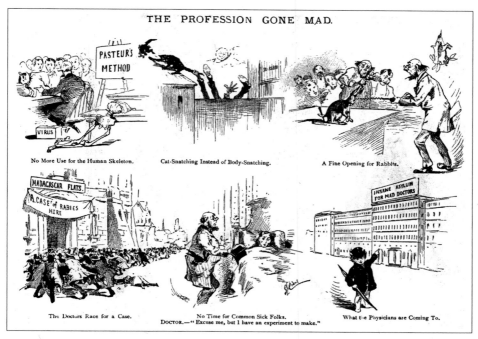

FIG. 30. "The Profession Gone Mad," *Puck* 18:462 (January 13, 1886), 314. Half-page cartoon by G. E. Ciani. Internal captions: (a) "No More Use for the Human Skeleton." (b) "Cat-Snatching Instead of Body-Snatching." (c) "A Fine Opening for Rabbits." (d) "The Doctors Race for a Case." (e) "No Time for Common Sick Folks. Doctor: 'Excuse me, but I have an experiment to make.'" (f) "What the Physicians Are Coming To—Insane Asylum for Mad Doctors." Author's collection.

way the epoch-making transition as medicine was being reconfigured by discoveries from the laboratory. Scenes show the traditional anatomy teacher's skeleton being cast aside in the medical lecture room, replaced by a box labeled "virus"; medical students engaged in "cat-snatching instead of body-snatching"; medical school demonstrators performing trephination on a live rabbit; physicians swarming to get a look at a case of rabies, the newly fashionable disease; and a doctor apologizing at a patient's bedside, "Excuse me, but I have an experiment to make."

As indicated by the prescience of *Puck*'s cartoonist, the Pasteur rabies-cure sensation was something more than a transitory fad for the new treatment of a frightening disease. Prior advances in medicine such as surgical anesthesia, antisepsis, identification of the microbes causing cholera and consumption, and the anthrax vaccine did not find strong traction in popular consciousness. In an unprecedented shift, the hydrophobia drama—because it captured the popular imagination—revolutionized medicine by disseminating a new image of the value of experimental research in medicine, helping to create a new expectation of continuing medical advances and implicitly encouraging public commitment to such research. But this change did not arise solely from Pasteur's work; there were several features of the climate of 1885–1886 that made such a frenzy about his achievement possible.

First, the media sensation was sustained and amplified by the pragmatic self-interest of editors competing for regular readers, entirely independent of this particular story. For the penny papers, vast numbers of readers were required, and any story that could engender daily curiosity about tomorrow's installment was a sure winner—and worth promoting. These editors boosted the rabies story not only by aggressively pursuing new angles and information but also by directly participating in the events themselves. The Paris correspondent for the *New York Herald* took an active role in making the news: for example, he showed Pasteur the "Hydrophobia Boom" cartoon from *Puck* and wired a report on his reactions back to New York. With the same technique that Joseph Pulitzer had used a few months earlier when his *New York World* sponsored a subscription campaign to raise funds for the base of the Statue of Liberty, James Gordon Bennett Jr. of the *Herald* coordinated a fund for sending the Newark children to Paris. Lists of donors created buyers for the papers, to see who gave, how much they gave, and whether anyone they knew might be immortalized. The papers did not limit the listings to major gifts but continued the names and amounts down through $4.20 from employees of the Domestic Manufacturing Company to the ten-cent donations by four-year-old Cora Syms and her six-year-old sister Ida.[51]

The papers also used the personal lives of the characters to entice readers into wanting more of the story. Readers came to know much about the Newark boys and their families. After a reporter visited one boy's home, readers were informed even that "a few cheap prints of sacred subjects hung on the whitewashed walls" (*New York Herald,* December 6). Once readers learned that Mrs. Ryan was pregnant, there was suspense about whether she might deliver en route to Europe or in France. Her baby was in fact born on the return voyage, after nearly a month of readers' anticipation. The papers then not only reported on Mr. Ryan's first look at his new son but quoted expert opinions on whether the boy, born in midocean on a French steamer, was an American or a French citizen. For the physicians and other middle-class players in the drama, such private information was held back and replaced with stories of their education and professional histories, their ambitions and achievements. But they too became celebrities, with their portraits appearing in papers and magazines, even if their home life was not made public and they could afford to refuse invitations to appear onstage in cheap theaters. Although many aspects of the rabies-cure coverage were adventitious, the editors were happy to exploit two inherent features of this story that were guaranteed to evoke strong human interest: children and dogs. Other selling points of the day were helpless victims, Good Samaritans, community fund-raising, a perilous voyage, a noble (and conveniently distant) hero, divided opinions among local authorities, and a potentially happy ending.

A second factor that contributed to the frenzy about this story was that the range of publications feeding this sensation crossed class lines, styles of writing, and genres. The story was carried in working-class and middle-class daily papers, in papers popular with immigrants and those favored by the native born, in the business papers that carried relatively little other news, and in the pictorials too. The quality of the papers ranged from the more serious *New York Tribune* and *New York Times* through the *Daily Graphic* and the sensation-seeking *New York World* to the salacious *National Police Gazette*.[52] But the reporting by these newspapers was not just human-interest storytelling. Substantive explanations of the rabies vaccine were available to a much larger audience than the readership of the era's monthly journals of ideas, such as *Atlantic, Century, Harper's Monthly, Littell's Living Age, North American Review,* and *Popular Science Monthly*. It is the broad popularity of the rabies-vaccine story that sets it apart from the public treatments of intellectual controversies in science such as Darwinian evolution that had been disseminated in elite periodicals but not in mass-circulation newspapers.[53] Furthermore, the attention to this case was not limited to news and feature articles. Cartoons, jokes, and political caricatures frequently incorporated the rabies-cure imagery, further confirming its vogue.[54]

A third factor in the popularity of this story was that not only did the coverage cross classes and genres, but it was also prodigious, with articles numbering in the thousands. In December 1885 and January 1886, there was at least one news article almost every day in each of the New York City papers and often four or more in the same paper—in addition to editorials, letters from readers, and related jokes and witticisms.[55] On at least two days, more than 10 percent of the *New York Herald's* space was devoted to rabies and its cure. Readers were so eager for the story that the *Herald,* so it claimed, was selling out by 9 A.M. In the month of December, the *Herald* (admittedly the most capacious in its rabies coverage) printed seventeen editorials, thirty-one letters to the editor, seventeen cable dispatches from Paris or London, and seventy-three news articles. In January, the *Herald* published ninety-eight distinct items. The same two months saw more than 130 items printed in Pulitzer's *New York World,* including at least two advertisements trying to ride the wave of hydrophobia excitement.[56] Of course, New York's *Courrier des États-Unis* gave the story full play. This fascination with Pasteur and his American patients sustained the breakthrough's high visibility for months, with effects persisting for years. Although the frequency of articles dwindled later in 1886, they did not disappear, rising again in the summer of 1887, when the British Commission presented a formal report on Pasteur's work, and especially in 1888, when the Pasteur Institute was opened in Paris. A later flurry of attention was prompted by Pasteur's seventieth birthday in 1892, and another by his death in 1895.[57]

A fourth factor in the story's popularity was that reports on the rabies discovery and the related American adventures were widely distributed. The enthusiasm for following the fortunes of the Newark boys spread across the continent (and beyond). Articles are found in small-town papers as well as in the big-city press, from Jacksonville, Florida, to Ottawa in Canada, and from Boston and Danbury, Connecticut, west to Nashville, Chicago, St. Louis, Los Angeles, and Honolulu.

Unlike other scientific advances, the rabies success and the associated images connecting medical practice with science and progress did not diffuse gradually from the small community of medical scientists. Rather, a very broad public grabbed it almost instantly. Without the intense cultivation of the story by the daily newspapers and the engaged response of their readers, the new treatment for rabies would probably not have changed expectations about medical progress. In time, those ideas might have made their way bit by bit into the general culture, as did awareness of ether anesthesia and the germ theory. But the newspaper writers and the graphic artists made it possible for the rabies-cure sensation to be disseminated effectively to distant regions and different social classes. Sustained repetition of the verbal and visual stimuli pressed this new picture of medical progress deeply into people's consciousness.[58]

The excitement about rabies shots and their life-saving potential prompted a significant outpouring a financial support. But, characteristically, the donations were directed at funding travel and patient care for American victims; for the first few years after Pasteur's breakthrough, people in the United States did not provide new investment for the institutions essential for the local production of this remedy. More time was needed for donors to rethink the longstanding assumption that charity should fund only care for the needy, not medical schools or laboratories, and to begin offering support to Pasteur Institutes on U.S. soil.

CHAPTER 4

POPULAR ENTHUSIASM FOR LABORATORY DISCOVERIES, 1885–1895

If the reports are to be credited, diphtheria will soon take its place beside small-pox and hydrophobia behind the victorious chariot of preventive medicine.

　　　　—Harper's Weekly, September 15, 1894

*T*HE DELUGE OF PUBLICITY about Pasteur and his Newark boys—hundreds of pictures, thousands of articles, live performances, and reenactments in wax—was not just a temporary flood that receded and passed into memory. Its consequences were many and lasting. It initiated a number of cultural developments, which in turn brought permanent changes to popular notions of medicine and to its images in the U.S. media. The "latest" remedies started to displace traditional medical care in popular writings and graphics; a concept of the medical researcher entered public awareness; and additional medical breakthroughs came to be expected. Biological fluids prepared in a laboratory (virus, lymph, serum, and organ extracts), together with the hollow needle and syringe used to administer them, began to displace the pulse taking and the consulting among doctors that formerly had dominated the iconography. The publicity about rabies shots also prompted new organizations and even entirely new organizational forms. Within four weeks of the Newark dog's rampage, plans for U.S. treatment facilities were announced in St. Louis, Newark, and New York City. Although these three initial ventures quickly disappeared, the public's newly raised expectation did not go away. People felt that American victims of dog bites should not be denied access to the life-saving treatment, and when new institutes opened in 1890, they received strong popular support.

Although the role of medical researcher came into American public consciousness through the publicity about Louis Pasteur, it was not limited to the great French scientist. In the late nineteenth century, the United States already had a few physicians who made their livelihood as researchers, though they were not familiar figures. The newspapers were fascinated by such research scientists as the veterinary doctor Frank Seaver Billings of Boston, who had received advanced bacteriological training in German laboratories. In December 1885, Billings happened to be in New York City and volunteered to accompany the Newark children to Paris. By coincidence, Billings's 450-page book, *The Relation of Animal Diseases to the Public Health, and Their Prevention,* which included a chapter on rabies, had just been published by the scientifically prestigious Appleton and Company.[1] In the newspapers, he was sketched as a typical physician with top hat and cane (see fig. 23 in chapter 3).

But as interesting to the press as any specific knowledge that Billings had was how laboratories defined his career. One New York paper portrayed Billings as "the first American who ever entered upon the study of medicine with the sole purpose of devoting his life to original research and the prevention of disease entirely regardless of making money" (*New York World,* December 10, 1885). Even surrounded by the media madness, Billings knew how to promote the scientific work he valued. Billings told the *New York Herald,* "I am sure [the wide publicity] will open up a new channel for original research and stimulate those who have been laboring zealously for a chemical laboratory on an extensive scale" (December 7, 1885). In the Gilded Age, being proclaimed "the first American . . . devoting his life to original research . . . regardless of making money" was a remarkable accolade. The notion of laboratory researcher that the press developed in its portrayal of Billings was further elaborated through lengthy reports about activities inside Pasteur's laboratory in Paris. Even when the portrayal of medical research was humorous, this image of the future of research could still make a strong impression, as in "The Profession Gone Mad" (fig. 30 in chapter 3).

The public, in fact, ran far ahead of the profession in its enthusiasm for rabies treatment, for microbes in medicine, and for optimism about a stream of new advances. During the 1880s, the medical profession for the most part did not share the public's unquestioning support of the rabies cure.[2] In fact, American doctors had uncertain and conflicted responses to bacteriological science in general, and many of them were hesitant to accept its potential contributions to medicine.[3] The hesitation among American physicians about bacteriology's value was probably due to how little it initially contributed to therapeutics.[4] Since rabies cases were so infrequent, physicians, even forward-looking ones, did not share the public's sense that the vaccine solved a major problem. But in the decade after 1885, the profession changed its mind about the rabies vaccine and about bacteriology in general.

As the public became familiar with laboratory research, people learned that such efforts needed financial support. Much of the initial willingness to contribute was based on the tradition of supporting needy patients through charity, such as the donations to send the Newark boys to Paris. And even gifts to build the Pasteur Institute in Paris, solicited after February 1886, tapped this philanthropic impulse rather than any commitment to research per se. But with excitement about the discovery and a growing hope for others like it, people came to see the value of investing in laboratory medicine. Indeed, taxpayer funding for diagnostic laboratories in the United States started in the years following this wave of popular enthusiasm for laboratory research. Other factors contributed to the trend, but it is striking that 1887 saw the establishment of the first federal public-health laboratory and two municipal labs and that by 1900, "many states and all of America's forty largest cities boasted such facilities."[5] A clear indication that some medical leaders saw a connection between popular enthusiasm and financial support for public laboratories is evidenced by the ways that the lessons of the rabies episode were used by Hermann Biggs, a leader of New York's public-health efforts from the early 1890s (heading, in turn, the city's laboratory, the city's entire health department, and the state's health department). Biggs exhibited a profound appreciation for public relations and cultivation of the public's support to ensure funding, especially in his work with the newspapers to promote introduction of the new diphtheria antitoxin in late 1894.[6]

Reporting of breakthroughs in the years following the rabies triumph followed patterns generated by the Pasteur boom. Once the template had been established, numerous features of the rabies triumph reappeared in later episodes. The primary character in all these episodes was the heroic and selfless scientist. By mixing images of Pasteur's genius, his special kindness to the young patients, and his role as benefactor to the human race, the reportage articulated a notion of medicine as characterized by progress, heroism, altruism, and public benefit. It is significant that, while the cartoonists and writers made great fun of the popular excitement, Pasteur himself was largely exempted from American mockery. Essential, too, were the worthy patients, many desperate enough to travel great distances for a miracle cure. Individuals were named, pictured, interviewed for the media, and sometimes even placed on exhibition. Children made the medical story more poignant, and that easy sympathy was frequently exploited by the press, physicians, and medical charities ever after.[7] Also involved were local physicians trying to replicate the work of the discoverers in order to provide treatment to Americans at home, and there were Good Samaritans, who helped pay for the Newark boys' steamer fares or who donated warm clothing for the boys' trip. Through the subscription campaign, hundreds, perhaps thousands, of unrelated individuals became active participants in the story. Finally, there were philanthropists, fund-raisers, and other advocates. Some contributed money, others used the power of the press to support the endeavor.

The animals used in the experiments constituted another important group of visible participants. In the rabies episode, their essential role was reported in ways that suggest that vivisection was not then particularly controversial for the American public at large. The animals, without being individualized like the patients, were not kept out of sight—not even the rabbits that were sacrificed to produce the therapeutic material. Illustrations of Pasteur's laboratory showed the caged rabbits and dogs and the operations performed on them, as did the portrayal of the Newark doctors trying their own experiments. The reports indicated that many animals lost their lives, sometimes to instruments and sometimes to the disease they had been given. A typical article in a morning newspaper, "In Pasteur's Laboratory: Watching the Inoculation of a Rabbit with the Virus," gave a straightforward narrative of how the animals were handled. The text described how the laboratory assistants grabbed the rabbit, trimmed the fur on its skull, tied it down, forced it to inhale chloroform, cut open the skin between the eyes, stretched the skin back with a piece of wire, and then augured a hole through the skull bone to insert a needle into the rabbit's brain (*New York Herald,* December 27, 1885). Similarly clinical accounts appeared in the *Chicago Tribune* (June 12, 1886) and elsewhere. The operation was pictured again and again in the popular press. In one widely circulated image, Pasteur and one assistant face the viewer across a bench on which another assistant, his back to the viewer, drills an opening in the skull of a rabbit stretched out on a slab (fig. 31). The caption informs the readers that the rabbit was anesthetized and not in pain.[8] Even the procedure of forcing healthy dogs to be bitten by rabid ones was described in the popular media. New rabbits were continually needed to produce the therapeutic substance used in the rabies shots and to serve as the culture medium for determining whether a dog that had bit someone was truly rabid. All this was regularly depicted in the daily papers without sensation or hint of scandal.

Through the rabies-cure enthusiasm, vivisection was presented in a positive light for a number of years before an antivivisection movement could gain much traction in the United States. From the outset, scientists among New York's physicians knew the importance of vivisection and how to argue publicly for its value. In discussing the proposed Pasteur Institute in late December 1885, Professor Adolph Corbett, to be superintendent of the new institute, told the *New York Herald* reporter,

> We will probably run against Mr. Bergh [who founded the American Society for the Prevention of Cruelty to Animals in 1866] when we get to work on the dogs and rabbits which are necessary to operate with. In that case we shall fight him. Mr. Bergh loves the animals, so do I, but I love the people more. We will kill as many dogs as are necessary. At the present time there are 150 patients under M. Pasteur's care. In my opinion the lives of all the loose curs in the world are as naught when the sacrifice can save those human beings.[9]

Even more than the easy popularity of such utilitarian arguments, it was the uncritical wave of enthusiasm for Pasteur's apparent triumph in saving children's lives that normalized the use of animals in medical research for Americans in general.[10] In

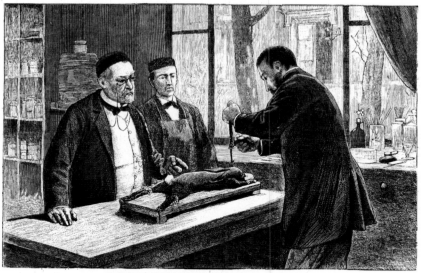
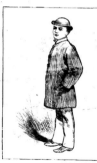
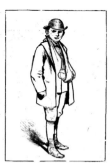
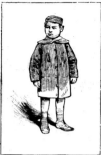

FIG. 31. "The French Chemist, M. Pasteur, Experiments on a Chloroformed Rabbit," illustration above a story entitled "M. Pasteur and His Patients," *Frank Leslie's Illustrated Newspaper* 61:1578 (December 19, 1885), 300. Full page. Author's collection.

the diphtheria-cure episode of 1894, horses displaced dogs and rabbits as the media stars, competing for attention with the dying babies who recovered quickly after treatment. Dogs returned as celebrated heroes in the insulin breakthrough in the 1920s and in the blue-baby operations of the 1950s and 1960s.

Alongside the flood of printed images of Pasteur and other researchers, one representation of the laboratory worker painted in France entered the iconography in the United States and gained a permanent place therein, "Pasteur in His Laboratory" (fig. 32). Louis Pasteur took time to pose for this oil portrait by Albert Edelfelt in 1885, even in the midst of the intense and secretive work on rabies.[11] The large canvas presents Pasteur leaning on a laboratory bench crowded with apparatus, holding a drying bottle in one hand, and contemplating the small piece of material suspended in the jar. Knowing viewers recognized the material as the highly infective spinal cord from a rabbit that had died of rabies and understood that this dried material was the potent, life-saving agent administered in rabies shots. Pasteur's facial expression is serious but not somber; he is thinking, perhaps about the risk of injecting lethal virus into persons or perhaps about the miraculous power found in a tiny piece of dried nerve tissue. He regards appreciatively the deadly biological material that has been transformed in his hands. This look of contemplative respect for a breakthrough remedy—expressed here for the first time in history—was to reappear in portraits of medical heroes again and again right through to our own day.[12]

Engraved reproductions of this painting may have appeared in French pictorials when it was first exhibited to acclaim at the Paris Salon of May and June 1886, but the earliest publication of it in the United States seems to have been a July 1890 center spread in *Harper's Bazar* with a report about rabies treatments in Paris and in New York City.[13] It was printed again in October of the same year on the cover of *Once a Week: An Illustrated Weekly*.[14] In honor of Pasteur's seventieth birthday, it was printed in January 1893 by *Frank Leslie's Illustrated Weekly*.[15] It was included in a long, remarkably well-illustrated article on Pasteur by Ida Tarbell in an early issue of the new *McClure's Magazine* in September 1893.[16] Two years later, in articles about Pasteur's death, *Harper's Weekly* published the image full page in October 1895, and the *Review of Reviews* did the same in November.[17] It was also included in a popular collection of short illustrated essays, *Great Men and Famous Women*, published in 1894.[18]

The image is historically significant far beyond the fact of its wide circulation during the 1890s. It pioneered an entirely new artistic vision of the scientist, and it created an iconography that continued to influence artists for several decades. Like Gustave Courbet and other realists committed to painting the "heroism of modern life," Edelfelt portrayed Pasteur in the manner of history paintings, a genre of oversized canvases, rich with emotion, meaning, morality, and heavy oil paint. These paintings typically celebrated a great scene from history, usually featuring a monarch or a military leader, often surrounded by numerous lesser figures in an out-of-doors setting. Edelfelt gave the form a new subject that clashed with the expectations of the older genre. Here was a man at work, with dirty hands, captured at a single

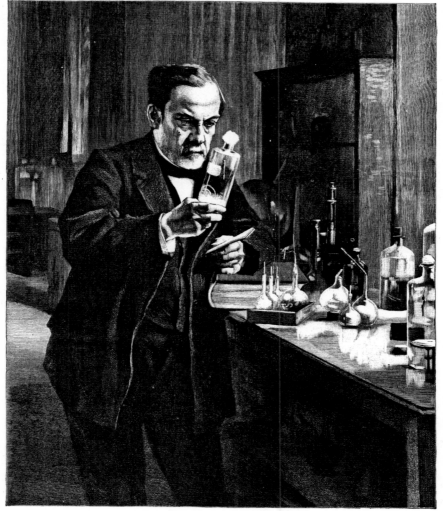

ONCE A WEEK

∴AN ILLUSTRATED WEEKLY NEWSPAPER∴

Vol. V.—No. 25.
Copyright, 1890, by P. F. Collier.
All rights reserved.

NEW YORK, OCTOBER 7, 1890.

$6.00 per Year.
INCLUDING LIBRARY.

PASTEUR IN HIS LABORATORY.

FIG. 32. "Pasteur in His Laboratory," *Once a Week: An Illustrated Weekly* 5:25 (October 7, 1890), cover (1). Neither Edelfelt as artist nor any engraver was credited in this publication. Author's collection.

moment, unposed, as if we just happened to walk in on him unnoticed. This deeply reverential portrayal offered a view of the character of medicine that persisted in the minds of viewers long after it was out of sight. Because of its great artistry, it was more memorable, once absorbed, than many ephemeral images in the newspapers and magazines. This celebration of Pasteur's new life-saving remedy was stylistically innovative in its time—despite its easy familiarity to modern eyes.[19] That the painting seems unposed, almost like a modern candid snapshot, should not keep us from recognizing the artist's powerful composition or from appreciating the innovative, even revolutionary, characterization of the scientist invented by Edelfelt.

Prior to about 1880, oil paintings of physicians were either genre scenes that told little stories—in which the physician was often examining the urine of a heartsick young woman or was fussing in the disarray of his alchemical workshop—or stiff formal portraits, in which no tools of the trade were in evidence.[20] Edelfelt in Europe and Thomas Eakins in the United States were the first to paint doctors at work in a grand, heroic mode. Edelfelt's pensive Louis Pasteur gave rise to a general image of the scientific healer, characterized by his contemplation of a vial of the precious, potent, and perhaps dangerous new fluid created by ingenious processes in a laboratory under the hero's personal guidance and genius. This pursuer of knowledge is observed meditating on the miracle product, not producing it. He is a thinker, not a cook. Somewhat like the older iconography of a physical scientist holding a terrestrial globe or a model of the heavens, this maker of medical miracles holds in his hands a sample that represents in miniature the enormous healing power that will in time spread around the world. The painting established a powerful iconography of posture and mood for "the great scientist." Edelfelt created an icon, an archetype that continued to serve as a model for artists, illustrators, photographers, cinematographers, and cartoonists over most of the twentieth century.

ORGANOTHERAPY MAKES THE HEADLINES

In early June 1889, when the multinational physician and physiologist Charles-Édouard Brown-Séquard announced in Paris that he had succeeded in effecting rejuvenation in men by injections of testicular extracts from animals, many aspects of the story captured widespread interest—not the least of which was that this elderly doctor tested the extracts on himself.[21] The research tapped popular curiosity about sex, masculinity, aging, and the use of animal extracts in humans. Brown-Séquard was then seventy-two years old, a member of the French Academy of Science, and a professor of medicine at the Collège de France. He was at the peak of a rather peripatetic career in which he had practiced medicine, taught in medical schools, and performed research in Boston, London, New York, Nice, Paris, Philadelphia, and Richmond, Virginia. Press coverage in the United States was sporadic until the complete text of his paper appeared in English translation in the *Scientific American*

Supplement for August 10, 1889.[22] News coverage then swelled, and it unfortunately came to include at least two reports of fatal outcomes at the hands of American doctors rushing to replicate the experimental treatment.[23] The weekly *Frank Leslie's Illustrated Newspaper* headlined its report "An Astonishing Medical Discovery" and cited experiments in the United States by former U.S. Army Surgeon-General William A. Hammond.[24] Hammond's work with testicular extracts appeared in professional journals, but he also disseminated his findings to a much broader public in the *North American Review*.[25]

The titillating imagery quickly seized the popular imagination and appeared in songs, comic poems, satires, and political caricature. Within two weeks of the first reports, the two leading magazines of political and social commentary employed the apparently well-known phrase "Brown-Séquard's Elixir of Life," in full-color, double-page center-spread cartoons about national politics. "Elixir of life" was not a new phrase; it had an established use among patent medicine makers and had appeared in political cartoons before. But a therapy that used piston syringes and hollow needles to inject tired men with juice from sexual organs gave the old alchemical term a comic new lease on life. Risqué jokes were irresistible. The *National Police Gazette* ran a news story, along with one of its outlandishly exaggerated illustrations, about a Muncie, Indiana, farmer whose young lambs had been disappearing. The first suspects were old men, supposed to have killed the lambs for their personal rejuvenation efforts. It was then discovered that the lambs had been killed by a very large snake. The image caption for this anaconda-like creature called it "a monster serpent in search of the elixir of life, and with no money to hire Brown-Sequard."[26] Before the end of the year, a song sheet entitled "Brown-Sequard's Elixir: The Greatest Comic Song of the Day" was published in Chicago and Cincinnati.[27]

At *Puck,* an independent magazine with Democratic leanings, Louis Dalrymple fashioned organotherapy into a lively attack on the Republican administration's new pension policy, by which James Tanner, the commissioner of pensions, had proposed using a government surplus to expand pension benefits for Civil War veterans and their relatives. Like the other political cartoons that used medical-breakthrough imagery, "It Beats Brown-Séquard" (fig. 33) is less interesting today for its role in partisan wrangling than for the evidence it provides of a mass familiarity with the latest headlined innovation.

Brown-Séquard's "elixir of life" showed up again a few days later in *Puck's* competitor, the Republican-inclined weekly *Judge,* in "Hopeless Cases," a center-spread caricature by Grant Hamilton (see color plate 7).[28] Here, the Brown-Séquard figure is Samuel Jackson Randall, a Democratic congressman from Pennsylvania, who had lost President Cleveland's favor two years earlier; he had been protectionist since the 1860s despite his party's distaste for that position. He is now well-supplied with two large tanks of "Protectionism" as an "Elixir of Life." But it is too late, he says, for this rejuvenation juice to revive the Democratic Party and its debilitated Free Trade policy. This up-to-date physician declares, "Take Them Away. They're Too Dead for Treatment."[29]

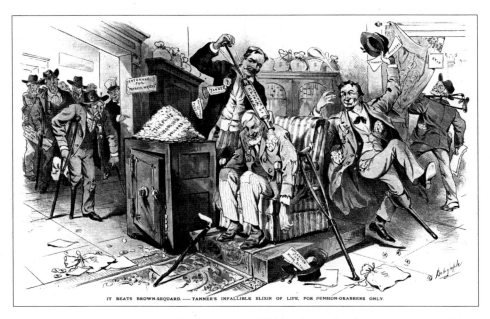

IT BEATS BROWN-SEQUARD. — TANNER'S INFALLIBLE ELIXIR OF LIFE, FOR PENSION-GRABBERS ONLY.

FIG. 33. "It Beats Brown-Séquard.—Tanner's Infallible Elixir of Life, for Pension-Grabbers Only," *Puck* 26:651 (August 28, 1889), center spread (8–9). Chromolithograph by Louis Dalrymple. Author's collection.

Notable, too, in these two political cartoons are the crude, but recognizable, depictions of the syringe with a hypodermic needle, not yet a commonly pictured device. When the hypodermic reappeared the following year in connection with Koch's tuberculin, it was portrayed more accurately (if still humorously enlarged). With respect to changes in medical iconography more generally, the seated figure was identified in 1889 as a physician by his medication bottle and syringe, not yet by a thermometer or stethoscope (both then in use), for their entry into popular imagery still lay in the future. The large comic syringes echoed the exaggeratedly large enema clysters that had been popular in caricature a century earlier.[30]

Whether or not partisan cartoonists and their readers deemed the new organotherapy effective, such images signaled widespread familiarity with the latest medical breakthrough. In fact, by mid-October, there had been so much excitement among the lay public that *Scientific American* felt it necessary to defend Brown-Séquard's character and his work against distortions and exaggerations in the popular press.[31] Another indication of just how quickly and widely the organotherapy craze spread was the large number of people who tried it. According to Brown-Séquard's biographer, by the end of 1890 "more than twelve thousand physicians were administering the extract to their patients."[32]

This kind of sudden, radical advance had long been unimaginable in medicine. Now it might be used by thousands of patients within months of the discovery. This pattern of fevered anticipation and recklessly rapid adoption was soon repeated

—and on a far greater scale—about a year later, when another European medical scientist captured headlines around the world with another injectable fluid, this one a purported cure for consumption: the German physician Robert Koch with his mysterious "tuberculin."

TUBERCULIN: ROBERT KOCH'S CONSUMPTION CURE

It would be hard to imagine a more significant or gratifying breakthrough than an injectable remedy for people faced with the lingering death of consumption, the greatest killer of the age. In 1890, Robert Koch proposed the use of his tuberculin lymph exclusively as a therapy; its value as a diagnostic test came only later, from observations made incidentally on the first cohorts of patients. For a while, the frenzy of an enthusiasm shared by the press and the public knew no bounds. Not only was tuberculosis a disease whose morbidity and mortality dwarfed that of rabies by many orders of magnitude, but its cure was at the hands of the great physician Robert Koch, whose discoveries about the etiological agents of anthrax, cholera, and tuberculosis had already carried him to the pinnacle of professional recognition internationally. If his name had not yet become the household name that Pasteur's was, it acquired that status in a flash. The excitement blossomed so quickly that it put the attention accorded Pasteur five years earlier into a shadow. If Pasteur was an experimentalist hero and a kindly gentleman who fussed over the children arriving for treatment, Koch was a St. George slaying the dragon of monstrous disease. Unfortunately for Koch and for the world, his tuberculin therapy was soon challenged as ineffective, and even harmful in some cases.[33]

For a few months, the media, the public, and the profession in the United States were captivated by what seemed to be laboratory medicine's crowning achievement. On November 15, 1890, the front page of the *New York Times* carried a translation of Koch's complete text from the *Deutsche medizinische Wochenschrift* of November 14 (received by cable). But this was not a big-city story only; it can be traced, for example, in Connecticut's *Danbury Evening News,* a paper appearing five times a week in a small city with fewer than three thousand listed taxpayers in 1885. Even without attempting to capture all the tuberculin coverage or the depth of the stories, the following selected highlights illustrate important themes and key events in this paper's coverage, such as the nature of the public's interest and the intense competition among cities and medical institutions to be the earliest participants.

NOVEMBER 17: The University of Pennsylvania is sending a doctor to Berlin.

NOVEMBER 18: Boston will have a Koch Institute.

NOVEMBER 22: "Will It Cure Cancer, Too? Professor Koch Looking for More Diseases to Conquer." (The article included a small portrait of Koch.) Pasteur sends Koch congratulations and is sent a vial of the lymph.

DECEMBER 4: New Haven receives a small portion of the lymph. "It is believed that the lymph is the first received and injected in America."

DECEMBER 5: Lymph is used in New Haven and its effects described.

DECEMBER 9: More tuberculin is received in New Haven.

DECEMBER 11: Danbury expects some tuberculin next week. The lymph is used in New York by Dr. Jacobi at Mount Sinai but earlier by Dr. Kinicutt at St. Luke's.

DECEMBER 12: A doctor in Paris prevents tuberculin's use at the Bichat Hospital.

DECEMBER 15: "Koch's Lymph at the Capital" (its use in Washington) and "Secrecy at Johns Hopkins" (doctors not revealing initial reactions of fourteen treated patients).

DECEMBER 18: The first Philadelphia injections. Lymph reported to be working well in New Haven.

DECEMBER 19: Lymph is expected in Danbury.

DECEMBER 30: The patients at Johns Hopkins are doing well.

JANUARY 12: The return of a New York doctor from Berlin with two bottles of lymph that he will use, but not on advanced patients.

JANUARY 15: "The Lymph [Is] Curing Lupus" at City Hospital in Worcester, Massachusetts.

JANUARY 16: "Koch's Cure Described: The Discoverer Tells the World All about It. Several Criticisms Answered. . . . While It Is Young, Yet Many Cures Have Resulted."

JANUARY 22: "Lymph for the President" (President Benjamin Harrison receives from the U.S. minister at Berlin five vials that are being distributed to hospitals in Chicago, Indianapolis, New Orleans, and Washington, D.C.).

Similar stories may be found in many papers.[34] The stacked headlines of one illustrated story in the *New York World* on November 26 used a recent death to pump up a sense of desperate need for the pursuit of tuberculin: "A Consumptive's Death. How Poor Jane Lee Yielded Yesterday Morning to the Great White Plague. The German Doctor's Remedy Too Late for Her. Pathetic Details of the Last Hours and the Death of a Charity Patient in the Consumptives' Ward on Blackwell's Island." A good example of how newspapers played up "firsts" and how they sometimes found a local dimension to a foreign story, which they otherwise had to report through the news in other papers, appeared in the *Rochester Post Express.* The article was based on private letters sent from Europe to American friends by a doctor from Albion, New York (a town about thirty miles west of Rochester): "The Koch Cure: How the Great German Physician Operates. Dr. William C. Bailey of Albion Writes of His Experiences in the Berlin Hospital. The First American to Witness the Operation" (December 11, 1890, 8).

Six months later, reflecting back on the previous winter's media coverage, the nationally recognized Chicago surgeon Nicholas Senn observed that "for days and weeks the public press devoted a liberal space to telegraphic messages, to editorials and messages from medical men, relative to the new treatment." He also claimed that "no other event in the world's history ever attracted so much attention and no discovery in medicine and surgery ever found such ready introduction and universal application."[35] Popular graphic images drew the public once again—and even more deeply this time—into an enthusiasm for laboratory research and science-based therapies.

U.S. papers and magazines frequently printed a rather engaging portrait of a handsome and younger-than-he-actually-was Robert Koch.[36] In some papers this image was paired with a rather lifeless sketch of the doctor in his laboratory. *Frank Leslie's Illustrated Newspaper* printed a full-page suite of images that combined these two images with four technical drawings labeled "fresh bacilli from the lungs of a consumptive patient, as seen under the microscope," "bacilli after two weeks' growth, under the microscope," "tube containing a 'culture' of tuberculous bacilli," and "tube containing 'culture' of comma (cholera) bacilli" (fig. 34). The page carried this firmly optimistic caption: "The Prevention and Cure of Consumption—Dr. Koch's Great Discovery."[37] Even though microscopes, specimens, and "cultures" had in 1890 not yet become routine aspects of medical training and practice, they were familiar to a broad segment of the public from parlor science activities, microscopical societies, and such cartoons as a cover of *Puck* that, earlier that same year, had portrayed a tiny President Benjamin Harrison under Uncle Sam's microscope.[38]

The tuberculin cure—like Pasteur's rabies treatment—quickly came to be represented as much by the lucky patients in their moment of celebrity as by the physicians involved. When an American patient was sent to Berlin for treatment with funds raised by *Frank Leslie's Illustrated Newspaper,* an artist recorded the steps taken to secure the life-saving intervention, starting with the patient's pretreatment examination in New York by Dr. George F. Shrady, a leading New York physician and editor of the *Medical Record* from 1866 to 1904. An inset portrait of the patient William Degan was given the same individuality and prominence as the physician's portrait.[39] Just a few days later, another pictorial paper, *Once a Week,* ran an article that included a drawing of a female patient with her back exposed to view, "Dr. Bergmann showing effect of lymph" (January 6, 1891, 11). This article reported that New York City then had 116 cases under experimental treatment at nine hospitals. It listed the hospitals and the numbers of cases, ranging from four to twenty-nine. It mentioned that five physicians had gone to Germany for training and returned on December 22 with enough lymph for an estimated thirty thousand inoculations. *Frank Leslie's* in due time (allowing for steamer travel across the Atlantic and back) provided the American public with a full-page illustration of the sponsored patient's treatment in Berlin (fig. 35).[40]

Without delay, political cartoonists grabbed new images from this "latest sensation," sometimes even jumping ahead of the news engravings, as they tapped the public's excitement about tuberculin as the greatest breakthrough of the era—and perhaps of all human history. *Puck's* leading artist, Joseph Keppler—possibly

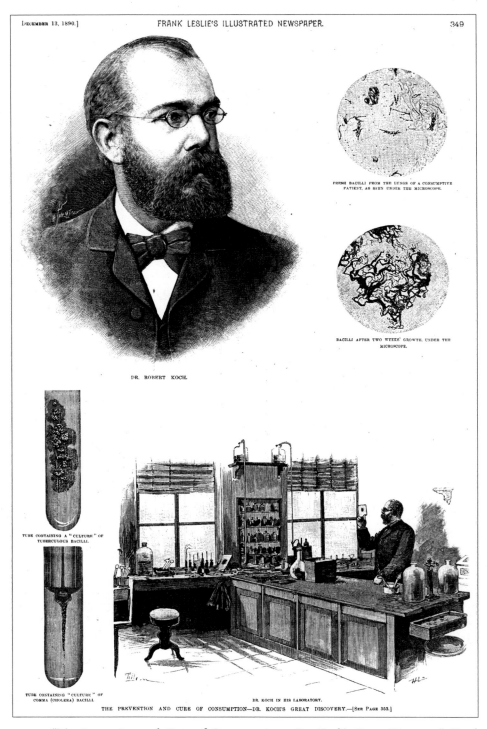

FRESH BACILLI FROM THE LUNGS OF A CONSUMPTIVE
PATIENT, AS SEEN UNDER THE MICROSCOPE.

BACILLI AFTER TWO WEEKS' GROWTH UNDER THE
MICROSCOPE.

DR. ROBERT KOCH.

TUBE CONTAINING A "CULTURE" OF
TUBERCULOUS BACILLI.

TUBE CONTAINING "CULTURE" OF
COMMA (CHOLERA) BACILLI.

DR. KOCH IN HIS LABORATORY.

THE PREVENTION AND CURE OF CONSUMPTION—DR. KOCH'S GREAT DISCOVERY.—[SEE PAGE 353.]

FIG. 34. "The Prevention and Cure of Consumption—Dr. Koch's Great Discovery," *Frank Leslie's Illustrated Newspaper* 71:1839 (December 13, 1890), 349. Author's collection.

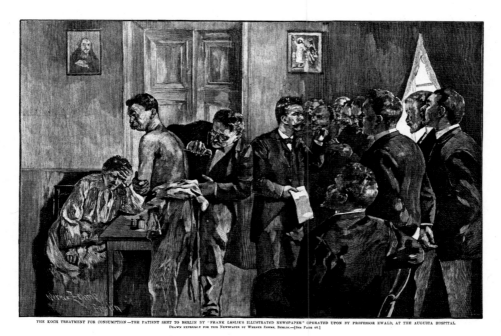

THE KOCH TREATMENT FOR CONSUMPTION—THE PATIENT SENT TO BERLIN BY "FRANK LESLIE'S ILLUSTRATED NEWSPAPER" OPERATED UPON BY PROFESSOR EWALD, AT THE AUGUSTA HOSPITAL.
Drawn expressly for this Newspaper by Werner Zehme, Berlin.—[See Page 46.]

FIG. 35. "The Koch Treatment for Consumption—The Patient Sent to Berlin by 'Frank Les-lie's Illustrated Newspaper' Operated Upon by Professor Ewald, at the Augusta Hospital, Drawn Expressly for the Newspaper by Werner Zehme, Berlin," *Frank Leslie's Illustrated Newspaper* 72:1848 (February 21, 1891), 47. Author's collection.

encouraged by the similarity of Robert Koch's oval face with full beard to that of Keppler's favorite target, James G. Blaine (referenced in the "Blainiac rabies" car-toon, in color plate 5, as well as in many other caricatures)—exploited the lymph cure for consumption in his center-spread political cartoon for the December 10 is-sue (probably printed a week earlier). In "A Bad Case of Consumption—Dr. Blaine Tries an Injection of His Reciprocity Lymph," the sick Republican Party elephant is surrounded by top-hatted doctors consulting on the case; one of them is timing the elephant's pulse with a watch in one hand and the animal's tail in the other. Those were stock images of medical caricature, but here they are pushed to the side by two important novelties: the hypodermic syringe (made popular via the Brown-Séquard elixir) and the injectable remedy ("Reciprocity Lymph") (see color plate 8).[41] The political issues of reciprocity, free trade, and protectionism were commonplaces of the era, but the latest therapy's bring-them-back-from-death's-door potential was quite new, echoing the miraculous rabies cure of five years before. To exaggerate the mysterious power of the lymph as well as Blaine's mercurial character (he is stand-ing on a "reversible platform"), the cartoonist garbs Blaine as a medieval wizard, in contrast to the recognizably contemporary physicians to his left and right.[42]

Widespread popular familiarity with the new lymph and with Koch as its inven-tor was indicated as well by *Judge* magazine's attack on problems in the Democratic

Party just a week later (see color plate 9).[43] Dressed in doctors' traditional top hats and armed with carefully depicted (if enlarged) syringes, Dr. Koch-Cleveland and Dr. Koch-Hill proffered competing therapies to revive the ailing Democratic Party tiger.[44] As with *Puck's* cartoon, the political issues were old hat ("humbug reform" versus "spoils system"), but the medical metaphor of "lymph" used to mock them was brand new.

By 1890, the new expectations of regular breakthroughs were already so firmly established that jokes could be made about them without conveying criticism. The following doggerel verses appeared under the title "Modern Medicine" in December of that year:

> First they pumped him full of virus from some mediocre cow,
> Lest the small-pox might assail him and leave pit-marks on his brow;
> Then one day a bull-dog bit him—he was gunning down at Quogue—
> And they filled his veins in Paris with an extract of mad-dog;
> Then he caught tuberculosis, so they took him to Berlin,
> And injected half a gallon of bacilli into him. . . .
> But his blood was so diluted by the remedies he'd taken
> That one day he laid him down and died, and never did awaken:
> With the Brown-Sequard elixir though they tried resuscitation,
> He never showed a symptom of reviving animation;
> Yet his doctor still could save him, (he persistently maintains,)
> If he only could inject a little life into his veins.[45]

Then, when disappointing results started appearing in January 1891, the humorists, journalists, physicians, and patients all turned against Koch. The *Danbury Evening News* was typical, reporting on January 23, 1891 (just one day after it heralded the delivery of five vials from Berlin to President Harrison), that people were calling Koch's lymph "a failure." William Degan, the consumptive whom *Frank Leslie's* sent to Berlin and the first American patient to be treated, was said to believe he derived no benefit from tuberculin and was in poorer health than when he went abroad. On February 3, the *Danbury Evening News* reported the death in New Haven of George M. Bradley, "the first person treated in America with Dr. Koch's lymph," and the near-death condition of "the son of Professor Blake" of Yale. Still, another Yale professor, Dr. Chittenden, who was in charge of these patients, defended the lymph as not to be judged by extreme cases. Two days later, the paper reported that a package containing lymph from Berlin had arrived in Danbury, that it would be discussed at a medical society meeting that evening, and that the lymph—almost as if it were an object of religious veneration—would be "on exhibition today at Reed & Co.'s drug store."

While everything had seemed so promising, most people were willing to overlook Koch's reticence about revealing the formulation of his tuberculin lymph and his rush to treat hordes of patients without preliminary studies on a limited number of them. When the lymph did not cure patients and sometimes aggravated their consumption, the media and the medical profession challenged Koch for being mercenary as well as for failing, and they accused him of inappropriately pursuing publicity and fame. Without admitting their own complicity in creating a sensation, papers started to offer comic put-downs such as the following quip: "A Voice from the Medical Limbo.—'Hello there, Koch's lymph! I'm expecting you.'—'Who are you?'—'I'm Brown-Sequard's elixir of life.'"[46] And the following January, in a back-page cartoon in *Judge* with seven vignettes entitled "A Chapter on Cranks," the artist Emil Flohri included as one of the scenes "Dr. Koch's Lymph for Consumptives" along with "the Brown-Séquard Elixir of Life," "Dr. Pasteur's Treatment for Rabies," and "Dr. Keeley's Bichloride of Gold" treatment for drunks, all under the rubric "Cranks who made it pay while it lasted."[47] From today's perspective, these innovations of Pasteur, Brown-Séquard, Koch, and Keeley were each quite distinct in origin, medical value, and intellectual achievement; yet this cartoon, despite its broad brush, indicates how breakthroughs were already coming to be seen by people as a continuous series.

SERUM TO SAVE SICK CHILDREN

By the summer of 1894, European results were accumulating to show that antitoxin injections for people suffering from diphtheria sharply reduced the mortality of this frightening childhood malady.[48] Like rabies vaccine, testicular extract, and tuberculin therapy, this antitoxin was an injectable biological product derived from laboratory experiments with small animals. But unlike those breakthroughs, this one earned permanent recognition by historians and the public alike as a major triumph over disease. Stimulating rapid recovery in mortally ill patients, especially children, was far more dramatic than explaining illnesses or even preventing them; and this therapeutic achievement was sudden and striking, often lowering case mortality from 50 to 15 percent. This antitoxin was built on the prior identification of pathogens, but that knowledge was taken in a new direction. Researchers manipulated animals' immune response to create a potent biological product, namely, blood serum (most effectively produced by horses) containing high concentrations of a diphtheria antagonist that, when injected into sick people, helped their bodies combat the disease. The cure was the result of collaboration and competition between French and German laboratories. The United States did not create the cure, but its medical scientists quickly found ways to manufacture it effectively.[49]

U.S. daily newspapers began to print encouraging reports of European trials of the new serum treatment in the summer of 1894. In mid-September, *Harper's Weekly* editorialized on "The New Remedy for Diphtheria."[50] This rather long and unillustrated piece established in firm and measured tones several key features that shaped the events to follow.

> A representative of the New York Board of Health [Dr. Biggs] has just returned from a trip abroad, made for the purpose of investigating a new German remedy that is said to be almost a certain cure for diphtheria. His report is so enthusiastic that our authorities are to be asked to establish a laboratory for the development of the remedy here. The outcome will be awaited with anxious interest by every one who truly understands how much is at stake.

The second paragraph argued the special urgency of this cause with revealing numbers and a picture of definite historical progress:

> Two years ago there was much ado because typhus fever seemed to have gained a foothold in the city. That much-heralded disease caused 40 deaths; diphtheria, unheralded, caused 1436. Last year there was no little apprehension in some quarters because small-pox was mildly epidemic in the city, claiming a few victims who by their folly or ignorance had invited it. Yet small-pox during the decade 1883–'92 caused only 335 deaths in the city; diphtheria caused 15,066. Thanks to sanitary science, typhus may be held at bay. Thanks to Jenner, the terrors of small-pox are only traditional. But the terrors of diphtheria are still real and ever-present.

The editorial then noted the discovery, ten years earlier, of the cause of diphtheria and explained that the bacilli produce toxins, which may be developed in media other than the human body, and that toxins, when attenuated, may be injected into animals whose bodies produce something now shown to cure cases of diphtheria in humans. "If the reports are to be credited, diphtheria will soon take its place beside small-pox and hydrophobia behind the victorious chariot of preventive medicine." In closing, the editor reminded readers not to let optimism go beyond actual achievement, as had sadly been the case with Koch's tuberculin.

News reports in the dailies continued sporadically through the fall. In November, *Scientific American* published a more substantial report whose three illustrations established the leading visual elements for all the successive depictions. The first image showed medical personnel injecting the remedy into the belly of a sick child apparently in a hospital setting (fig. 36). A second image portrayed white-coated laboratory workers surrounded by flasks and tanks. In the third drawing, a docile and dignified horse was patiently allowing its blood to be drawn (fig. 37).

None of the participants in these scenes was identified, nor was a specific hospital, laboratory, or city named. Though generic (perhaps created by American artists merely from verbal accounts), these pictures were to become iconic. The stream of brief newspaper accounts widened in early December, when the *New York Herald* began an aggressive campaign in support of funding (both public and private) to set up a laboratory and stables needed by the Health Department for the production of

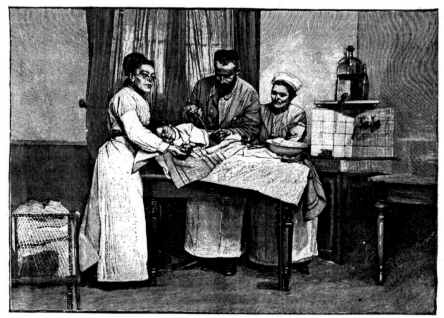

THE NEW CURE FOR DIPHTHERIA, CROUP ETC.—INJECTING THE SERUM.

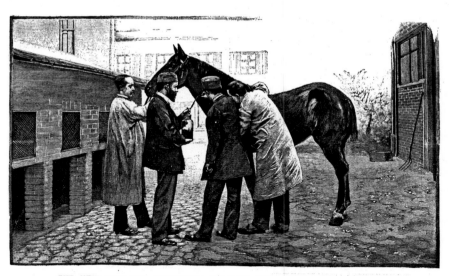

THE NEW CURE FOR DIPHTHERIA—DRAWING THE SERUM FROM THE HORSE.

Top: **FIG. 36**. "The New Cure for Diphtheria, Croup, etc.—Injecting the Serum," *Scientific American* 71:20 (November 17, 1894), 308. This image also appeared in the *New York Herald* (December 11 1894), 3; in *Review of Reviews* 11:1 (January 1895), 4; and in *Leslie's Illustrated Weekly* 80:2053 (January 17, 1895), 46. Author's collection. *Bottom:* **FIG. 37**. "The New Cure for Diphtheria—Drawing the Serum from the Horse," *Scientific American* 71:20 (November 17, 1894), 309. This image also appeared in the *New York Herald* (December 12, 1894), 3; and in *Leslie's Illustrated Weekly* 80:2053 (January 17, 1895), 46. Author's collection.

antitoxin. The *New York Herald* was the newspaper that had led the pack in coverage of the Newark boys' trip to Pasteur's laboratory in Paris back in 1885. By 1894, changes in printing technology allowed daily newspapers to run pictures that were wider than one column.[51] This development had two effects, providing a new hook for quick emotional engagement and making possible much larger graphics in the dailies to compete with those in the heavily illustrated weeklies.

On Monday, December 10, the *Herald* published five pictures in an article that covered five columns of a six-column page. Opening the piece, a tall stack of headlines announced the issues and pumped up the excitement:

ANTI-TOXINE FOR THE POOR.
Popular Subscription Started by the Herald to Provide Dr. Roux's Great Remedy for Diphtheria for the Public.
HEADS THE LIST WITH $1,000.
Public Invited to Join in the Work of Supplying the Health Restoring Fluid.
PHYSICIANS APPROVE THE PLAN.
Drs. Curtis, Edson, Shrady, Gibier, Jacobi, and Loomis Indorse [*sic*] the Herald's Enterprise.
NEED OF SERUM URGENT.
Many Lives Will Be Saved If It Can Be Brought Within the Reach of All.

A two-column-wide portrait of Dr. Émile Roux dominated the page (fig. 38), supplemented by four other single-column images: Professor Emil Behring, M.D., "In the Laboratory" (a man standing at a bench covered with glassware), Dr. Cyrus Edson, and Dr. Paul Gibier. Because the first two pages of the *Herald* carried only classified ads, page 3 was equivalent to the front page of other newspapers.

The following day, December 11, the *Herald*'s mass audience was presented with the sketch that had earlier been seen only by the more restricted readership of *Scientific American*: "Inoculation with Anti-toxine" (the same image as in fig. 36). This print was four columns wide (about seven inches by ten) and placed at the top of page 3 next to another batch of self-promoting headlines:

ALL EAGER FOR ANTI-TOXINE.
Enthusiastic Support of the Herald's Project for Manufacturing the Great Diphtheria Remedy in This Country.
UNIVERSAL COMMENDATION.
Physicians and Other Scientists Approve the Enterprise in Flattering Terms.
IT MEANS A SAVING OF LIFE.
Leaders in Medicine Pronounce the Undertaking One of Commanding Importance.
OTHER CITIES APPLAUD IT.
Prompt Assistance Means Early Success, and Money Is Imperatively Required.

On the next day, the *Herald* reprinted the horse picture from *Scientific American* (same image as in fig. 37) over the caption "Taking the Serum from a Horse," again

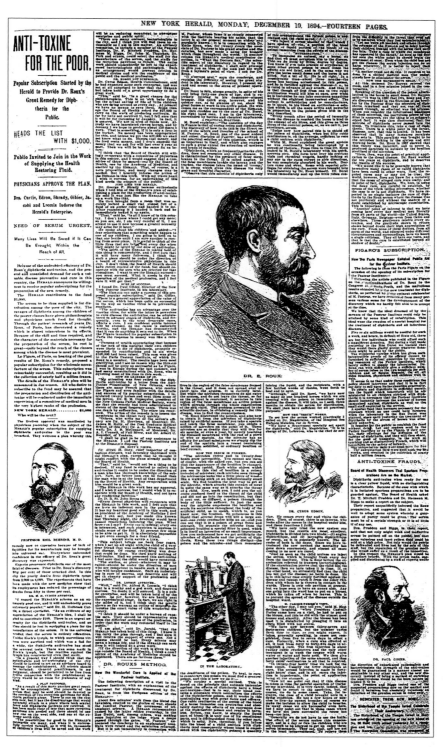

FIG. 38. "Anti-toxine for the Poor," *New York Herald,* December 10, 1894, 3.

in four-column width at the top of page 3, with headlines proclaiming "Anti-Toxine Is Greatly Needed. A Chorus of Approvals Everywhere. . . . Physicians Greatly Hampered by Their Inability to Obtain the New Cure."[52]

The frequent reiteration of horse pictures suggests that they were especially engaging.[53] But even if horses heightened the emotionalism of the pictures, didacticism was present as well. The public was served numerous images of serious men handling the precious serum and manipulating elaborate glassware in settings that nicely mingled hectic activity and scientific order. In some, there were impressively neat rows of flasks; in others, the important work took place on benches crowded with apparatus in less discernible order. "Separating the Serum from the Red Corpuscles of the Blood" was the caption for the *Herald*'s picture on the following day, December 13, a caption that encouraged the public's curiosity about the underlying components of an apparently homogeneous fluid. Then, after three days without illustrations, the horses returned on December 17 in three new images about the preparation of the serum and the care of the horses, with further horse pictures on the twentieth and the twenty-third, the latter in an article whose headlines encapsulate the key dimensions of this dramatic story: "Life Saved by Anti-Toxine—The Remedy Reduces the Death Rate from Fifty to Fourteen Per Cent. . . . Doctors Actively at Work—Bacteriologists Who Supervise the Herald Fund Busily Engaged in Producing Curative Serum" (*New York Herald*, December 23, 1894).

January 1895 saw a flood of new and repeated images that sustained a high level of excitement about the antitoxin. When the U.S. edition of the monthly *Review of Reviews* opened its first issue of the year with "The Progress of the World," its very first entry was "A New Medical Discovery." This article included a portrait sketch of "Professor Roux, Discoverer of Anti-toxine" and a picture entitled "Inoculating a Diphtheria Patient," which reprinted the image of the child's inoculation that had already appeared in *Scientific American* in mid-November (fig. 36) and in the *New York Herald* in mid-December. And this picture was to be republished again shortly in *Leslie's Illustrated Weekly* on January 17, where it was joined by the drawing of a horse providing serum (fig. 37), likewise printed earlier in both *Scientific American* and the *Herald*.[54]

On January 5, 1895, *Harper's Weekly* ran a full-page article with four photographs: "How Antitoxines Are Developed" (fig. 39). This page exhibited the new graphic devices and iconography that came to have prominence in magazine images for decades, as unsigned photographs replaced the dramatic engravings of artists' sketches, which had long dominated popular pictorial media. Winslow Homer, Frederick Remington, Thomas Nast, and their colleagues had virtually defined the Victorian newsmagazine's visual style. The images in figure 39 are the first nineteenth-century photographs in this book—appropriately so, since half-tone photographic prints became common only during the 1890s. Although photographs were not entirely new in these magazines in 1895, they were beginning to displace drawings and they eventually came to dominate reportorial images and magazine covers, just as they do today.

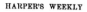

HOW ANTITOXINES ARE DEVELOPED.

The new treatment of diphtheria is a practical application of the latest advances of experimental bacteriology. The general facts upon which it is based are briefly these: Certain bacteria, when developing in the organism of an animal or man, produce an albuminoid poison called a toxine, which, circulating in the blood, causes disease. For example, the Klebs-Loeffler bacillus, growing in the throat of a child, generates a toxine that produces the systemic condition called diphtheria.

If some of these bacteria be removed from the organism and placed in artificial media, such as broth, under proper conditions they will grow and multiply and produce the same toxine as before. This toxine may now be separated from the bacteria by filtration, and if introduced into an organism by inoculation it will produce the disease as readily as if it had been formed in the organism. But the virulence of the disease thus produced will vary with the quantity of the toxine injected. Moreover, if the first dose given is so small as to produce only slight illness, a larger quantity may be introduced a few days later without producing a corresponding effect; and progressively larger doses may be administered from time to time, until at last the animal receives with impunity doses many times larger than could possibly be borne at first.

In the case of the diphtheria toxine, for example (obtained, as has been said, by growing the diphtheria bacillus in meat broth), if fifteen drops of the filtrate containing the toxine be injected into a vein of a horse, the animal will be severely poisoned. But by repeating the injection from time to time in progressing doses, at the end of three or four months the animal will bear a dose of two hundred times the original quantity. In other words, the animal has become immune to the disease.

If now a vein of the immune animal be opened and some blood withdrawn, the serum of that blood (the other constituents being removed) may be injected into the sys-

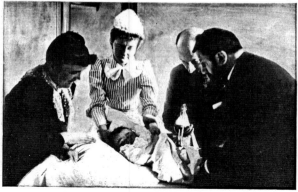

INOCULATING A CHILD WITH ANTITOXINE

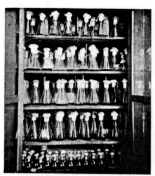

INCUBATOR CONTAINING 180 ERLENMEYER FLASKS.
Each flask contains Colonies of Diphtheria Microbes in various stages of Development feeding upon sterilized Chicken Broth.

tem of another animal or a human being without ill effect, and the animal or human being thus inoculated becomes immune to the disease, in virtue of the inoculation. More than that, if the organism inoculated had already acquired the disease, the inoculation, within reasonable limits, is curative. For example, if a child has been exposed to diphtheria, inoculation with the serum of a horse rendered immune to diphtheria as above described will prevent development of the disease. At a later stage inoculation tends to cure the disease.

These are the facts as applied in the new serum treatment of diphtheria.

Exactly what happens in the system of the animal during the process of its becoming immune, no one at present knows. The toxine as it is injected is in some way rendered harmless, but whether by transformation of the toxine itself, or by the secretion of an antidotal substance, is still in doubt. The latter hypothesis seems to most investigators more probable.

But in either case it is convenient to speak of the antidotal substance which the serum of the immune animal contains as an antitoxine. This word, like its antithesis toxine, is a generic term. There are as many toxines and antitoxines of this series as there are forms of germ disease, though most of them have been but little investigated.

The special investigations into the nature of the diphtheria toxine and the practical development of its antitoxine have been going on for several years. The original investigators, Behring and his associates, in Koch's laboratory in Berlin, were extremely conservative in making announcement of their discoveries. Their experience with tuberculin had warned them of the danger of premature announcements.

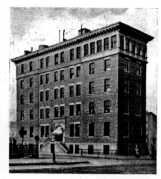

PASTEUR INSTITUTE, WHERE ANTITOXINE IS MADE
IN NEW YORK.

They therefore kept their own counsel till they felt very sure of their results.

Since their discoveries were made known their experiments have been repeated elsewhere, notably by Dr. Roux and his collaborators at the Pasteur Institute in Paris, who confirm Behring's claims in all essential particulars. So large a mass of evidence has accumulated that apparently it is no longer in question that the new remedy has some potency. Individual physicians have become enthusiastic over the new treatment, and municipalities have made appropriations for the development of the remedy. New York, for example, recently appropriated $30,000 for this purpose.

It is confidently believed by those best qualified to judge that the results will justify this confidence. At the same time it should be understood by every one that, great as is its ultimate promise, the new serum treatment of disease is still in its infancy. To judge from the editorial comment of the best medical journals, the attitude of the medical profession as a whole toward the new treatment of diphtheria is at present one of anxious expectancy rather than of certitude.

HENRY SMITH WILLIAMS, M.D.

NATURE'S ART.

How strange it is that Nature should
fashion till complete
The lissom silken lily so delicately
sweet;
And then the self-same dainty and
subtle art employ
The lily's chaste perfection of beauty
to destroy!

R. K. MUNKITTRICK.

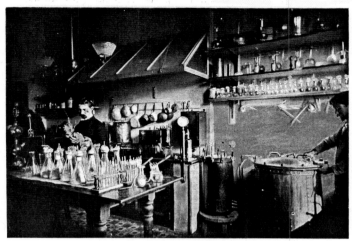

LABORATORY WHERE ANTITOXINE IS MADE.
Showing "Autoclaves" in which Chicken Broth is sterilized, and Operator filling Flasks with Serum.

FIG. 39. Henry Smith Williams, "How Antitoxines Are Developed," *Harper's Weekly* 39:1985 (January 5, 1895), 8. Full page with four uncredited photographs. Author's collection.

Three of these photographs showed already-familiar scenes that were similar to wood-cut images that had appeared in the *New York Herald* and other publications: male physicians inoculating a child with a female nurse's assistance, ordered ranks of Erlenmeyer flasks (given their formal name), and a laboratory worker with flasks, tanks, and sterilizing equipment. Although photographs can sometimes bring us closer to reality, these early magazine photographs are less engaging and less memorable than the engravings they were replacing.[55]

The fourth image, likewise, was traditional in appearance, just a six-story building of undistinguished architecture. But its caption offered a clue to what an innovation it was: "Pasteur Institute Where Antitoxine Is Made in New York." For the first time in the United States, the new therapies were connected to a major investment in infrastructure, in this case a large building, independent of any medical school or drug company, solely devoted to biomedical research and development and supported by an enthusiastic public, philanthropic gifts, and sales of the new biological remedies. The story of this pioneering organization, founded and directed by Dr. Paul Gibier, is examined in chapter 5.

HOW LABORATORY THERAPEUTICS INCREASED MEDICINE'S PRESTIGE

By early 1895, a family magazine of middle-class leisure time was calmly discoursing about toxins, antitoxins, incubators, Erlenmeyer flasks, autoclaves to sterilize chicken broth on which colonies of diphtheria microbes feed, and serum extracted from horses. It was also inviting readers to admire (and perhaps to consider supporting) a substantial building devoted exclusively to this new kind of life-saving work. The daily papers, reaching further down the range of social class than the weeklies, showed many of the same images and used the same vocabulary, although they worked more horses into the visual mix. This was a historically new lexicon for medical reportage, drawn more from the laboratory than from the clinic and based on the midcentury achievements of cell theory and bacteriology and their powerful offspring, germ theory and immunology. Some of this lexicon was more than ten years old, but it achieved its new visibility and social power from the intense enthusiasm connected with breakthroughs in the decade starting with the rabies announcement of 1885. It seems likely that this enthusiasm for innovative therapeutic interventions may have had a wider and deeper effect on U.S. culture than just making people familiar with injections for hydrophobia, consumption, and diphtheria. The series of advances helped to establish permanently in mass culture two new intertwined notions: medicine is scientific, and medicine makes progress. Research had become visible; medical innovation was now a public thrill.

Printed materials can take us only part of the way to an understanding of what the public thought. Even if the pictures were likely to help shape public attitudes, they cannot—by themselves—reveal people's ideas and feelings. Only other kinds of sources can overcome the inherent limitation of printed images and articles. More-private sources such as letters and diaries might help, but people's actions are even better evidence of their thoughts and beliefs. Several events bore witness to such actions. Tens of thousands of people—and perhaps far more—paid admission fees to enter a museum or a theater to see Pasteur in wax or Pasteur's patients in the flesh, confirming a mass involvement in the rabies-vaccine excitement. When hundreds of individuals, perhaps even thousands, mailed in their contributions large and small to the newspaper campaigns to send the Newark boys to Paris and then later to establish diphtheria-serum production facilities, their actions acknowledged how the articles and pictures had moved them to action. When twelve thousand American physicians started providing patients with an injection of animal-testicle extracts of questionable safety and value within eighteen months of its introduction, they were responding to an irresistible popular enthusiasm for the newest product of the medical laboratory.

These episodes of popular excitement surrounding two enduring medical advances and two partial failures have not received much attention in the standard accounts of nineteenth- and early-twentieth-century U.S. medicine, perhaps because some of the discoveries that garnered the headlines lacked the intellectual significance that most historians have used as the criterion for medical landmarks. Another reason that the 1890s popular enthusiasm for laboratory medicine has not been fully appreciated is that historians of medicine largely depend on the documents created by the medical profession itself, and the physicians of the era did not entirely share the public's excitement or bring the new techniques quickly into their practice. For example, in 1903, when a Boston physician examined the acceptance of laboratory research by physicians, he noted with disappointment "a lack of sympathy and frequently, even, a feeling of hostility between the laboratory worker and the general practitioner." He blamed much of the indifference on commercialism, and he found many in the profession lacking a respect for their younger colleagues and for the new procedures and equipment.[56] Modern scholars, in neglecting these media episodes, have overlooked a significant mechanism by which the general public came to replace an attitude of cynical disdain about medicine's pretensions with an unalloyed enthusiasm and a passion for more and bigger discoveries. Although historians have recognized for some time that the medical profession gained substantial cultural and social authority around the turn of the twentieth century, the role that widespread popular excitement about laboratory discoveries played in bringing this about has not received its due.[57]

The specific breakthroughs whose imagery has been documented here seem likely to have been crucial stimuli to public acclaim for medicine. Additionally, they show us what kind of science played this role, what the general public got excited about, just when the shift occurred, and what particular features of medical research were foregrounded in the transition. Although the general public's new enthusiasm in the 1880s and 1890s for sudden, headline-grabbing therapeutic advances was not the only factor in establishing the broad cultural authority that medicine seized and held for most of the twentieth century, it deserves a place of recognition alongside such factors as the rise in medical philanthropy, the growth of knowledge in physiology and other basic medical sciences, and the general expansion of the profession's surgical and therapeutic powers.

CHAPTER 5

CREATING AN INSTITUTIONAL BASE FOR MEDICAL RESEARCH, 1890–1920

The gift is a handsome brood mare, which has thrice won prizes at horse shows and which Mr. West has placed at the doctor's disposal for experimental purposes. Mr. West also granted the use of sixty stalls in the Morton Stables, which the doctor will fill with horses to be inoculated for test purposes and to increase the supply of antitoxin.

—New York Daily Tribune, January 3, 1895

*I*SOLATED BREAKTHROUGHS, sporadic and unconnected, represented the first wave of medical discoveries that entranced the American public. Between 1885 and 1895, rabies shots, organ extracts, tuberculin, and diphtheria antitoxin all emerged from European laboratories and crossed the Atlantic to great acclaim. How did Americans start to do it for themselves? How were intermittent foreign advances superseded by an infrastructure that could generate them continuously? How did the United States establish institutions of research and discovery like those in Paris and Berlin? And how were the new research institutions pictured in the mass media?

The initial hurried attempts to establish U.S. Pasteur institutes in 1885 quickly failed because the public was then not yet ready to redirect its medical charity from patient care to laboratory work. But just a few years later, when the notion of medical progress had become more widely grounded, Paul Gibier, a French-trained engineer and physician, emerged as the United States' first scientific impresario, a commanding presence who was good at the science but also able to encourage popular interest in laboratory work and to cultivate social and financial support for his enterprise. Months before Robert Koch announced tuberculin and years before Roux and von Behring perfected antitoxins for diphtheria and tetanus, Gibier was single-handedly building a new kind of institution, an independent laboratory with the capacity for research, development, and production of the new biological cures. His New York Pasteur Institute pioneered key features of the modern biomedical industry.

These institutional changes were more gradual than the first breakthroughs, but they were no less revolutionary. Newspaper and magazine coverage of the New York Pasteur Institute (NYPI) shows how the general public became involved with this new kind of research institution. Pasteur institutes, initially founded and funded in response to popular demand for rabies treatment, helped to create a familiar public face for the new medicine. This image was laboratory-based medicine, and it was expected to be an ever-changing medicine, continuously improved by novelties and advances. It was modern medicine, up-to-date medicine.

In 1890, the United States was home to few biomedical laboratories. Only after the turn of the century did the laboratory become a characteristic feature of medical schools, drug companies, and health departments. Although the laboratory in time came to serve all aspects of medicine and public health, its image in popular culture around the turn of the twentieth century was largely animated by the public's appreciation for the life-saving Pasteur treatment. From 1890 into the 1920s, hydrophobia's special place in popular consciousness gave the work of the NYPI a national prominence in the mass media that other ailments and other discoveries did not always receive. Soon after the opening of the institute in New York, illustrated articles in the *Los Angeles Times* (fig. 40) and in *Once a Week* (fig. 41) ensured its immediate national visibility. The latter article offered a portrait of Gibier, a scene with Gibier giving an injection, a view of the laboratory with a framed portrait of Louis Pasteur on the wall, and illustrations of scientific equipment.

Simultaneously with the rise of the biomedical research laboratory during the 1890s, a new photographic vision of medicine was being fashioned. Magazines and newspapers started to replace line engravings with photographs using the new halftone screening process that permitted high-speed mechanical reproduction. Prior to this development, photographs could be printed on book pages and as cabinet cards and cartes de visite but not in newspapers and magazines. Halftone photographs were far cheaper than line engravings, and they also facilitated the success of a new publication invented in the 1890s, the magazine supplement included in Sunday newspapers. This first generation of magazine photographs lacked the theatrical staginess and the dramatic narratives that characterized the engraved news

A TREATISE ON RABIES.

Pasteur's Pupil, Dr. Gibier, Discusses the Subject.

THE AMERICAN INSTITUTE

Dog-killing Is a Blunder—How to Act After Being Bitten—Cauterization Deprecated—The Injection Exhilarates

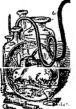

HILE in this country on a professional mission during a part of the years 1888 and 1889, my attention was frequently attracted to publications in the newspapers stating that hydrophobia had occurred at certain places, and that the persons who were the victims had been bitten weeks before by animals not then known to be rabid. The story was invariably the same: The dog summarily killed, the wound either roughly cauterized or neglected, and the fatal sequel. It was the frequency of these cases that first suggested to my mind the idea of establishing in this country an institute modeled after that of my old teacher, the distinguished Pasteur in Paris.

Returning to France I passed several months there, where I studied with M. Pasteur the question of establishing an institute in America. On December 1, 1889, I again came to America; the institute project now fully matured in my mind. My first care was to take this house, and, strangely enough, on the very day I was installed I was prostrated by la grippe, and was for fifteen days my own patient. The institute furnished, I next established a laboratory, a task that occupied much time. My instruments I had long ago. They are of Pasteur's own invention and have been used in the work a long time. The chief delay was in the time consumed in making the preparations for inoculation. I found it necessary to spend two months in the preparation of the virus, in its various cultures and different degrees of strength. In February the institute was formally opened.

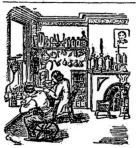

In the laboratory.

Soon patients began to come in from

morphine, and it gives the same sensation, except that it does not put the patient to sleep.

I have had patients from many States —from Texas, Missouri, Maryland, New Hampshire, New York and even from Canada. Many of them are "poor patients." For such cases, when they come from distant points, the cities usually pay; but here in New York the treatment is gratuitous.

No rule can be laid down for telling whether a dog has true hydrophobia or not in the early stages. A dog is dangerous five, six or eight days before he begins to show the symptoms of rabies, and even at that stage he can communicate hydrophobia. Cases have been known where experimentalists have inoculated some dogs with hydrophobia with the syringe or lancet, and after two or three days their saliva has been tried with a view to determining its virulence. Sometimes it was demonstrated that even before they began to show any evidence of hydrophobia the saliva contained the deadly germs of rabies.

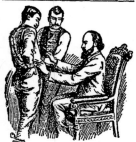

Inoculating with the virus.

When a person has been bitten by a dog, the sore should not be cauterized. The cautery sometimes makes bad wounds, which are difficult to heal, and it produces inflammations. The wound should be washed out freely with plenty of water and treated with antiseptic dressing. It is a blunder to kill the dog; such a course is revengeful and brutal. Some people I have treated only because they have killed the dog, when perhaps it was not really mad. The doubt, however, remains, and in such cases makes treatment imperative. The popular fallacy which leads to the slaughter of the dog is due to superstition, and most people still believe that with the death of the animal the venom dies also. I cannot qualify such foolishness. A few days of waiting would have shown whether or not the dog was really mad—the wound being dressed meanwhile as I have suggested—and if, after being watched, the dog showed signs of hydrophobia, then the treatment could be had without further delay. It is only a trifling burden for fifteen days, when it is all over.

As an illustration of the scepticism this institute has had to encounter I might mention one case in point. Judge Masterson of Texas was bitten, and by the advice of some friends, came East for treatment. Here he met other friends, some of them in the profession, who gravely urged him to go to Pasteur at once. Still in doubt he cabled to Paris, and the reply he received from Pasteur was: "Go and be treated by Gibier."

When this institute was established a few months ago I knew not whether it would be successful or otherwise, but the system has met with encouragement beyond all expectation. There are some people who have urged me to make a business of the institute; some who want to make it a hospital, to re-

FIG. 40. "A Treatise of Rabies. Pasteur's Pupil, Dr. Gibier, Discusses the Subject," *Los Angeles Times*, July 6, 1890, 10 (detail).

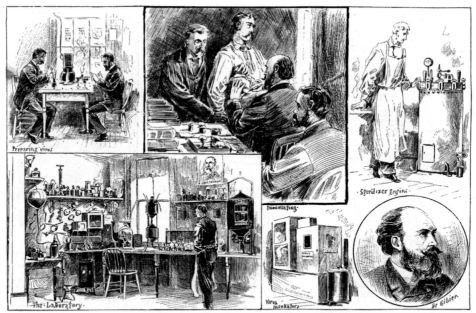

NEW YORK—THE PASTEUR INSTITUTE FOR TREATING PERSONS BITTEN BY DOGS.

FIG. 41. "New York—The Pasteur Institute for Treating Persons Bitten by Dogs," *Once a Week* 6:3 (November 4, 1890), 12 (lower half). Author's collection.

sketches that had flourished for half a century. Whatever authenticity and accuracy these early photographs brought to the stories, they did not make the pages vibrant, and readers of this book may well find this chapter's illustrations far less enticing than those in the preceding chapters. I have not chosen dull or muddy examples; these are typical. Some of the contrasts between the styles of the old and the new reproduction processes are easily observable in newspaper and magazine images of the NYPI at the beginning of the decade (in figs. 40 and 41) and at middecade (in fig. 39 in chapter 4).

THE FIRST FREE-STANDING MEDICAL RESEARCH ORGANIZATION IN THE UNITED STATES

The NYPI's history illustrates the changing character of popular images of medical progress from 1890 to World War I. By an odd twist of fate, the story of the U.S. Pasteur institutes began in France even before Pasteur had publicized his rabies work. Born in 1851, Gibier had been a mechanic in a machine shop, served in the French cavalry in Africa, and worked as a clerk for a railroad company before he changed careers and earned a medical degree at the University of Paris. The engineering and management skills he acquired early were essential to making his institute a success.

His 1884 doctoral thesis on rabies in animals was supervised by a friend of Louis Pasteur's.[1] Shortly after completing his degree, Gibier was commissioned by the French government to investigate, first, "the organization of laboratories for medical research" in Germany and, second, outbreaks of epidemic disease in Cuba and elsewhere.[2] Because ships from Cuba were barred by Florida during the yellow-fever epidemic, Gibier traveled via New York City to investigate yellow fever in Florida in 1888.[3] Apparently, he liked what he saw on his detour, for he chose to settle in New York City the following year.

When Gibier opened the first facility in the United States to produce rabies virus and to deliver the Pasteur treatment effectively to the needy patients who came from near and far, not only did it flourish, but it set precedents for expanding biomedical research more generally.[4] He came to the task with an unusually rich experience in medical microbiology, not to speak of his mechanical and organizational skills, sharpened by what he had observed in German laboratories. Gibier had exceptional proficiency in laboratory manipulations. There were as yet no standard methods for the culturing of microbes or the production of sera and antitoxins and few standardized reagents and pieces of equipment on which he could depend.[5] Even though he had to invent and improvise techniques and procedures, he was consistently successful. Gibier's well-equipped laboratory and his highly skilled staff were able, for example, quickly to perform experiments on samples of Koch's lymph immediately upon its arrival in the United States.[6]

Not only was Gibier a technically adept medical scientist, but he was also a successful spokesman for the new approaches in medicine. In addition to articles in the medical press, he published popular accounts of the Pasteur treatment and Koch's tuberculin for a lay public in the *North American Review*.[7] The annual statistics of patients Gibier had treated were routinely printed not only in daily newspapers and medical journals but in such magazines as *Scientific American, Manufacturer and Builder,* and *American Rural Home*. Another indication of his institute's success is the amount of real estate he accumulated. He started in a house in Greenwich Village but quickly moved to a larger building on Twenty-third Street to house his residence, offices, and animal facility. By early 1892, he was seeking philanthropic support for the construction of a much larger building uptown on Central Park West. Among the celebrities who helped with fund-raising were the famous actress Sarah Bernhardt and the symphonic conductor Walter J. Damrosch. The building's formal dedication in October 1893 was celebrated by a *New York Times* article with a large drawing of the structure (the same building pictured in fig. 39 in chapter 4).[8] In 1896, Gibier purchased a large farm about thirty miles northwest of the city, where he raised experimental animals and operated a sanatorium.

Gibier's reputation as a socially prominent intellectual was such that the *New York Times* published a feature article in December 1893, illustrated with a handsome portrait drawing and crowned by an extended headline, "An Hour with Paul Gibier: The Fashion of Specializing in Art and in Books; His Library Room; Theory of Temperaments; Application of the Discovery Made by Pasteur to a Lesson in the Scientific Religion of Intelligent Selfishness; Poverty as a Culture Medium of Microbes; A Persuasive Christmas Sermon."[9]

In order to stimulate laboratory medicine in the United States, Gibier began publishing a quarterly medical journal in 1893, the *New York Therapeutic Review,* the title of which later changed to *Bulletin of the New York Pasteur Institute.* This journal carried translations of French and German medical articles, studies prepared by Gibier and his colleagues, reports on the patients treated for rabies, and a significant amount of advertising of medical products and devices for the practitioner. When Gibier's Pasteur Institute started producing antitoxins and other serum remedies, they were advertised in his journal (fig. 42).[10] Thirteen biologics were being produced by Gibier, and of the group, all except smallpox virus, tuberculin, and mallein had been developed in his laboratory. These new products established this Pasteur Institute as far more than a rabies treatment clinic; it was an independent facility for biomedical research and development, unprecedented in the United States and unique until the founding of the Rockefeller Institute for Medical Research after the turn of the twentieth century. In the mid-1890s, Gibier's institute also provided vital help to Walter Reed and his colleagues with their research on rabies and diphtheria. On request, Gibier sent Reed antitoxin samples as well as cultures of especially virulent germs after Reed's attempt to produce antitoxin failed. And in 1894, when an army physician named James Carroll cut himself while dissecting a rabid rabbit in Reed's research laboratory, Reed sent Carroll to Gibier for rabies treatment.[11] Throughout the 1890s, dog bites remained a newsworthy item in daily papers, and the press also reported on the treatments, especially when the patients traveled some distance to New York or Chicago, the only rabies clinics in North America before 1897.[12] For ordinary citizens, the Pasteur treatment for rabies remained a fascinating miracle and the most familiar example of modern laboratory medicine until it was joined by the success of diphtheria antitoxin.

In late 1894, when diphtheria antitoxin needed to be manufactured on the American side of the Atlantic by using animals to grow the serum, Gibier's institute already had in place the expertise, the equipment, the animal facilities, and the skilled personnel that allowed him to produce substantial quantities of the first antitoxin made in the Americas. By the end of the year, Gibier's diphtheria antitoxin had been in use for several weeks as the only such product made in the United States or Canada, distributed as widely as New Orleans, Milwaukee, Los Angeles, Toronto, and Montreal. New York's famous Health Department laboratories had not yet been able to produce any, and the city's horses were "ready for their first bleeding" only in the middle of February.[13] Nonetheless, the Health Department has almost always received undeserved credit as the pioneers.[14]

While the life-saving antitoxin for diphtheria was at the peak of its publicity in the first week of January 1895 (the same week as the *Harper's Weekly* story pictured in fig. 39 in chapter 4), a report in the *New York Daily Tribune* epitomized the connections being developed between laboratory research and the experience of people far from the laboratory. This article exemplifies a number of the elements in our story:

TUBERCULOSIS.

We beg to inform the Medical Profession that the Sanatorium of the New York Pasteur Institute is prepared to receive patients affected with TUBERCULOSIS, especially of the lungs.

The treatment consists principally in the application of the antiseptic method associated to the injection of combined antitoxins (Tuberculosis, Streptococcus and Staphylococcus.)

Products of the New York Biological and Vaccinal Institute.

LIST OF PRICES:

DIPHTHERIA ANTITOXIN DOUBLE (Gibier's).
For malignant as well as ordinary cases:
1 vial, 20 c. c., 3000 units $4 00
1 vial, 10 c. c., 1500 units 2 25
1 vial, 5 c. c., 750 units 1 25

SEPTICÆMIA ANTITOXIN (Streptococcus).
For use in case of Erysipelas, Pyemia, Septicæmia, etc.
1 vial, 25 c. c $5 00

SYPHILIS ANTITOXIC SERUM (From the horse).
Prepared according to the formula of Prof. Richet and Hericourt.
1 vial, 25 c. c $5 00

TETANUS ANTITOXIN (Liquid form for human being).
1 vial, 25 c. c. (1 to 1,000,000) $5 00

ANTI-VENOMOUS SERUM (Calmette's).
1 vial, 10 c. c., for one case $2 00

ERYSIPELAS and PRODIGIOSUS TOXINS.
For injections in Sarcoma and other malignant growths.
1 vial, 25 c. c $3 00
1 special Syringe, 3 c. c., in a metallic case 2 50

EXTRACTS OF ANIMAL ORGANS (Brown-Sequard's Method.)

TESTICLE EXTRACT.
1 vial, 25 c. c $2 50

GRAY MATTER.
1 vial, 25 c. c $2 50
1 special Syringe, 3 c. c 2 50

LIQUID VACCINE VIRUS (In sealed glass tubes.)
2 vaccinations, (1 tube) .... $ 25
5 " " 45
10 " " 75
20 " " 1 25

LIQUID VACCINE VIRUS ON IVORY POINTS (New, patented.)
1 ivory point, in a sterilized glass tube .... $ 15
2 " " in separate tubes 25
5 " " 60
10 " " 1 00

BIOLOGICAL PRODUCTS FOR VETERINARY USE.

TETANUS ANTITOXIN (Dry form.)
1 vial, 3 grams $3 00

TUBERCULIN (Ready for use.)
1 vial, 25 c. c., ten injections $3 00
1 vial 2¼ c. c., one injection 50

MALLEIN (Ready for use).
1 vial, 25 c. c., ten injections $3 00
1 vial, 2¼ c. c., one injection 50

New York Biological and Vaccinal Institute,
Pasteur Institute Building, 1, 3, 5 and 7 West 97th St., New York, N. Y.
THE G. F. HARVEY CO., Saratoga Springs, N. Y., Sole Agents for the United States and Canada, and LEHN & FINK, Wholesale Druggists, New York.

FIG. 42. Full-page ad offering tuberculosis treatment and an array of serum therapies, *Bulletin of the New York Pasteur Institute* 5:4 (December 1897), vi. Author's collection.

the emotional power of these treatments, the kind of appreciation they could engender, and the public's awareness that further progress depended on financial support.

> Gratitude Shown in a Practical Way. . . . Dr. Paul Gibier of the Pasteur Institute, who has been interested recently in tests and experiments with antitoxin in cases of diphtheria is greatly elated over a gift which has been made him by C. G. West of the Morton [Street] stables. . . . The gift is a handsome brood mare, which has thrice won prizes at horse shows and which Mr. West has placed at the doctor's disposal for experimental purposes. Mr. West also granted the use of sixty stalls in the Morton Stables, which the doctor will fill with horses to be inoculated for test purposes and to increase the supply of antitoxin. . . .

The stalls are placed at the doctor's disposal as a thank-offering by Mr. West, who . . . lives at Greenwich, Conn., with his wife and eight children. One of the latter, a boy of six years, was treated by Dr. Gibier for hydrophobia two years ago in the old institute in West Tenth St. The child improved under Dr. Gibier's care and was finally cured. Six weeks ago, the boy was taken sick with diphtheria, as was also his younger brother. The two were treated by [a doctor in] Greenwich, who advised Mr. West to see Dr. Gibier and secure some antitoxin. This was done. The two sick children, their parents, and the six other children were inoculated. The two that were ill began to improve immediately, and were soon well. The eight other [family] members, although constantly exposed, showed no signs of having contracted the disease even in the mildest form. . . .

Dr. Gibier will begin purchasing more horses at once, and place them in the stable. He already has forty in a private stable.[15]

This kind of publicity about bringing children back from death's door had such an impact that a bill was introduced in the New York State legislature in 1895 to support Gibier's rabies treatments. The expense of more than a dozen daily injections plus three weeks of housing for out-of-town patients had put the miracle cure beyond the reach of many people, despite the public's clamoring for the treatment. Gibier could provide free shots to the indigent and the working poor, but he could not afford to subsidize their travel or housing. The state budget would now cover transport "to New-York [City] at public expense [of] persons bitten by rabid animals or otherwise exposed to infection with rabies, for treatment at the New-York City Pasteur Institute. The sum of $10,000 a year for five years is to be paid to the institute by the State for the care of such rabies patients."[16] Such legislation was unusual, and this annual allocation was remarkably large. But the public saw the need as pressing since, as everyone now knew, rabies was treatable, and without treatment it was uniformly fatal.[17]

The very same year that the New York legislation was passed, Gibier started distributing a second kind of antitoxin to combat the often fatal tetanus, or lockjaw. "Tetanus Cured by Antitoxin" read a headline in the *New York Tribune* on October 31, 1895. This story of another scientific miracle cure told of a boy in Pennsylvania to whose doctor Gibier had shipped the new remedy. "Within hours its effect was noticed. . . . The patient's recovery was then rapid." Gibier explained to the reporter that this was the third case in humans that the antitoxin had cured, and he denied any significance to the case of a Brooklyn youth who had died of tetanus a few days earlier, explaining that it "was a test case in no sense [because] the disease had advanced so far that nothing could have saved the boy."[18] In his own practice, Gibier was using tetanus antitoxin imported from Europe, and he was selling doses to other physicians at a price of five dollars a vial.[19] The city's Health Department first made its tetanus antitoxin available in July 1896.[20]

Month after month, Gibier's research continued to draw attention through substantial feature articles in general-interest magazines, as well as through its regular mention in the dozens of news reports in the daily press about dog-bite victims arriving for treatment. For example, in January 1896, *Metropolitan Magazine* ran a substantial article that emphasized the search for new understanding rather than clinical care, "The Defenders of the Human Body and Their Foes. What Is Being Done at the New York Pasteur Institute to Enlarge Our Knowledge of Health and Disease."[21] Some of the included photos were those also used in Gibier's annual reports. Among the subjects pictured in this article's numerous photographic illustrations are found the doctor in his laboratory, microbes beneath the microscope, raising bacilli by the billions, patients awaiting inoculation, an inoculation to cure hydrophobia, and a convalescent patient.

In January 1898, the *New York Times* Sunday magazine published "The Pasteur Institute Zoo," with agreeable pictures of Gibier's animals, looking content, although the text made clear that, though some of the animals were receiving medical treatment to prevent rabies, others were sacrificed for research.[22] Several of these images reappeared the following year in a London magazine (fig. 43) and again five years after that in *Broadway Magazine*.[23]

The Pasteur Institute was the most visible U.S. producer of the "biologics"—the new living remedies entirely distinct from the dead vegetables and minerals in the

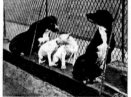

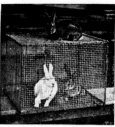
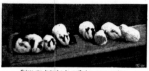

FIG. 43. Photographs captioned "Four valuable dogs in course of inoculation," "Prize rabbits sent to the Institute to be inoculated," "Valuable sheep under treatment for the prevention of lockjaw," and "Guinea pigs destined to be sacrificed as martyrs to science," in J. Montgomery McGovern, "Martyrs of Science," *Royal Magazine* 1:6 (April 1899), 540–541. Author's collection.

traditional pharmacopoeia. In addition to the antitoxins for diphtheria and for tetanus, the first wave of biologics in the 1890s included antivenom for snake bites (sold
by Gibier's institute though not produced locally); sera to combat streptococcus,
syphilis, and tuberculosis; and organ extracts from animals' testicles and thyroid
glands. Not only were these sera and extracts the first important animal products
introduced into medicine after cowpox virus; they also required entirely new kinds
of laboratory equipment, expertise, and activities. Expensive facilities and animals in
great numbers became essential for the experimental process of discovery, for testing
of quality, and for producing the actual injectables. These medications—especially
the injections for diphtheria and tetanus—were fundamentally different from the
old remedies in another way: they could effect rapid, visible, and dramatic cures.
And they undeniably saved lives. Even cowpox, supremely valuable as a preventive,
did not save lives in a visible way. And almost everything else in the doctor's bag
could provide only a modest adjustment in a patient's condition, perhaps relieving
pain while the body healed itself. But in many cases, after an injection of antitoxin,
parents and doctors could literally watch a dying child recover within hours.

The energy and the visibility of Gibier (and of his colleagues and imitators)
played a significant role in popularizing the new vaccines and serum therapies across
the United States and Canada. In time, pharmaceutical companies assumed production of antitoxins and the rabies vaccine. Their advertising began to boast of the importance of their scientific laboratories for ensuring potency, purity, and novelty.[24]
Health departments also started producing their own diphtheria antitoxin and often
sold it for a profit. Serum therapies are today only a small fraction of our medical
armamentarium, but until the first antibiotics became available in the 1930s, serum
therapies were a leading element of advanced medical care, shortening illness and
saving lives, especially for pneumonia.

A remarkable decade of achievements by Gibier closed abruptly with his premature death in June 1900. He was famous enough that the news of his fatal carriage
accident ran at the top of page 1 in both the *New York Tribune* and the *New York
Times*. After Gibier's death, the Pasteur Institute managed to maintain its public
service for another eighteen years, and it continued to receive wide publicity about
its physicians and their work. Gibier's nephew George Gibier Rambaud, a physician, took over management of the institute, reducing its scope by selling the upstate property and refocusing more exclusively on rabies treatments. Rambaud became a nationally recognized authority on rabies, and his work garnered significant
publicity.[25] Two of Gibier and Rambaud's New York co-workers spread the gospel
by moving west in 1900 and opening their own Pasteur institutes in Pittsburgh (Dr.
Aime Leteve) and St. Louis (Dr. Carl Fisch), thereby reducing travel distances for
many dog-bite victims. Rambaud closed the New York institute in September 1918,
when he left for active duty overseas as a major in the Army Medical Corps.[26]

Over the course of the institute's twenty-eight years, it had provided the Pasteur
treatment to roughly four thousand patients.[27] Although the NYPI closed for World
War I and its achievements were largely lost to history, the institutionalization of

research that Gibier pioneered on the city's West Side rose to even greater heights in a competing enterprise over on the East Side. Exactly one year after Gibier's death had been page 1 news on June 2, 1900, the same newspapers' front pages carried reports of a new advance in medical research. In 1901, however, the advance was not a single discovery but rather a well-funded campaign to produce discovery. John D. Rockefeller was setting up the Rockefeller Institute for Medical Research (RIMR) as a laboratory exclusively devoted to research. Patient care was to be incidental to its purpose and undertaken only when it could foster experiment-based scientific knowledge. To emphasize this mission, the new institute titled its periodical the *Journal of Experimental Medicine.* Although the RIMR was hardly alone in creating for the United States a laboratory-based medicine characteristic of the twentieth century, its leadership proved pivotal. Early illustrations in the mass media echo the pictorial coverage of the NYPI and show how the RIMR and the NYPI together helped to establish the twentieth century's imagery of an institution-based enterprise for biomedical research in the United States.

For the opening decade of the new century, these two pioneering research centers were treated by the press in a remarkably similar fashion. But by the time of World War I, the older institution had largely lost its purpose when new technologies of production allowed pharmaceutical companies to package preserved rabies vaccine for sale to family doctors. And once the RIMR had enlarged its facilities and opened its research hospital in 1910, its accomplishments and reputation blossomed, far outpacing that of the NYPI.[28]

A SECOND INSTITUTE FOR MEDICAL RESEARCH

The name Rockefeller easily drew media attention to the young institute, but its scientific achievements gradually displaced a focus on the founder. Perhaps most important among the news reports in the institute's first decade were those on serum therapy for cerebrospinal meningitis. "A Cure for Meningitis," read the bold headline on page 1 in the *New York Times* of August 6, 1907, followed by this subhead: "Discovered by Dr. Flexner, Head of the Rockefeller Institute." The *New York World* put it a little differently: "Cure Is Found for Meningitis with John D.'s Aid."

In fact, this particular story was far more complicated. Simon Flexner was then traveling in Europe and could not make the announcement himself; there were only three cases, treated in Ohio. And Flexner never took credit for discovering the serum, which had been developed by others. Flexner's significant innovation was to inject the serum not into muscles but directly into the spinal column. He was able to develop such a method by using primates in his experiments, a very expensive operation that was made possible only by the good funding at the RIMR and that was not yet widely available to scientists elsewhere. Because the mortality rate of meningitis was highly variable, studies were not able to establish how effective this serum was, yet it seemed to reduce the fatality rate by as much as half.[29] And nothing would do a better job until the introduction of sulfa drugs in the 1930s.

With a small number of patients, an absent hero, and a complex narrative, this meningitis serum treatment did not become a big media event in the manner of the 1890s breakthroughs. Still, the news did reach its single most important observer. A stack of headlines summarized the page 1 story:[30]

> Rockefeller Gives Another $500,000.
> This Sum to Be Used for Hospital for Treatment of Unusual Disease.
> Due to Flexner's Genius.
> Gift Made in Recognition of Discovery of Meningitis Cure.
> Building Near the Rockefeller Institute.

And although cerebrospinal meningitis serum did not get Flexner's picture into the papers, other news from the RIMR did do so before the end of the year.

At the other institute on the other side of town, George Rambaud turned out to be as photogenic as his uncle, and he encouraged the publication of photographs of his work in newspapers and magazines. Photo spreads were becoming more popular

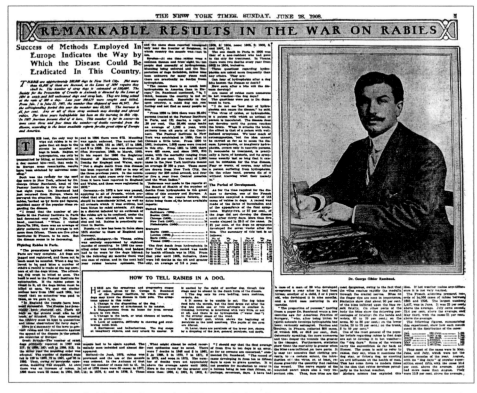

FIG. 44. "Remarkable Results in the War on Rabies," *New York Times,* June 28, 1908, Sunday magazine, 5.

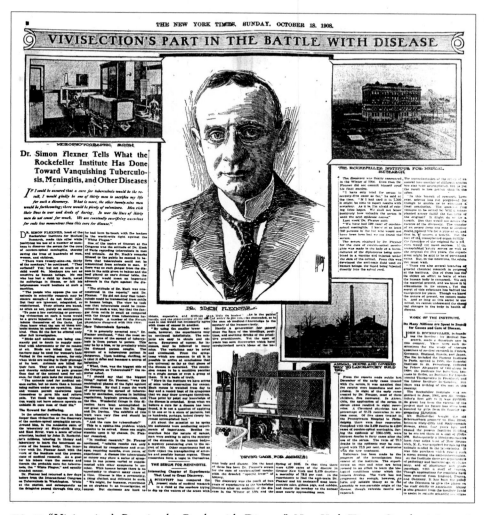

FIG. 45. "Vivisection's Part in the Battle with Disease," *New York Times*, October 18, 1908, Sunday magazine, 2.

in many magazines, and the Sunday *New York Times* often printed large articles accompanied by several halftone photographs. These venues repeatedly featured one of the institutes or the other. In 1908, for example, "Remarkable Results in the War on Rabies," a large article illustrated with a photograph of institute director Rambaud at his desk, argued that muzzles and dog licenses could overcome the rabies problem (fig. 44). The subtitle read, "Success of Methods Employed in Europe Indicated the Way by Which the Disease Could Be Eradicated in This Country." Just a few months later, an article with a very similar layout featured RIMR director Flexner for his active role in publicly defending medical experiments using animals (fig. 45). A large center drawing of Flexner was surrounded by images (clockwise from upper left) of the microphotographic room, the RIMR building, the animal

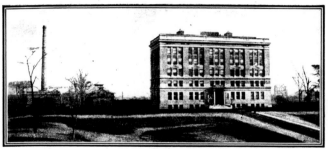

Power house.   Animal house.   Main laboratory.   Site of new
hospital.

THE ROCKEFELLER INSTITUTE FOR MEDICAL RESEARCH, SIXTY-SIXTH STREET AND AVENUE A, NEW
YORK CITY.

THE ROCKEFELLER INSTITUTE FOR MEDICAL RESEARCH.

BY HERBERT T. WADE.

THE extraordinary and practical success that has attended the work of well-endowed or government-supported institutions for the scientific study of disease and the systematic test of new methods for the treatment of such maladies as have hitherto resisted the efforts of physicians and surgeons is one of the most striking and promising features of present-day medicine. In the United States the most important of the few institutions of this kind is the Rockefeller Institute for Medical Research, founded in 1901 by Mr. John D. Rockefeller. Under this endowment there is maintained in New York City a well-equipped medical laboratory where a staff of trained investigators, free from the cares of routine practice, hospital work, or teaching, are concentrating their entire attention upon researches which deal with the prevention and cure of disease. As in other scientific institutions, where effective organization and adequacy of material equipment are most essential, so at the Rockefeller Institute everything has been arranged in order that experimental medicine may be prosecuted under conditions most productive of good results.

Within little more than half a century there has been a great revolution in medical ideas and methods, so that to-day the aver-age man, whose interest in medicine has been said rarely to extend beyond the prompt relief of his own ailments or those of his family, is quite unable to appreciate the bearing of modern medical science on his own welfare and that of the world at large. And it must be confessed that there are also physicians who still find it impossible fully to realize and appreciate what important results have been and are being secured from the research laboratories and the intimate connection existing between scientific medicine and investigation and the prevention and cure of disease, notwithstanding the brilliant record made in the prevention or control of such epidemics as plague and yellow fever, and in coping with other infectious diseases. But in medicine, as everywhere, the scientific method to-day is supreme, and though the practicing physician occupies as important and honorable a position as ever, yet in his efforts to cure and prevent disease he has become more and more dependent upon the labors of the scientific investigator. In other words, the laboratory worker must discover and, in many cases where scientific methods and special technique are required, prepare the tools which the practicing physician uses with such great and tender skill.

FIG. 46. Photograph of new campus, in Herbert T. Wade, "The Rockefeller Institute for Medical Research," *American Review of Reviews* 39:2 (February 1909), 183. For a copy of this article, I am grateful to Leslie Bailey of Orangeburg, South Carolina.

house with the covered way to the laboratory building, and a drying cage for animals. Metaphors of war and battles were joined with powerfully suggestive words such as "success," "eradication," and "results" in many of these articles, continually reinforcing the picture of medicine as now being about big triumphs, overshadowing its traditional focus on individual patient care.

A few months later, a photograph of the RIMR's new building opened a general article in the *American Review of Reviews* about the institute's activity (fig. 46). As with the Pasteur Institute building erected in the prior decade, the substantial and expensive edifice was an important symbol of the magnitude and permanence of the investment in the experimental laboratories housed therein. But what the public saw was not limited to exteriors. In some magazines, readers were invited to look inside the laboratories and view technicians at work (fig. 47).

Dr. Alexis Carrel, an eccentric French surgeon who had come to the RIMR in 1906, was performing amazing feats of transplantation, successfully moving quite a variety of limbs and organs from one animal to another. The photographs in a seventeen-page article in *McClure's Magazine* began with the scientists and then proceeded to close-ups of the experimental animals. Readers were first shown the directors of the Rockefeller Institute; the scientific laboratory (external view of the main building); a formal portrait of Dr. William H. Welch, president of the board of directors; a formal portrait of Dr. Alexis Carrel, experimental surgeon; the central chemical laboratory; and Flexner's private laboratory. After such a prosaic beginning, there followed examples of the freakish animals that Carrel was creating to explore the power of his new techniques—all made possible by his breakthrough method for cutting blood vessels and sewing them together again to reestablish circulation to the severed parts. His work on suturing vessels was honored three years later with the Nobel Prize.

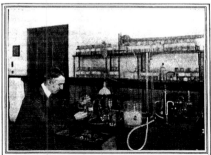

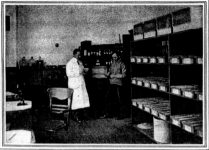

FIG. 47. "Room for the Experimental Study of Cancer" and "The Physical Chemical Laboratory," in Burton J. Hendrick, "Work at the Rockefeller Institute: The Transplanting of Animal Organs," *McClure's Magazine* 32:4 (February 1909), 376–377.

If readers of *McClure's Magazine* were so inclined, they could examine photographs of a dog that had both of its kidneys removed and one put back; Cat Number 6, which had both kidneys removed and the kidneys of another animal transplanted into its body; a composite blood vessel; another composite; a dog onto which had been transplanted the ear, part of the scalp, and other sections of a second dog; a leg that, though it looked as if nature made it, was really composed of parts of two hind legs of two different dogs; and the bacteriological preparation room. As this experimental surgery offered no obvious cures, it again confirms that the public was becoming more comfortable with the idea that medical research can be worthwhile even if the applications are not immediate and even when animals' bodies are being manipulated in rather grotesque ways.

Still, cures were always more popular than basic research, especially when they helped children. "Blindness Vanishes before the March of Modern Science" proclaimed a six-column banner headline in the Sunday *New York Herald* of December 5, 1909. What the headline announced was a substantial article that opened with three cross-section diagrams of eyeballs of the normal, the near-sighted, and the far-sighted eye. Just below the diagrams were photographic portraits of Dr. John Herbert Claiborne, an eminent professor of diseases of the eye, and Dr. S. Josephine Baker, physician and director of New York City's new Bureau of Child Hygiene.[31] The subheadline provided a more modest and more accurate report of the situation: "Advances in Treatment of Ophthalmia and Trachoma Controlling These Diseases: Child Victims Fewer"; but the main rubric evoked the era's common notion of progress from science ("the march") and the routinely high expectations ("blindness vanishes"). In 1909, Baker was already rather famous, and she knew how to court publicity that would support children's health and welfare. The *Pittsburgh Post* devoted most of a page of its Sunday edition of July 14, 1912, to a story about Baker's work in New York City, with seven photographs under a headline printed in red ink: "How a Woman Saves a City's Babies." In stories like these, the Sunday papers brought to ordinary readers a depth of coverage that had earlier been found only in magazines. The new Sunday supplements were also bringing what might have been local stories to audiences across the nation, such as Baker's innovative child-hygiene agency in New York City. Another example of a story moving from local to national prominence was that of the Mayo brothers' clinic in Rochester, Minnesota. The *Detroit Free Press* of February 3, 1907, opened its Sunday magazine with a four-color front-page story and five illustrations celebrating "The World's Surgical Centre: An American Country Town."

In 1911, rabies once again secured a place in the Sunday magazine of the *New York Times,* with an article based on new data collected in a federal report (fig. 48). This time, the page offered an image of Pasteur as well as one of Rambaud, thereby helping readers connect the present workers with the great successes of the past.[32]

Later in the summer of 1911, it was polio that earned Flexner and the RIMR another full-page feature in the Sunday *New York Times*: "Fighting the New Scourge of Infantile Paralysis" (fig. 49). This story likewise highlighted links to prior dis-

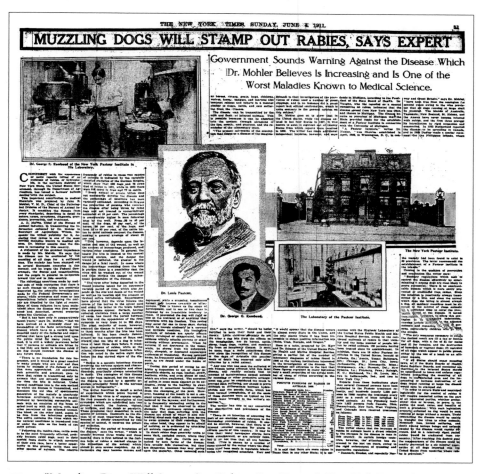

FIG. 48. "Muzzling Dogs Will Stamp Out Rabies, Says Expert," *New York Times,* June 4, 1911, Sunday magazine, 11.

coveries in the growing chain of triumphs. Five photographs called attention to the new hospital devoted strictly to clinical research as a complement to the already established laboratories in the original building. Infantile paralysis was a new disease at the time, rising to significant incidence in the early years of the twentieth century, with notable outbreaks in most years in one locale or another. Physicians borrowed etiological notions from diseases such as cholera and typhoid fever, assuming infantile paralysis arose from urban filth; they blamed crowded living conditions and immigrants' poor hygiene. Modern knowledge sees it quite differently, however, attributing the rise in cases of paralysis to improving levels of hygiene rather than the reverse. Apparently, in prior eras with dirtier water supplies, most infants and children were exposed to the virus at an early age and developed subclinical infections that protected them from later attacks. As new generations of children were starting to grow up more hygienically—and thus without a protective early exposure—they

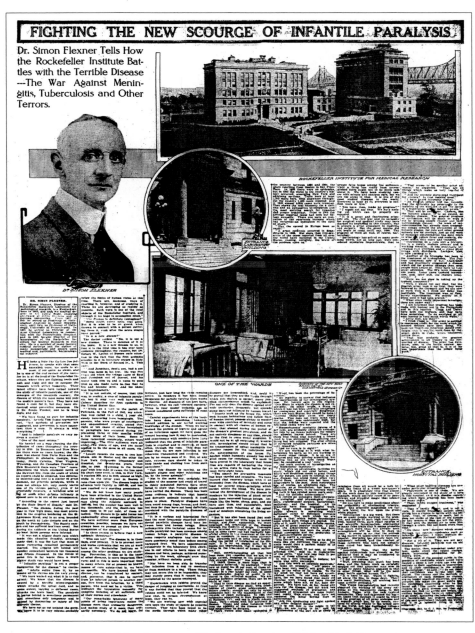

FIG. 49. "Fighting the New Scourge of Infantile Paralysis," *New York Times,* August 20, 1911, Sunday magazine, 3.

began to suffer from the more serious paralytic form when they did get sick. It was this unexpected and counterintuitive etiology that made polio such a perplexing disease in the early twentieth century.

Scientists felt a particular urgency about trying to control infantile paralysis far beyond the number of cases because it arrived just when major strides were being made against infectious diseases in the laboratory and when the media had gotten the public so engaged in following the progress of science. Flexner hoped his successful approach to cerebrospinal meningitis would be applicable to polio and began experiments on monkeys. In time, he and his colleagues did manage to establish polio infection in monkeys and find ways to transmit it from one to another. Although some animals build an immunity after an exposure, Flexner found no large animal that might produce immune serum as horses did for diphtheria antitoxin. And the virus could not yet be cultivated outside the animal body. Perhaps because of Flexner's energetic public activities defending vivisection in medical research and also because of the succession of important breakthroughs over the previous twenty years, the press sometimes took his polio work as being closer to a cure than it was.[33] In the interview that forms the bulk of this article in the *New York Times,* Flexner acknowledged the public's desire for miracle cures, and he took pains to emphasize that, despite his general confidence in the continuing progress of research, prevention was still the only effective way to combat this particular disease.

ACCUMULATING ADVANCES BRING HISTORY TO THE FORE

Twenty-five years after the rabies breakthrough, one important effect of such recurring reports on biomedical research—both the news of sudden breakthroughs and the more routine explorations of laboratory activities—was the establishment of a "long view" of medical progress. In this perspective, medicine was seen as evolving systematically, and the list of achievements as growing ever larger. A good illustration of this emerging retrospective view may be found in "Marvelous Preventives of Disease," a 1913 article in *World's Work: A History of Our Time,* a richly illustrated monthly magazine (fig. 50). Written by Leonard Keene Hirshberg, a physician who frequently contributed to popular magazines, the story opened with a long subtitle: "How we may now be made invulnerable to the attacks of typhoid fever, bubonic plague, and cerebro-spinal meningitis—how Memphis saved itself from an epidemic —the beneficent work of Drs. A. E. Wright, Noguchi, Haffkine, and Sophian, and of other pioneers of preventive medicine." Despite the international scope of the names in the heading, the article was illustrated with photographs of unidentified laboratory workers, a row of calves with cowpox, a horse, and several familiar images of the New York Pasteur Institute.

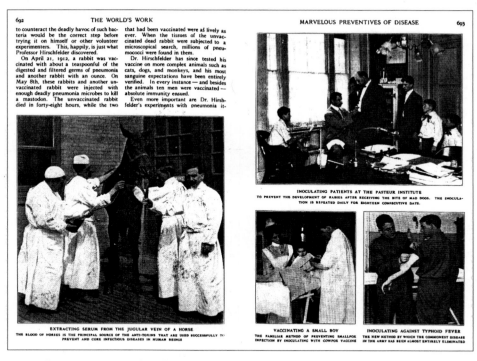

FIG. 50. "Extracting Serum" and other photographs, in Leonard Keene Hirshberg, "Marvelous Preventives of Disease," *World's Work* 25:6 (April 1913), 692–693.

In the very same month, *Leslie's* magazine paraded the accumulating medical triumphs and pictured the institutions that were now creating the new cures and preventions. "Diseases Already or Almost Conquered" opened with an editor's headnote touting "the most notable victories of scientific medicine against epidemics and scourges" and heralding another article to follow soon on "The Yet Unconquered Diseases."[34] Such articles were not studies in the history of medicine per se, but they were part of a new consciousness that saw contemporary medical research, even when it was not yielding big breakthroughs, as part of an advancing tide of victories over diseases just like the pioneering triumphs over smallpox, rabies, and diphtheria. The *Leslie's* article opened with a large photograph of the buildings of the Rockefeller Institute. Portrayed on each side were Dr. Charles W. Stiles of the hookworm campaign and Dr. Jesse W. Lazear, "who lost his life in the final victory that made possible the eradication of yellow fever." At the bottom of this page, *Leslie's* ran the same photograph of Rambaud inoculating rabies patients at the New York Pasteur Institute that had appeared in *World's Work*. That this picture of Rambaud was recycled again and again until 1931 points to the iconic status of rabies shots as the paramount cure developed in the laboratory, even at a time when a biomedical industry was growing far beyond its humble origins in simple injections of dried spinal marrow.

A few months later, when a prominent Rockefeller Institute scientist, Hideyo Noguchi, announced that he had identified the germ that causes rabies, it predictably made front-page news. The *New York Times* asked rabies expert Rambaud for comments, and he chose his words carefully: "If this report [had] emanated from any other source than Dr. Noguchi, I would be inclined to discredit it. . . . [But] if Dr. Noguchi has succeeded, as there is every reason to believe he has, in isolating the germ of rabies, he has made an important contribution to medical science."[35] Journalists were now playing a more active role, asking Rambaud for his expert opinion, not about a published scientific paper but about a reporter's summary of another scientist's work. Rambaud was also quoted in magazine stories in the *Independent* and in *Outlook*.[36] Other reports, not mentioning Rambaud, appeared in *Harper's Weekly* and *World's Work*.[37] During the month of September, the *New York Times* ran five different articles about Noguchi's "discovery."

That Rambaud of the Pasteur Institute answered cautiously was a good thing since Noguchi of the Rockefeller Institute turned out to be wrong about the rabies germ. But although Noguchi's rabies discovery was not sustained, the media's burst of enthusiasm about it indicated that rabies had not lost the public's interest even at a time when wider access to rabies shots was reducing some of its terror. The episode also made clear that the Lower West Side's modest institute under Rambaud's leadership was still a match for its younger, richer, and more corporate rival on the Upper East Side.

Some years later, when Noguchi had achieved even greater popularity in the media, he claimed an even more important triumph: an identification of the germ behind the deadly epidemics of yellow fever. Again, he was unfortunately wrong. Yet the momentum of accumulating biomedical discoveries was strong enough that such big mistakes, even coming from the highly visible Rockefeller Institute, posed no challenge to a now uncontestable picture of institutionally produced medical progress.[38]

PART III

MEDICAL HISTORY FOR THE PUBLIC, 1925–1950

CHAPTER 6

THE MASS MEDIA MAKE MEDICAL HISTORY POPULAR

The strange, throbbing excitement found in the realm of research . . .
—*Newsweek* on the film *The Story of Louis Pasteur,* February 15, 1936

[*The film* Madame Curie] *makes the quest for knowledge a romantic and thrilling pursuit.*
—*New York Times,* December 17, 1943

BY THE EARLY 1920s, new medical discoveries had become routine in newspapers and magazines. Single advances each received less notice than in the past. Even stories that made front-page news, like insulin injections for diabetes in 1922, did not generate sustained waves of excitement. Discoveries were no longer met with the grand enthusiasm that had characterized an earlier generation's response. No breakthroughs galvanized the nation. Had regular medical progress become so well established in popular culture that people were taking it for granted? What might have brought about a decline in the level of excitement about medical research?

No single cause seems likely to account for this large, if quiet, shift in media attention and popular feelings, but several factors seem to have played a role. The technical aspects of medical science were becoming far more complex and thus harder to convey to the general public. Because medical research, like all of science in the post–World War I period, was becoming more corporate in structure, it had fewer charismatic individuals who could draw attention to themselves. More research projects were becoming collaborative enterprises, and with teams there was often no single discoverer about whom to tell a story. As universities, research institutions, medical centers, and pharmaceutical companies grew in size and number, the sites of research activity became more numerous. As scientific knowledge accumulated, advances were more likely to be made through incremental steps than sudden bursts of novelty. Big stories were harder to find. Individual scientists were less likely to be known to the reporters and to the public. No longer could reporters simply drop by the New York Pasteur Institute or the Rockefeller Institute to take the pulse of medical progress. As the doctors became more numerous and less differentiated, their personalities and the human elements in the research work became less accessible. Individual patients also disappeared from most stories, whether out of privacy concerns or because the newer studies were using larger data pools and were replacing anecdotes with statistics.

Serum therapy, for example, was a significant advance for pneumonia patients, but it lacked an easy-to-capture simplicity and resisted popularization. For the first four decades of the twentieth century, the identification of pneumonia's bacterial strains and the production of typed serums formed a large part of the activity of advanced medical care.[1] Rapid typing of the patient's strain was essential since only a serum prepared for that specific strain would have an effect. Such bench work occupied much of the attention of the leading hospitals, doctors, and medical scientists for two generations. It was important research at the time, especially at the Rockefeller Institute's hospital, though it was not generally appreciated by the public because there were so many variables in its use in patients and it had no singular moment of success that might generate publicity.[2] Similarly, the story of infantile-paralysis research in the 1920s and 1930s was not an easy one to tell. The advances in typing of polio strains and in developing tissue-culture media, though scientifically important, did not usually grab headlines.

Another obstacle to science popularization in the 1920s was that the use of chemical weapons in World War I had given chemistry a bad name, and the battlefield poisons cast doubt over science in general. In fact, American scientists became so anxious about declining public respect and support that they demanded their professional associations take action to restore their status. Along with other initiatives, this worry led to the creation of Science Service in 1921, which provided news releases to the media and promoted public education.[3] Concern also prompted grand plans for new science museums to stimulate the public's curiosity.

Yet even if reports of medical discoveries were losing their cachet for the general public, images of medical progress did not entirely disappear from popular consciousness during this lull. Newspapers and magazines in the 1920s continued to run stories like those of the prior decades. In some of these stories, however, one can discern two elements that became more prominent over time. Writers were more frequently bringing historical figures into the story, and the photographic images were getting clearer, sharper, and more dramatic. Consider, for example, a two-page article, "All the Health in the World," in *Collier's The National Weekly* in 1922. In that era, *Collier's* was a large-format magazine, with a cover price of five cents and a large circulation of about one million. The color illustrations of fashionable women that graced most of its covers confirm that it served a wide readership. The first page of this story immediately established the importance of John D. Rockefeller and Louis Pasteur as individuals who had set things in motion, and it linked them to contemporary medicine (fig. 51). "The former contributed to the

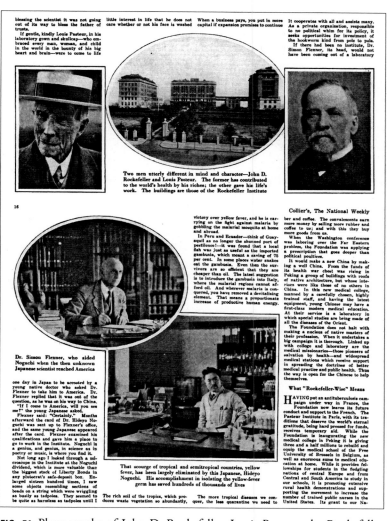

FIG. 51. Photographs of John D. Rockefeller, Louis Pasteur, the Rockefeller Institute, Simon Flexner, and Hideyo Noguchi; details from Frederick Palmer, "All the Health in the World," *Collier's The National Weekly* 70:18 (October 28, 1922), 15–16. Author's collection.

world's health by his riches; the other gave his life's work." Notice how the phrasing "gave his life's work" hints at personal devotion and sacrifice, with science seen as a worthy calling. Centered between the two men's portraits were photographs of the large buildings of the institute, which emphasized the physical continuity of science from the past into the present. The second page of the article was dominated by two well-composed black-and-white portrait photographs of men at work: Rockefeller Institute director Simon Flexner at his desk and researcher Hideyo Noguchi at a lab bench. These photographs were quite different from the staid, even lifeless portrait photographs common before the 1920s. Despite a lack of motion, these sharply lighted still images, in which each man's figure is poised for motion, suggest a kind of dramatic action, almost as if they are stills taken from a moving picture. Furthermore, by keeping the men's figures small within the frame, these photographs draw viewers into the settings, making us think as much about the institute and its science as about the individuals portrayed. Among many achievements mentioned in the article is the claim that Noguchi's work had largely eliminated yellow fever in tropical and semitropical countries.

SCIENCE REPORTING TURNS TO HISTORY

Just how writers and reporters actively brought history into science popularization during the 1920s may be seen in two books for the general public by Henry Smith Williams, a physician and well-established science writer. *The Story of Modern Science* was published in 1923 as a set of ten octavo volumes, mostly text but with photographs on glossy paper clustered at intervals. The tenth volume was devoted to "Man and the Magic of Medicine." Williams opened this volume with Edward Jenner's discovery of vaccination and ended the first chapter with an explanation of preventive inoculation and serum therapy, a century of progress that made the past relevant to the present.[4] Eight years later, *The Book of Marvels* by Williams had a quite different format that resembled a magazine, with two columns of text interrupted by numerous photographs. This book's subject was the scientific progress of the first third of the twentieth century, based on a *Popular Mechanics* poll of experts who picked the seven main advances of the early twentieth century: telegraph, telephone, airplane, radium, antiseptics and antitoxins, spectrum analysis, and the X-ray. Despite the twentieth-century orientation of the book as a whole, both of the featured advances in medicine dated from the nineteenth century, suggesting that—at least for the general public—there were no recent "marvels" in medicine to report. Williams highlighted the importance of the institutions of research with a section about the Pasteur Institute in Paris (fig. 52), but the illustration used was, again, the twenty-year-old photograph of New York's Dr. Rambaud giving a rabies shot.[5] The rhetoric of magic and marvels, with its invocation of a romantic past, illustrates the nervous striving for popular interest that characterized science writing at this time.

88

THE BOOK OF MARVELS

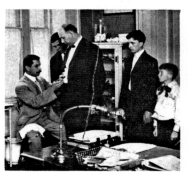

ANTI-RABIES INOCULATION

The Pasteur Institute

REPORT comes from the Pasteur Institute in Paris that a method has been found of developing the germs of tuberculosis through successive cultures until they lose their virulence. There is substantial reason for believing, however, that the germs that have become incapable of menacing the life of an animal are potent to give the animal immunity against tuberculosis.

Should it be possible to make application of this method to the human subject, the importance of the discovery is obvious. But it represents the application of an old method rather than the discovery of a new one. In point of fact, it was by similarly attenuating the virulence of a disease germ that Pasteur himself made the memorable demonstration of the possibility of giving protective immunity as long ago as 1881.

In that year Pasteur demonstrated that he could protect sheep and cattle against anthrax by inoculating them with a vaccine secured by the cultivating of the anthrax bacillus. Twenty-five sheep and goats and five cattle were given a preventive inoculation

ANTI-SERUM TO COUNTERACT HOG CHOLERA

and subsequently they were inoculated with active virus as were a similar number of animals in an adjoining pen. Two days later all the unprotected animals were dead or dying. The protected ones were well, and so continued.

Pasteur's treatment of hydrophobia followed; and the method of immunization by inoculation with dead germs has become familiar more recently as applied to typhoid fever and some other maladies.

The method has even been extended to tuberculosis, but not to the entire satisfaction of the medical profession. It is to be hoped that the new Pasteur Institute experiments point the way to the development of a completely satisfactory immunizing method that will be another step towards robbing tuberculosis of its terrors. Our pictures show an inoculation against rabies at the Pasteur Institute, and animals used in preparing antitoxic serums.

Turn About Is Fair Play

NOT many years after my graduation in medicine, I had opportunity to make an experiment which many of my colleagues thought foredoomed to failure.

A partially tamed black-tailed deer in the park at Bloomingdale Asylum (then located where Columbia University now is) ran amuck and attacked an attendant, who defended himself with a rake handle and, striking out vigorously, broke one of the animal's front legs.

My experiment consisted in setting the bone, with application of a plaster of Paris bandage.

This would have been a simple and familiar experience in case of a human patient.

But a deer's leg is so slender and fleshless a member, and the animal itself so far from docile under treatment, that the chance of getting a successful union of the fractured bones seemed more than doubtful.

Nevertheless I thought the attempt worth making. Assisted by my young colleague, Dr. Richard R. Daly (now a noted

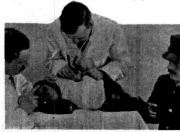

A CHIMPANZEE UNDER TREATMENT

specialist of Atlanta, Georgia), I tied the animal cowboy fashion, and applied the bandage liberally, until the damaged member was held securely in a plaster cast almost as hard as stone.

When, after a suitable interval, the splint was cut away, it was at once apparent that the procedure had been an entire success.

The bones had "knit" perfectly, the leg had not shortened, and only a small nodule, hardly to be noticed by the casual observer, gave evidence of the former injury.

The buck was presently transported to the Bronx Zoological Garden, where it spent the remainder of its life with companions of its species, able to run and jump with the best of them, and in nowise handicapped.

Recollection of this almost forgotten experience came to mind when I saw a photograph showing a group of students at the Pennsylvania Veterinary School in the act of applying bandages to the legs of injured dogs.

The conditions under which they are working are very different from those under which Dr. Daly and I worked forty years ago; yet there is no difference in principle.

We had no glass-topped operating table, and our facilities for practising asepsis were not up to the modern standard; but the result proved that our technique was adequate. The antisepsis, even of that day, was a thoroughly practical method.

FIG. 52. Photographs of antirabies inoculation, a chimpanzee under treatment, and antiserum to counteract hog cholera in Henry Smith Williams, *The Book of Marvels* (New York and London: Funk & Wagnalls, 1931), 88. © 1931. Used by permission of Weekly Reader Corporation. All rights reserved. Author's collection.

Medical history was then an unfamiliar subject; its appeal to the public was untested. But it offered a promising approach for writers, editors, and scientists troubled by the public's weak engagement with science. Reaching beyond the little nuggets of medical history in contemporary magazine stories, writers started going fully into the past. Telling stories of medical history overcame some difficulties found in presenting contemporary medical progress in popular forms. The science involved was simpler, making it more accessible to readers. Writers could dramatize sympathetic victims of disease without invading patients' privacy. They could choose stories in which the doctor's quest always met success. In looking back in time, it was easier to sort out the good guys from the bad guys, and it was possible to turn their struggles into morality tales. In prior eras, individuals had played bigger roles than in the corporate settings of the twentieth century. The doctor hero from history could be constructed as a complete personality, unlike the living scientists, who rarely exposed the personal side of their creative work to reporters. And the same features that made a story easier for a writer to tell could also heighten a reader's personal involvement with the characters. Although some editors and writers initially took up medical history strategically as a form of science popularization, the public turned out to like what they read and made the subject wildly popular.

Paul de Kruif, a maverick medical scientist at the Rockefeller Institute, took the lead as one of the science writers who started out providing accounts of contemporary medical research and then gradually brought more and more history into them. But he would not be remembered today if he had not written a book that was entirely historical. That book, called *Microbe Hunters,* offered vigorously dramatic storytelling with emotionally charged prose. It made de Kruif a household name and sparked a flood of writing about medical history.

De Kruif's education and early experience had provided a solid intellectual base in medical research and a wealth of insights into the laboratory life of leading scientists, both of which contributed to the creation of his enduringly successful book. After completing a Ph.D. in bacteriology in 1916 at the University of Michigan under mentors who were champions of scientific medicine, Victor Vaughan and Frederick Novy, de Kruif entered war service and developed an antitoxin for gas gangrene, a life-threatening wound infection common in trench warfare. With boundless energy and great scientific promise, he joined the staff of the Rockefeller Institute in 1920. There he carried out important work on variation within bacterial species and the characterization of strains and types. But a passion for writing and a rebellious streak opened new avenues for his career that prompted an awkward separation from the institute. A series of articles that he wrote about contemporary medicine appeared anonymously in *Century* magazine in 1922 and were then collected and published in a book under his name later the same year, *Our Medicine Men.* Although the Rockefeller Institute was not named in the book, an account of conflict, pettiness, and crassness among researchers and clinicians seemed to reflect poorly on his home institution and led to his departure.[6]

Our Medicine Men, along with a series of articles in *Hearst's International* about such breakthroughs as insulin for diabetes and sunlight for rickets, alerted others to de Kruif's talents.[7] Morris Fishbein of the American Medical Association introduced de Kruif to the famous writer Sinclair Lewis, who was seeking help with the medical elements in a novel he was writing. The author and his new collaborator worked beautifully together on all aspects of the book's content: science, settings, and characterizations. Once again, the Rockefeller Institute was not named, but it was clearly parodied as the McGurk Institute (both in the novel and in the later film). Unfortunately for de Kruif's writing career, he and Lewis failed to agree on how he was to be publicly credited. De Kruif's name was not on the title page of *Arrowsmith* in 1925, even in a subordinate fashion. When *Arrowsmith* won the Pulitzer Prize for fiction, Lewis refused the prize, an action that further eclipsed possible public notice of de Kruif's essential contribution to the book. Then in late 1925 and early 1926, *Country Gentleman* published a series of five articles by de Kruif, illustrated with drawings, about historical episodes of medical discovery (fig. 53).[8]

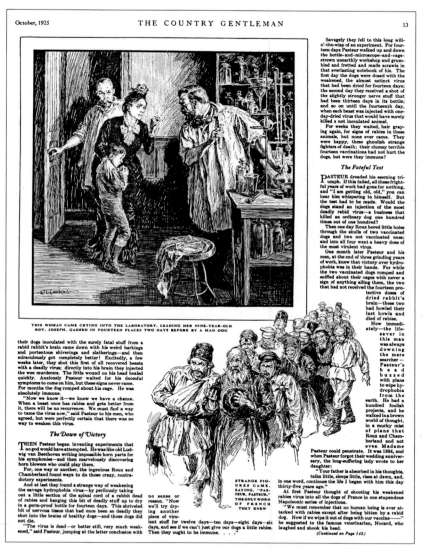

FIG. 53. An illustrated page from Paul de Kruif, "Pasteur and the Mad Dogs," illustrated by R. L. Lambdin, *Country Gentleman* 90:36 (October 1925), 13. © 1925 SEPS: Licensed by Curtis Publishing, Indianapolis, Ind. www.curtispublishing.com. All rights reserved. Author's collection.

This series was de Kruif's first venture in writing history, and its spectacular success not only shaped his career but also contributed an important new element to U.S. culture. When the articles were expanded into the book *Microbe Hunters* in 1926, they quickly captured a wide and enthusiastic readership.

De Kruif animated his stories from the laboratory with clear delineation of character, lively details of personal life, and imagined conversations. The pace was fast, the language often colloquial. There were no academic formalities here; these were adventure stories, and they could almost have been about frontier explorers, cowboys, or big-game hunters. The excitement of the chase gave the book its often breathless tone as well as its title metaphor. The opening of the chapter on Robert Koch illustrates characteristic features of the book's style:

In those astounding and exciting years between 1860 and 1870, when Pasteur was saving vinegar industries and astonishing emperors and finding out what ailed sick silkworms, a small, serious, and nearsighted German was learning to be a doctor at the University of Göttingen. His name was Robert Koch. He was a good student, but while he hacked at cadavers he dreamed of going tiger-hunting in the jungle. Conscientiously he memorized the names of several hundred bones and muscles, but the fancied moan of the whistles of steamers bound for the East chased this Greek and Latin jargon out of his head.

Koch wanted to be an explorer; or to be a military surgeon and win Iron Crosses; or to be a ship's doctor and voyage to impossible places. But, alas, when he graduated from the medical college in 1866 he became an interne in a not very interesting insane asylum in Hamburg. Here, busy with raving maniacs and helpless idiots, the echoes of Pasteur's prophecies that there were such things as terrible man-killing microbes hardly reached Koch's ears. He was still listening for steamer whistles and in the evenings he took walks down by the wharves with Emmy Fraatz; he begged her to marry him; he held out the bait of romantic trips around the world to her. Emmy told Robert that she would marry him, but on condition that he forget this nonsense about an adventurous life, provided that he would settle down to be a practicing doctor, a good useful citizen, in Germany.

Koch listened to Emmy—for a moment the allure of fifty years of bliss with her chased away his dreams of elephants and Patagonia—and he settled down to practice medicine; he began what was to him a totally uninteresting practice of medicine in a succession of unromantic Prussian villages. . . .

But Robert Koch was restless. He trekked from one deadly village to another still more uninteresting, until at last he came to Wollstein, in East Prussia, and here, on his twenty-eighth birthday, Mrs. Koch bought him a microscope to play with.

You can hear the good woman say: "Maybe that will take Robert's mind off what he calls his stupid practice . . . perhaps this will satisfy him a little . . . he's always looking at everything with his old magnifying glass. . . ."

Alas for her, this new microscope, this plaything, took her husband on more curious adventures than any he would have met in Tahiti or Lahore; and these weird experiences —that Pasteur had dreamed of but which no man had ever had before—came on him out of the dead carcasses of sheep and cows. These new sights and adventures jumped at him impossibly on his very doorstep, and in his own drug-reeking office that he was so tired of, that he was beginning to loathe.

"I hate this bluff that my medical practice is . . . it isn't because I do not *want* to save babies from diphtheria . . . but mothers come to me crying—asking me to save their babies—and what can I do?—Grope . . . fumble . . . reassure them when I know there is no hope. . . . How can I cure diphtheria when I do not even know what causes it, when the wisest doctor in Germany doesn't know? . . ." So you can imagine Koch complaining bitterly to Emmy, who was irritated and puzzled, and thought that it was a young doctor's business to do as well as he could with the great deal of knowledge that he had got at the medical school—oh! would he never be satisfied?

But Koch was right. What, indeed, did doctors know about the mysterious causes of disease? Pasteur's experiments were brilliant, but they had proved nothing about the how and why of human sickness. Pasteur was a trail blazer, a fore-runner crying possible future great victories over disease, shouting about magnificent stampings out of epidemics; but meanwhile the moujiks of desolate towns in Russia were still warding off scourges by hitching four widows to a plow and with them drawing a furrow round their villages in the dead of night—and their doctors had no sounder protection to offer them.[9]

Microbe Hunters remains in print to this day. Its success catapulted de Kruif to celebrity status as a leading writer (with appropriately high compensation). It was probably his dramatizing style that made these stories so readily adaptable for plays, puppet shows, feature-length movies, radio dramas, and comic books. His book helped reshape popular culture by making medical history and laboratory science exciting for readers and viewers, and his style encouraged imitations in various media. A small indication of the personal renown he achieved beyond his books and articles is his place as a celebrity expert on the popular radio show *Information Please,* on which he appeared with Clifton Fadiman, Oscar Levant, and others. And in the typical way that media reports reinforce one another, this otherwise invisible appearance on a radio program was recorded visually in a national magazine's photo feature, "*Life* Goes to a Broadcast of 'Information Please.'"[10] More important than de Kruif's personal fame, however, was how his book turned the world's attention to the exciting stories found in medical history.

WHAT DE KRUIF WROUGHT

Microbe Hunters initiated a sustained wave of mass-media interest in the subject. There had been, of course, a few earlier books for the layman about medical discovery, as well as the novel *Arrowsmith*. A two-volume biography of a recently deceased physician received the Pulitzer Prize for Biography in 1926 (*The Life of Sir William Osler* by Harvey Cushing).[11] Nonetheless, *Microbe Hunters* was the major stimulus to popularizing the subject. *Microbe Hunters* was even serialized in daily newspapers for an even broader readership within months of its publication in hardcover.[12]

Publishers quickly began to add similar titles. *Triumphs of Medicine* by H. S. Hartzog Jr. appeared in 1927. Arthur Selwyn-Brown's *The Physician throughout the Ages* came out in 1928. That same year, de Kruif's *Hunger Fighters* was published, with a striking set of woodcuts by Bertrand Zadig. That book dramatized a dozen research triumphs in biology and medicine, concluding with the epidemiology of pellagra uncovered by Joseph Goldberger, G. H. Wheeler, and Edgar Sydenstricker. The next year saw the appearance of two different editions of the same book by Samuel W. Lambert and George M. Goodwin, one titled *Minute Men of Life: The Story of the Great Leaders in Medicine from Hippocrates Down to the Present Day* and the other *Medical Leaders from Hippocrates to Osler.* Grove Wilson's *The Human Side of Science,* also published in 1929, bore a portrait of English surgeon Joseph Lister as its frontispiece. An especially successful work of 1929 was Howard W. Haggard's *Devils, Drugs, and Doctors: The Story of the Science of Healing from Medicine-Man to Doctor.* This often-reprinted work was the first of four thick books on medical history by this prolific author, a Yale physiology professor.

Rapid growth in popular medical history began in the 1920s, peaked in the 1930s, and declined a little in the 1940s. My examination of this unprecedented surge of general books published in the United States for adult readers counts seven books in the decade ending in 1909, four in the 1910s, and then twenty-six in the 1920s. The count rises to thirty-nine in the 1930s and decreases to twenty-three in the 1940s. These conservative numbers undercount the popularity of the subject among readers since my tabulation omits reprints and revised editions as well as single-subject biographies and local history studies. These books regularly carried seductive and romantic title words such as "triumphs," "master-minds," "leaders," "pathfinders," "heroes," "stalkers of pestilence," "riders of the plagues," and "partners in progress."

MEDICAL HISTORY IN THE NEWSPAPERS

In the 1920s and 1930s, books were hardly the only medium for medical history stories. U.S. daily newspapers and their weekly pictorial supplements published their own explorations of medicine's history in addition to the reporting of medical news. Three examples may indicate the character of this exotic presence in the dailies and their more expansive weekend editions. In 1926, the *Boston Evening Transcript* devoted most of a weekday page to illustrations for an article, "Dressing the Surgeon—Past and Present," portraying medical museum pieces as a fashion show (fig. 54). In 1934, the *Albany Times-Union* headlined a substantial illustrated article as follows: "Doctors in Olden Times: Almost Unbelievable Things the Medical Men of Earlier Centuries Did to Cure Their Patients Believing That a Toad Has a Magic Stone in Its Head, That Insane People Were Afflicted by Evil Spirits and That

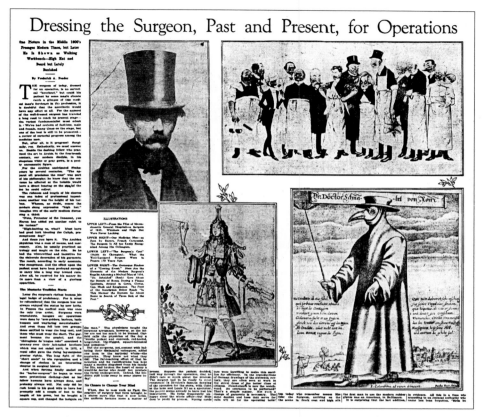

FIG. 54. Frederick A. Fender, "Dressing the Surgeon—Past and Present, for Operations," *Boston Evening Transcript,* November 17, 1926, 8. Four images show a photo of a bearded man in a top hat; a costume with large beak to protect against the plague; a caricature of a group with aprons, saws, knives, and such; and an early engraving of a man decorated with surgical instruments. © 1926. All rights reserved. Author's collection.

Sneezing Cleaned the Brain."[13] In 1939, a four-color cover feature in the *American Weekly,* "How Healing Began: Tomb Pictures Prove Ancient Priests Made Medicine Help Their Religion," offered several illustrations from ancient Egypt.[14] As stories like these indicate, medical history during the interwar years was not an esoteric scholarly topic confined to university libraries and the shelves of humanistic physicians but something exotic and intriguing that ordinary Americans might peruse at the breakfast table.

On some occasions, newspapers chose to report recent medical advances in the same biographical style popularized by the stories of de Kruif. For example, a series of twelve long articles about current and past research at the National Institute of Health ran weekly in the Sunday edition of the *Washington Evening Star* in early 1937. Written by Lucy Salamanca, these articles each described the work of one "G-Man of Science," including a woman scientist in one story.[15] Most of the illustrations were photographs of white-coated figures in laboratory settings. The headline's metaphor tapped the popular passion in the 1930s for G-Man stories, prompted by James Cagney's starring role in the film *G-Men* of 1935.[16] An advertisement from Metropolitan Life Insurance Company that same year drew on the same metaphor, using "G-Men of Medical Science" to headline an ad that appeared in popular magazines. The image was of a white-coated man looking into a microscope; the text explained the contributions of Edward Jenner, Louis Pasteur, and Paul Ehrlich, and it mentioned the use of pneumonia typing for the production of sera. It also pointed to the recent successes in controlling diabetes with insulin and pernicious anemia with liver extract. It cited a rise in life expectancy since 1900 from forty-nine years of age to sixty-one. The company's goal was to promote the value of "warmly cooperating with health officials, physicians, civic organizations and hospitals that bring these great discoveries to you and your neighbors."[17]

Late-nineteenth- and early-twentieth-century scientists and doctors dominated much of the popular medical history at the beginning of the 1930s, but attention gradually grew to include earlier figures. Sometimes these earlier figures were Americans who were being publicized by medical groups or by local history efforts. For example, in 1933 the *New York Times* reported that physicians were celebrating the hundredth anniversary of William Beaumont's book *Experiments and Observations on the Gastric Juice and the Physiology of Digestion,* which had recently been reprinted for modern readers in an edition that included an essay on Beaumont by William Osler (1929).[18] Besides Beaumont, the other American figure who gained new prominence through a chauvinistic effort to find early American heroes was Dr. Ephraim McDowell. An unusual article called attention to him through a commemoration of his most famous patient. According to an Associated Press report of 1935, the citizens of Danville, Kentucky, erected "a monument to the pioneer heroine of a remarkable scientific drama staged here 126 years ago in the office of a daring frontier surgeon," Dr. Ephraim McDowell. Mrs. Jane Todd Crawford had "made medical history in 1809 by submitting without an anesthetic to the world's first ovariotomy." The report noted that "never before has the patient of a surgical operation been so honored."[19] These two short articles might seem minor, but they point to the stirrings of a wider effort to insert McDowell and Beaumont into the increasingly settled canon of major medical heroes. Both of these doctors, if less famous than Louis Pasteur or Walter Reed, came to be widely celebrated alongside them in the main cluster of medical history images in the 1930s and 1940s.

MEDICAL HISTORY ON THE STAGE

The general public's enthusiasm for medical history stories went far beyond newspaper stories, hardcover books, paperbacks, and the new "pocket books" that became extremely popular in the 1940s. Stories and characters from medical history, often borrowed from the books of de Kruif, migrated widely into the performing arts. Dramatizations of medical history were more common on the screen than on the stage, but playwrights did not ignore the subject. The most important of these plays was Sidney Howard's *Yellow Jack: A History,* a dramatization of the human experiments with volunteers used to test the theory of mosquitoes as the vector of yellow-fever transmission, based on the Walter Reed chapter in *Microbe Hunters.* A hardcover edition of the drama was published in 1933. It played on Broadway in 1934, and a film version was released a few years later.[20] Paul de Kruif received formal credit in both instances for collaboration with Howard, but he denied any role in either dramatization in an article he published at the time of the film's release.[21]

De Kruif's work also inspired various productions of the Federal Theatre Project, a New Deal agency funded from 1935 to 1939 by the Works Progress Administration. The project sponsored hundreds of new plays and productions all across the nation, both as professional shows and as community theater. For example, in 1939 some of de Kruif's popular stories were brought to the stage as a puppet show for adults, *Men against Microbes.*[22] A loud refrain of "Science marches on!" bracketed scenes from various epochs, starting with the invention of the microscope in the seventeenth century by Anton van Leeuwenhoek toiling alone in his eyeglasses workshop. "SCIENCE MARCHES ON!" Pasteur saves Joseph Meister from rabies. "SCIENCE MARCHES ON!" Walter Reed confirms by experiment that mosquitoes are the vector for yellow fever. "SCIENCE MARCHES ON!" Several other Federal Theatre Project plays promoted medicine and public health within agit-prop performances called "Living Newspapers." Sometimes historical figures were included, such as Fritz Schaudinn, Paul Ehrlich, and August von Wassermann in the antisyphilis play *Spirochete* by Arnold Sundgaard. The Living Newspaper series featured other health-related productions such as *Hookworm, Milk,* and *Medicine Show.* The plays promoted health improvement using discoveries already made and helped citizens understand the scientific approach of observation, hypothesis, and experiment.[23]

SCREEN RE-CREATIONS OF MEDICAL HISTORY

During the 1930s and 1940s, the whole nation was going to the movies, it seemed, and people in all social classes were captivated by Hollywood's flickering images. In President Franklin Roosevelt's second inaugural address in 1937, he famously observed, "I see one-third of a nation ill-housed, ill-clad, ill-nourished." But it was also true that one-third of the nation entered a movie theater every week.[24] In these two decades when movies were extremely popular, a great number of films took up medical themes, often featuring the history of medical research.[25] These films were often set in exotic locales such as the jungles of Africa, Central America, or, closer to home, the Rocky Mountains. Medical figures from history were especially important in a genre of biographical dramas, known as "biopics."[26] Following the success of the 1931 film version of the fictional *Arrowsmith,* adapted by Sidney Howard from Lewis's novel, Americans flocked to see historical doctors in films. *The Prisoner of Shark Island* (1936) celebrated the heroic actions of Dr. Samuel A. Mudd, a prisoner himself, in managing the care for yellow-fever victims in a prison off the coast of Florida. Mudd had been convicted of aiding the escape of Lincoln's assassin, John Wilkes Booth. Although he has never been acquitted, this film and other popular accounts of the era portrayed him as innocent. In film and in reality, he received clemency for selfless medical services he rendered under extremely arduous conditions.[27]

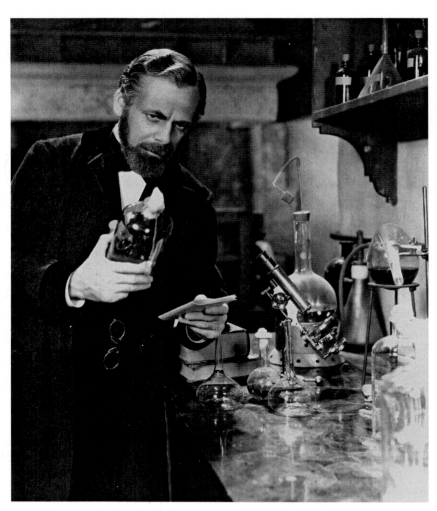

FIG. 55. Publicity still from *The Story of Louis Pasteur* (1936). Paul Muni as Louis Pasteur holding the spinal cord from a rabid rabbit in a drying bottle, posed as in the painting by Edelfelt. © Turner Entertainment Co. A Warner Bros. Entertainment Company. All rights reserved. Courtesy of the Academy of Motion Picture Arts and Sciences.

The Story of Louis Pasteur also premiered in 1936.[28] Although the Warner studio did not expect much from this film and it was offered to theaters at a lower-than-usual royalty rate, it became a national and international success.[29] The film even played in China the year of its U.S. release.[30] Because of the studio's low expectations, old sets has been reused to keep the budget down, and the studio initially released the film as the second feature on double bills. When the film caught on, the studio improved publicity and distribution.[31] This film set a high standard for making science popular; it prompted a wave of medical history biopics; and it became a model against which others came to be judged (fig. 55).

The screenplay for *The Story of Louis Pasteur* invented some characters, especially an antagonist named Dr. Charbonnet (a pun on the French word for anthrax, *charbon*), and modified the chronology of certain events. A review in *Time* magazine asserted that the accurate parts on anthrax and rabies were so good that audiences would not mind an invented villain.[32] *Louis Pasteur* succeeded in bringing to life a number of important issues: the iatrogenic sources of puerperal sepsis; the germ theory as implausible but ultimately convincing through experiments and microscopic images of bacteria (shown on screen); the critical importance of controls in experiments; the essential role of animal experiments; Pasteur's many battles with conservative physicians; the core ideas of immunization employing weakened disease agents; the public's interest in new medical discoveries; the Joseph Meister case, which forced Pasteur to apply his rabies vaccine earlier than he had planned; the significance of the public support Pasteur received from Sir Joseph Lister; and the many accolades Pasteur received by the end of his life.

As in many other biopics, the script for *Louis Pasteur* calls for the protagonist to give a public speech in a formal setting, a device that helps the theater audience merge with an onscreen audience to experience a direct connection to the hero. The film ends in the Sorbonne's amphitheater at a gathering in Pasteur's honor near the end of his life.[33]

Close shot Pasteur. He starts to speak.
PASTEUR: "I—I have no words to express—"
His voice falters. He stops. The ovation dies down rapidly. There is complete silence. Pasteur
    gains possession of himself, looks up at the gallery.
Full shot gallery, which is crowded with the young medical students of France. . . .
Close shot Pasteur. He slowly looks over the auditorium, his eyes filled with tears of emotion.
    He lifts his head toward the gallery.
PASTEUR (addressing his remarks to the students, his voice ringing with conviction): "You
    young men—doctors and scientists of the future—do not let yourselves be tainted by
    a barren skepticism, nor discouraged by the sadness of certain hours that creep over
    nations. Do not become angry at your opponents, for no scientific theory has ever
    been accepted without opposition. Live in the serene peace of libraries and laboratories. Say to yourselves first: 'What have I done for my instruction?' and as you gradually advance: 'What am I accomplishing?,' until the time comes when you may have

the immense happiness of thinking that you have contributed in some way to the welfare and progress of mankind."[34]

In an unsigned review, *Newsweek* made two key observations about the plot and
the values embedded in the film: "For the sake of congealed drama they have passed
over some of Pasteur's important scientific contributions—the preservation of wine
and beer. But the incidents they have used convey the strange, throbbing excitement
found in the realm of research."[35]

Scenes of the public test of Pasteur's anthrax vaccine on a farm at Pouilly-le-Fort
and of the treatment of Joseph Meister were often featured in publicity stills, and
they seem to have worked their way deep into public consciousness. The film greatly
exaggerated coverage of the anthrax trial in 1882 by the French and the international
press. No doubt the filmmaker assumed it would have happened that way because of
all the publicity that surrounded the rabies vaccine in 1885 and later breakthroughs.
A similarly anachronistic portrayal of great public enthusiasm for medical discovery
appeared a few years later in another Hollywood film, *The Great Moment,* about the
1846 discovery of ether anesthesia.

The popularity of *The Story of Louis Pasteur* prompted many other films like it,
both biopics and fictional dramas. The following year, a newspaper review of *Green
Light,* another film about medical scientists, opened with a comparison that it was
"as inspiring as *The Story of Louis Pasteur.*"[36] In *Dark Victory,* a fiction film released
in 1939, Pasteur's name is invoked for the image of a selfless devotion to research,
and historical breakthroughs are mentioned as touchstones of monumental achievement. When a successful brain surgeon explains to a colleague in general practice
why he is abandoning a profitable practice and building a small laboratory on his
farm in Vermont, the plan receives a puzzled response:

GENERAL PRACTITIONER: Don't tell me you've been bitten by the bug for scientific research?
SURGEON: Something like that.
PRACTITIONER: On what?
SURGEON: Cells. Brain cells. Why do healthy cells go berserk—grow wild? Do you know?
PRACTITIONER: No. I—
SURGEON: Neither does anyone. We call them tumors—gliomas—cysts—cancers. We op-
erate and try to cure with the knife when we don't even know the cause. People put
their faith in us because we're doctors and . . . well, you can tell the boys they can split
up my practice—and welcome.
PRACTITIONER: Well, shine my golden halo—you and Pasteur!
SURGEON: Probably you're right. But someday somebody's going to discover a serum that
will be to these growths what insulin is to diabetes—what antitoxin is to diphtheria
—and really earn his title of Doctor of Medicine.[37]

For Warner Brothers, known perhaps too well as a producer of gangster films, *Pasteur* was part of a strategy to alter its image with more respectable subject matter.[38]

With William Dieterle as director working with Paul Muni as star, the idealistic biopic came into its own. Of course, the genre was not limited to the work of Dieterle and Muni or to Warner Brothers. But they were central. After playing Pasteur, Muni played Émile Zola (1937) and then Benito Juarez (1939), both under Dieterle's direction. Dieterle was also the director of *Dr. Ehrlich's Magic Bullet* (1940).[39] After *Pasteur*, Warner Brothers quickly produced *The White Angel* (1936), with Dieterle directing Kay Frances as Florence Nightingale.[40] This story of how Nightingale created professional nursing as a respectable occupation for women in Great Britain centered on her determination in facing down reactionary opponents and her selfless devotion to wounded soldiers even at great personal cost.[41] Her heroism also entailed the social and personal sacrifice of remaining unmarried. But by the end of the film, like all the medical and scientific heroes of the biopics, she had not only triumphed over ignorance but also given an inspiring speech and received accolades from the establishment.

Before 1936 was over, a historically oriented fiction film, *White Legion* (also released under the title *Angels in White*), offered the public several more medical heroes. The story takes place in 1905, the era of Walter Reed's breakthrough on yellow-fever transmission. In this romantic drama with interspersed comic scenes, four doctors from New York join the fight to control the yellow fever that was holding up U.S. construction of the Panama Canal. Though the film's narrative is scientifically and historically jumbled, some of the characters resemble medical scientists with whom the public would have been familiar. The film tapped the public's growing curiosity about medical history, and it honored the spirit of medical research undertaken at significant risk to person and reputation by selfless doctors. Inter alia, this film makes reference to the human experiments done by Walter Reed and his colleagues, the utility of spraying oil on stagnant water to control mosquitoes, human vivisection, variation among different disease infections in creating immunity against a second attack, and the exceedingly dangerous "healthy carrier." The team includes an unmarried woman doctor, who might have been modeled on Louise Pearce of the Rockefeller Institute.[42] Another scientist is an Asian doctor, "Dr. Nogi," clearly a stand-in for Hideyo Noguchi of the Rockefeller Institute, who had pursued the yellow-fever germ in Central and South America and then in Africa, where he had died of the disease in 1928. Noguchi was far better known among the general public than Pearce, but the daily press had reported on her work as well as on his.[43]

In 1937, Errol Flynn starred as Dr. Newell Paige in *The Green Light*. Based on a novel by Lloyd C. Douglas, a Congregational minister and prolific author, the screenplay is a religiously oriented romance about medical personnel. The story is entirely fictional, but the film's second half, in which medical research becomes central to the plot, has a substantial basis in historical fact. Dr. Paige, innocently and unfairly discredited in his medical practice, moves to the Bitterroot Valley of Montana to join a colleague who has undertaken dangerous research on Rocky Mountain spotted fever, a tick-borne lethal disease with characteristic skin lesions.[44] This setting is historically correct as a site of important research on the disease. Unable to separate the virus from the ticks, Paige's unorthodox approach is to try to make a vaccine by allowing an extract of ground-up ticks to age (just as Pasteur attenuated rabies virus by drying an infected piece of bone marrow for three weeks). Paige tests the vaccine on himself and refuses any medical intervention that would destroy the value of the experiment. This single trial by a scientifically inexperienced surgeon is portrayed as the breakthrough that led to a vaccine whose widespread use overcame local suspicions about the research center and brought much credit to the research work of the Public Health Service. Even rather mediocre romance films such as this one employ tropes from the medical history biopics, such as the medical maverick who risks personal sacrifice for the good of science, and they mention names of historical figures to enhance their story's verisimilitude. In a closing scene in which Dr. Paige is given credit for the new vaccine, he pushes the praise aside and attributes the success to predecessors in this research, naming Hideyo Noguchi, Roscoe Roy Spencer, and Ralph Robinson Parker. The latter two scientists were, in fact, central figures in the work of the Bitterroot Valley laboratory; Noguchi had merely attended a conference there in the spring of 1923, though this visit received much attention at least in the local newspapers.[45]

Similarly, *The Crime of Dr. Hallet,* another fictional romance (this one about an exotic disease in Sumatra that the film calls "red fever"), mentions historical persons such as Walter Reed and his colleagues James Carroll and Jesse Lazear to give it authenticity. As in several such films, the research involves experiments to transfer some kind of immunity either for prevention or cure, based on the models of serotherapy known from diphtheria antitoxin and pneumonia sera. For these scientists, as for pneumonia researchers in general, the problem is to distinguish various subtypes of one species of bacteria. Another plot element in this film was also common to a number of these films, namely, a scientist's testing the new product on himself secretly so his colleagues could not stop him. But in *Dr. Hallet* (and also in *White Legion*), experimental injections are also used to save the life of a spoiled society girl who had been hostile toward the medical researchers, thereby securing a kind of moral triumph on behalf of medical progress.

In 1938, Hollywood released a movie version of the Broadway play *Yellow Jack,* a fact-based dramatization of nontherapeutic experiments on humans with a screenplay credited to Edward Chodorov and Paul de Kruif. Then, with war clouds gathering on the horizon in 1939, RKO Radio Pictures premiered *Nurse Edith Cavell,* a film about a British nurse in World War I who was executed in Belgium by the Germans in 1915 for aiding soldiers who had escaped from German prison camps. In contrast to the other films, however, Cavell's heroic stature is based on the personal risks she takes and on her martyrdom as a patriotic woman executed in wartime, rather than on any particularly medical elements in the story.

As the international conflict grew more intense and many people in Hollywood were gearing up for a war against the Nazis, Warner Brothers created a biopic about Paul Ehrlich, a German Jew, whose numerous contributions to modern medicine at the turn of the twentieth century had been monumental. He had played key intellectual roles in the development of diphtheria and tetanus antitoxin. His theory of how the body produced resistance or immunity to the assaults of disease shaped a major research program. He succeeded in synthesizing an organic molecule containing arsenic that could kill invading microbes without damaging the host's body. Ehrlich was honored with the Nobel Prize in 1908, and his work was well known to specialists. Although his story had been told in a chapter of de Kruif's *Microbe Hunters,* his name had not become familiar to the American public. Ehrlich's rich life provided this studio, known for films about Louis Pasteur, Zola, and Juarez, the opportunity for a successful biopic with a strong statement against intolerance.

Released in 1940, *Dr. Ehrlich's Magic Bullet* became Hollywood's single most important exposition of medical history. The film garnered an Academy Award nomination for best original screenplay. Ehrlich was played by Edward G. Robinson, a film star who could lure crowds to his films (fig. 56). The struggle that leads to the discovery of "606," or Salvarsan, by Paul Ehrlich and its acceptance by a grateful world anchors a story that manages to dramatize several distinct historical developments from the 1880s into the 1910s. In many scenes, the characters' dialogue provides the audience with enough information not only to care about the search for solutions but also to understand how the breakthroughs worked. The account is moderately correct in scientific terms, even while it is historically misleading when it places events out of sequence and thereby falsifies cause and effect among the discoveries and insights.

The underlying unity in Ehrlich's historical achievements was to find chemical explanations of biological phenomena. He produced new understanding of how the body creates internal immunity when invaded by foreign particles, and he engineered a new approach to finding chemical compounds that can be applied in the body to target specific germs precisely. The film version dramatizes both kinds of discoveries, mixing together Ehrlich's early steps toward a chemical science of immunology with his research on how biological organisms react to individual chemical compounds, especially the newly discovered aniline dyes. This film offered the general public a remarkably rich dramatization of scientific conceptions and of the processes of laboratory research and discovery. Syphilis, as the disease defeated by Ehrlich's "magic bullet," ties the film together without overshadowing Ehrlich's work on tuberculosis, snakebite, and diphtheria.

In the film, when Ehrlich explains his work on staining to a colleague, the audience learns about the peculiar affinity of dyes for specific cells that makes them stand out visually from surrounding materials. When Robert Koch presents his finding that the tubercle bacillus causes consumption and faces many skeptics who cannot find it under the microscope, he is forced to acknowledge that seeing the germ is very difficult for all but a few experts. A young Ehrlich, then unknown, impetuously suggests that it should be possible to make the bacillus visible by staining it. A rather skeptical Koch tells him that if he can do that, it will be a great contribution to medicine. When Ehrlich succeeds, after a lucky accident caused by his wife, we learn that this discovery transforms Koch's identification of the germ from a mere

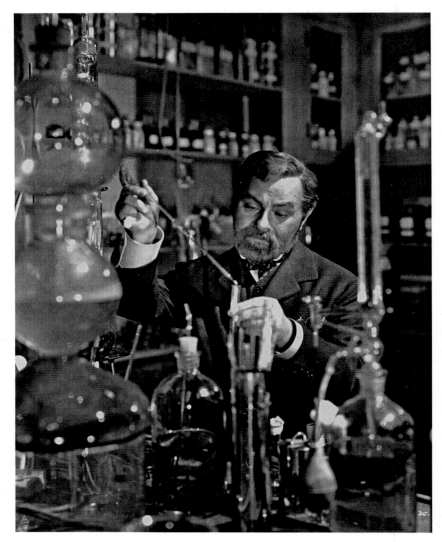

FIG. 56. Publicity still from *Dr. Ehrlich's Magic Bullet* (1940). Edward G. Robinson as Paul Ehrlich using a pipette. © Turner Entertainment Co. A Warner Bros. Entertainment Company. All rights reserved. Author's collection.

scientific achievement to something useful. Once ordinary practitioners can use the stain to examine specimens from their patients, an important diagnostic tool has been placed in their hands. We also learn that high government officials greet practical advances such as this one far more enthusiastically than they do purely intellectual ones.

In the film's version of events, Ehrlich gains a key insight into how the body acquires immunity to disease while in Egypt convalescing from the tuberculosis he acquired working with the germs in his laboratory. When a child suffering from a snakebite is brought to him, Ehrlich inquires why the child's father, who was bitten far more badly, is not as sick. He is told that the father's first snakebite years earlier had made him quite sick but that each successive bite thereafter had a milder effect. This observation helps Ehrlich imagine that the blood's chemistry had somehow been changed by a first encounter with chemicals in the venom and had acquired a new property of being resistant to it. He then speculates that a body's becoming immune is due not to a qualitative change of the blood in general but to a new chemical entity circulating within the blood. He further imagines that, just as this kind of chemical assault by the venom stimulates new chemicals in the blood, the assault by a microbe or its toxin might have the same effect. This reasoning leads him to try challenging experimental animals first with mild and then with stronger extracts of the diphtheria microbe as a way to get their bodies to produce the chemicals that offer immunity. This leads to a plan to transfer the chemical immunity that is found in the blood serum of horses exposed to diphtheria into the bodies of sick children, thereby helping them throw off the disease. This work introduces antitoxins into medical practice.

Ehrlich's success in finding chemical compounds that attach to certain microbes as stains also leads him to search for a destructive chemical compound that will attach only to a specific microbial invader within the body and not affect the body's cells. Many drugs were known to kill germs in a laboratory dish, but they were also lethal to host organisms. So Ehrlich embarks on a search to create minute modifications in chemicals, with the hope that in time he may find one that retains the power to kill microbes without also damaging the microbe's host animal. Other scientists scoff at his search for such a "magic bullet" and he loses his funding, but he continues on his own by family sacrifice and the help of loyal assistants. The microbes that they study are a group called trypanosomes, and they test many chemicals on mice infected with trypanosomes in a series of different drugs that runs into the hundreds. Each test requires scores of mice and other laboratory animals. Eventually, one of Ehrlich's customized organic compounds containing arsenic shows positive results as well as safety. It is number 606 in the series of tested compounds. Then, when the germ causing syphilis is identified as a spirochete, Ehrlich notices its resemblance to his trypanosomes. He becomes optimistic that his drug might cure syphilis, so he tries to find funding to test it on humans. But he finds no support for research that might benefit stigmatized syphilitics until he meets Franziska Speyer, an independent-minded and wealthy widow who becomes fascinated by Ehrlich's clear explanations of his ideas and vows to fund his research on this untouchable subject. When it comes time to test the new remedy, deformed and sick men in the syphilis ward are hesitant to volunteer for testing of Ehrlich's new drug until one of them who has been blinded from the disease steps forward as the first volunteer. Then others follow his lead. Excitement rises—both inside the film and in the theater—as gradual recovery is photographically illustrated from the blind patient's viewpoint and as the blurred images seen become clearer and clearer as the drug performs its miracle cure.

Many other scenes with suffering patients raise the emotional stakes for viewers, including the suicide of a young patient after being told by Ehrlich at the beginning of the film that because of his syphilis, "marriage is out of the question." Before a trial of the diphtheria antitoxin, parents desperate with fear for their children's survival force their way into the hospital while doctors debate whether or not it is humane and ethical to withhold a likely remedy from the patients in a control group. When one child in the test group dies, Ehrlich breaks the protocol and moves a boy from the control group to that bed so he can receive the life-saving serum.

The film ridicules both the conservative sexual attitudes that had almost prevented the search for a cure of venereal disease and Germany's anti-Semitic and racist attitudes that inhibited the careers of Paul Ehrlich, a German Jew, and Sahashiro Hata, a Japanese scientist in his laboratory. As in the Pasteur and Nightingale films, speeches addressed simultaneously to characters in the film and to people in the theater intensify viewers' emotional engagement. In a courtroom scene, Ehrlich is forced to defend himself because some of his patients died in treatment, and he addresses the jury with eloquence and passion. The historical Ehrlich had died in 1915, but when the cinematic Ehrlich addresses a group of colleagues from his deathbed, the message is attuned to the world in 1940:

> The magic bullet will cure thousands. The principle on which it works will serve against other diseases, many others, I think. But there can be no final victory over diseases of the body unless the diseases of the soul are also overcome. They feed upon each other, diseases of the body, diseases of the soul. In days to come, there will be epidemics of greed, hate, ignorance. We must fight them in life as we fought syphilis in the laboratory. Fight. Fight. You must never, never stop fighting.

The film was well received by the press and the public. *Life* magazine gave it an impressive four-page spread with seven large publicity stills and a close-up of the germs for syphilis, diphtheria, and tuberculosis (fig. 57).

Paul de Kruif felt initially that he had been unfairly denied credit for the story, which was in fact derived partly from his "Magic Bullet" chapter about Ehrlich's work in *Microbe Hunters*. Then he decided that the film was so inaccurate that he did not want any association with it, and he demanded that his publisher replace the new cover on its Pocket Book edition, which was touting the relationship of the film with the book.[46] Indeed, the cover design made "Dr. Ehrlich's Magic Bullet" seem to be the book's title (see color plate 10). Special activities increased attendance and stimulated public involvement with the film and the struggle of science to conquer venereal disease. For example, the Good Housekeeping Club Service helped women's clubs across the country promote viewings of the film.[47] An edited version of the film was prepared for venereal disease education by the U.S. government during World War II. Omitted by the government were some scenes with Ehrlich's family, some of the interpersonal quarrels, and the suicide of a man facing a hopeless

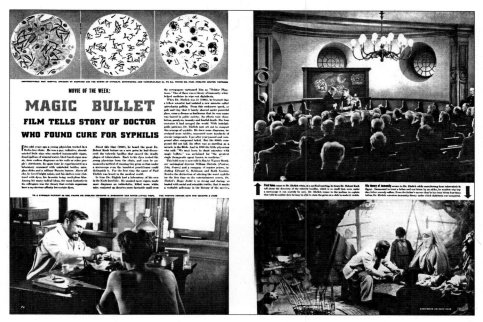

FIG. 57. Splash pages, "Movie of the Week: Magic Bullet. Film Tells Story of Doctor Who Found Cure for Syphilis," *Life,* March 4, 1940, 74–75. Reprinted with permission of Time, Inc. Movie publicity photographs by Mark Elliott 1940 © Turner Entertainment Co. A Warner Bros. Entertainment Company. Microscopic illustrations from Muir's Bacteriological Atlas © 1937. All rights reserved. Author's collection.

diagnosis of syphilis. Still, the story was not reduced simply to facts of biology and medicine; much of the historical narrative remained.[48]

The same year that *Magic Bullet* was released, the United States Film Service released *Fight for Life,* a feature film that dramatized a campaign to reduce infant and maternal mortality by means of up-to-date obstetrics training combined with pre-natal care and home delivery of normal births. Though the film has a documentary feel and the medicine is accurate, the story line is fiction, and the film played in regular movie theaters, not in art houses. Based on part of a book with the same ti-tle by Paul de Kruif, the film was directed by Pare Lorentz, an innovative and politi-cally engaged documentarian best known today for three New Deal films. Lorentz also directed *The Plow That Broke the Plains* (1936) and *The River* (1937), both with scores by Virgil Thomson. *The City* (1939) was co-written by Lorentz and Lewis Mumford and scored by Aaron Copland. *Fight for Life* received an Oscar nomina-tion for Louis Gruenberg's music.[49]

In 1943, MGM's *Madame Curie,* based on the biography written by Eve Curie, one of Marie's daughters, cast Greer Garson in the leading role of Marie and Walter Pidgeon as her husband, Pierre.[50] The family had wide public renown, even in the United States. Not only had Marie and Pierre shared a Nobel Prize in 1903, but

Marie was awarded a second Nobel in 1911. Their daughter Irène Joliot-Curie and son-in-law Frédéric Joliot-Curie shared a Nobel Prize in 1935. Marie was not a physician, of course, but from the first news of her isolation of radium at the beginning of the century, the discovery had been regarded as a medical advance because it was immediately applied as an experimental cancer therapy. Directed by Mervyn LeRoy, the film clearly places itself into the pattern set by Dieterle's *Louis Pasteur* and *Magic Bullet*. Partly a romance, it is largely an appreciation of science. Technical concepts discussed by characters educated the theater audience. As in the other films, scientists have to challenge social restrictions while overcoming nature's tenacity in hiding its secrets. But arduous work by Marie and Pierre, based jointly on knowledge and inspiration, pays off. Their 5,677 extractions from tons of pitchblende—an obvious parallel to Paul Ehrlich's testing of 606 different arsenical compounds—yields a discovery that thrills both the community of science and a broad public.

Employing a familiar strategy, director LeRoy used the applause of a gathering inside the film to help the theater audience identify with a celebration of the hero. In Marie Curie's climactic scene, she tells a huge crowd of dignitaries and students assembled in her honor, "Science has great beauty and—with its great spiritual strength—will in time cleanse this world of its evil, its ignorance, its poverty, diseases, wars, and heartaches."

Critics agreed that these films were more than entertainment, more than interesting stories. They were an admirable expression of rationalism and humane values. The *New York Times* reviewer of *Madame Curie* explained it this way: "Whether the film is entirely a picture of the Curies as they were and whether its scientific data are precise is beside the point. The important thing is that it expresses the spirit of science honestly and that it makes the quest for knowledge a romantic and thrilling pursuit."[51]

A year after *Madame Curie* appeared, Paramount released *The Great Moment* by Preston Sturges, a leading director, based on a popular 1938 book, *Triumph over Pain* by René Fülöp-Miller.[52] The medical hero is William T. G. Morton, the American dentist who gave the world pain-free surgery. In this version, Morton is given credit over Charles T. Jackson, the chemist who taught him about ether, and Horace Wells, the chemist who had tried it first but without clear success. As in several other medical history movies, the discovery is made by a maverick, whose persistent experiments (many on himself) finally confirm his great idea and whose determination overcomes social and material obstacles that might have held another person back. The title refers to a controversy within the film about whether Morton will withhold the identity of his anesthetic chemical to ensure personal financial gain. If he keeps it secret, he will be violating medical ethics and the compound could not be used by other doctors since they are required to eschew secret remedies. When faced with the situation of a young patient who would have to be operated on in great pain without the anesthetic, Morton rises to the occasion and—in his great moment—decides to reveal the nature of his remedy, thereby putting the patient's needs and humankind's benefit ahead of his own. Once again, American audiences could admire both the process of discovery and the selflessness of a medical researcher. This film was probably used in classrooms as well.[53]

Although this film did not strive for historical accuracy to the extent that the other biopics did, one particular historical error is revealing. The movie's opening title sequence as well as later scenes show crowds of people with banners celebrating Morton's triumph over pain. But in 1846 and for some years thereafter, his new technique received little press coverage, no general popular acclaim, and no consensus in the profession about its value. The filmmaker's use of this historically incorrect imagery illustrates again how the rabies breakthrough engendered the widespread assumption that great medical advances were always recognized quickly and applauded by the general public.

Alongside these medical heroes from the past, a few contemporary medical celebrities were given feature-length biographical treatments in the 1940s. In 1944, Cecil B. DeMille produced *The Story of Dr. Wassell* about a doctor on the Pacific front during World War II, with Gary Cooper in the title role. Then in 1946, *Sister Kenny,* starring Rosalind Russell, saluted a contemporary pioneer of polio therapy.[54] This triumphant biography of the heroic Australian "bush nurse" closely resembled the medical history films of the era. Kenny's struggle to win a fair hearing for her therapeutic innovations, though not a matter of science, paralleled that of the laboratory researchers. Kenny is frustrated by medicine's helplessness in the face of infantile paralysis (as Pasteur had been with childbed fever and Ehrlich with syphilis), but she tries whatever new treatments she can imagine and carefully observes the results, gradually forming a theory about what works best. The application of her approach in numerous difficult cases appears worthwhile, but she cannot get enough attention from doctors to put her ideas to a real test with numerous patients. She is scorned and rejected—as a nurse, as a woman, as a person from the bush, as a provincial. But she persists, sustained emotionally by grateful ex-patients and their parents. She even leaves Australia, hoping to get a fairer hearing in England, but she again meets unthinking resistance. Finally in the United States, she finds enough open-minded physicians who will test the technique as applied to patients by her and by those she has trained. Eventually her unusual method is recognized and appreciated. Like the cinematic exemplars of Pasteur, Ehrlich, and Curie, Kenny too gives a speech for which the moviegoers could mentally merge into the audience of her enthusiastic supporters within the film.

Hollywood in the 1930s and 1940s screened many fictional doctors along with these contemporary figures and those from medical history. But the "real doctors" seem to have made a more lasting impression, partly because of the studios' well-publicized research activity in support of historical accuracy and authenticity. Even if the studios pursued period detail in costumes more thoroughly than they did in other aspects of the dramatizations and even if the background research was highly publicized as a marketing ploy, the audiences and the critics liked the verisimilitude and they accepted modest deviations from truth.[55] Moviegoers' connection with the greats of medical history was reinforced as they repeatedly encountered the same stories in radio, magazines, and advertising. Louis Pasteur and Walter Reed especially, but also Paul Ehrlich, Florence Nightingale, and Elizabeth Kenny, were portrayed again and again in various popular media.

In these films, the cinematic heroes struggle to conquer both the unknown secrets of small-scale nature and the obscurantist resistance of small-minded opponents. All are active doers. They are shown in the settings of laboratories and clinics, with scientific equipment, assistants, and many experimental animals. In a few of the weaker movies about doctors, scientists, and inventors, the hero is depicted only as a tinkerer or fix-it man whose successes spring from personality, and the science is left unexplained.[56] But in the main, the scientists from history are portrayed as deep thinkers, as people who used observation to figure things out. Their breakthroughs were not sudden, mysterious insights but the outcome of thoughtful reasoning, contemplation, imagination, and personal vision. Some of the most iconic visual images are of scientists who could ignore their surroundings and mundane existence, often with a faraway look, as they focus their thoughts on the mysteries of nature (as in figs. 55 and 56). Directors and cinematographers seem to have fully appreciated the power within Edelfelt's painting of Pasteur, and they re-created it on the big screen for Pasteur but also for other scientists. In a few scenes, this deep mental concentration is portrayed as a sympathetic form of absent-mindedness in the heroic scientist, but more often it is used to exemplify a spiritual dimension in these otherwise materialistic quests for a cure.

THE BIOGRAPHICAL PICTURE OF MEDICAL PROGRESS

Purveying medical history primarily through the stories of individuals was not without consequences for popular conceptions of the past. One important effect of a biographically oriented medical history was that it confirmed the optimism that every problem has a solution. In biographies, there is a built-in bias toward success since the figures are chosen after-the-fact, by virtue of their having triumphed. Setbacks and detours are, of course, part of the dramatic narrative, but none of the stories ends in failure—or fails to end. Such a neat story is a great contrast to the messy realities of medical research playing out in real time, with no sure forecast of the outcome. It is also quite different from accounts in scholarly history, which often focus on a problem or a disease, creating a narrative in which characters enter and exit for a variety of reasons without dramatic unity. In real life, triumph may elude the researchers or it may take a different form from what they had sought. And it might even be produced by one of the minor characters. A good dramatist can sometimes overcome such distractions, but the task is easier if a single person is at the center of things. Moreover, it is easier to develop in the audience a "rooting interest" in a single lead character than in a team or an impersonal quest.[57]

Work at the frontiers of knowledge is too complicated for easy presentation in biographical format. The fits and starts, those steps that are not clearly forward or backward, cannot be captured in short biographies, and such features of medical development were often left out of the popular accounts. Such complexities are neatly illustrated by research at the Rockefeller Institute. For example, Hideyo Noguchi time and again seemed to be on the verge of a major breakthrough or to have made one. Sometimes the results got into the newspaper; always they were carefully watched and vetted by Simon Flexner; and sometimes they were praised and pumped to the press by Flexner. But repeatedly they did not pan out as great advances, even if some aspects of the results were useful within the field. Noguchi, like many others, erroneously claimed to have found the yellow-fever germ. Noguchi, like a few others, claimed in error to have found the rabies germ. Noguchi was recognized for having found the trachoma germ; but this discovery, too, was discarded as a mistaken interpretation some years later. Similarly, Flexner's substantial work on meningitis and poliomyelitis was productive in technical advances not easily intelligible to the public, without ever achieving the kind of singular breakthrough that earns acclaim within the profession and celebrity outside it.[58] In many ways, this mix of success and failure, with many false hopes and wrong turns, is far more typical of laboratory life than are the neater stories of triumphs such as rabies shots, diphtheria antitoxin, and Salvarsan. Significantly, with the advantage of hindsight and the ability to take the long view, even the errors made by figures such as Pasteur are trumped by the historical recognition that ultimately he was "right" and his detractors were wrong.

Medical history, especially in the semidramatized biographical mode that started to become so popular in the 1920s, could not help but carry an air of triumph. Progress seemed inevitable. De Kruif may have been a rebel in the laboratory, cynical about human nature, frustrated by second-rate colleagues and the efforts of administrators such as Flexner to have his scientists produce regular results to share with the press, but he had devotion to the ideal of research—as well as a passion for knowledge and the excitement of research. And it was his stories that gave the public a supply of heroic exemplars of science, which shaped popular notions of medical progress. Though de Kruif may not have approved of boosterism, or practiced it intentionally, his writings delivered it—shaping public consciousness about the worthiness of biomedical research, sparking imitators galore, drawing young people into scientific careers, and making *Microbe Hunters* required reading for generations of high school students.

Another effect of the rise of medical history stories was to elide a differentiation between present and past. Current advances were seen as just part of one long story, and their makers were just the latest in a great tradition. A second important elision was made by the two founding books of this movement, *Arrowsmith* and *Microbe Hunters*. Both the realistic novel and the novelistic history seemed to reduce the gap between fact and fiction. Although *Arrowsmith* was a novel and always recognized as such, its protagonist became real to Americans, partly through the novelist's craft and partly because when portrayed by an actor in the film, he was no less "real" than the actual historical figures such as Pasteur and Nightingale also played by actors on the screen. *Microbe Hunters* was not fiction, as readers knew. But de Kruif's construction of dialogue in private scenes that would not have been documented in historical sources gave his prose the sensibility and the tonality of fiction.

With this blurring of lines, made-up characters and actors alike were taken for medical scientists. A photograph of an actor who portrayed Paul Ehrlich—not a photograph of the real Ehrlich—was used for a while on the cover of *Microbe Hunters* (color plate 10). Conversely, readers of at least one edition of *Arrowsmith* found between its covers several black-and-white photographs of the very real Ronald Colman and Helen Hayes where one might have expected an artist's depiction of wholly fictional characters (fig. 58).[59]

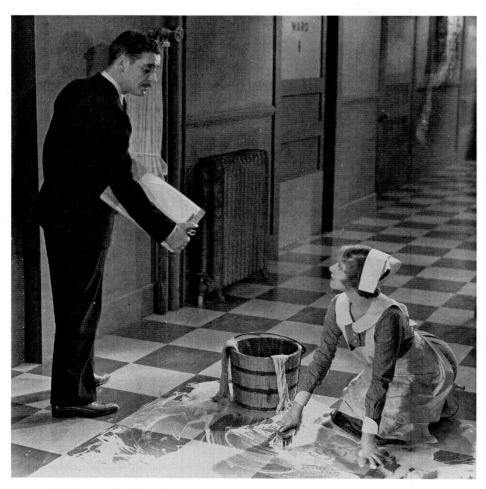

FIG. 58. Publicity still of the characters Leora Tozer and Martin Arrowsmith, as played by Helen Hayes and Ronald Colman, at the moment they first meet in the film *Arrowsmith* (1931). Photograph © 1931 Samuel Goldwyn Company. All rights reserved. Author's collection. This image was also printed in an undated edition of Sinclair Lewis, *Arrowsmith* (New York: Grosset and Dunlap, n.d.), facing 130.

Sometimes writers employ a biographical approach to draw readers into the interior of personality; alternatively, some writers use it as a unifying thread for the narrative of sequential actions. Medical history biographies in this era more commonly pursued the latter course. And these stories, by centering themselves on a step-by-step narration of what happened rather than on a psychological explanation of why things happened, naturally drew readers into the active process of research and those procedures covered under the traditional rubric of scientific method: guesses, hypotheses, evidence that favors one or the other, and the experimental trials that can establish the truth of a discovery and win over doubters.

CHAPTER 7

"AND NOW, A WORD FROM OUR SPONSOR"

MAKING MEDICAL HISTORY COMMERCIAL

Many men have forgotten Joseph Lister's work in antisepsis. Few now know the meaning of "to listerize" and of "listerism," words brought into the language as a tribute to him.
—*Time* magazine, 1927

Experience is the Best Teacher. . . . Rudolf Virchow (1821–1902) proved it in pathology. Experience is the best teacher in smoking, too. . . . More doctors smoke Camels than any other cigarette.
—R. J. Reynolds magazine ad, 1947

OVER THE SAME DECADES that medical history came into prominence in books and films, commercial enterprises began to exploit images of doctors from the past. Large corporations sponsored hundreds of radio programs that dramatized medical history; insurance companies produced information booklets and magazine advertising that featured stories of medical heroes; and businesses of all sorts drew on the cachet of medical progress to promote their own products. Sometimes the print ads and pamphlets sold specific products; more frequently they served as "image advertising" intended to burnish a corporation's general reputation for integrity and scientific dependability. These appearances were myriad, diverse, and sometimes odd. Examples were everywhere, but they were ephemeral and are not widely known today. Together they reveal something of popular attitudes between the wars, even if they were individually less artistic and far less enduring than de Kruif's books or Dieterle's films.

MEDICAL HISTORY ON THE RADIO

In the 1920s, radio became a medium of unprecedented power to connect millions of listeners with the same experience at the same moment. Radio was an instant success all across the United States. It is sometimes thought that compared to film, radio drama was weak or incomplete because it lacked visual content. Yet radio often created an even stronger connection with an audience than did film because it forced a listener's brain actively to create visual images, conjuring up scenes, for example, of ball players, characters in a radio drama, or a president chatting with millions of citizens from his living room. Though its nature was ethereal, radio's bond with the public was very strong. In the 1930s and 1940s, radio's sound pictures of medical progress resonated fully with the visual images circulating in other media.

Until the rise of television in the 1950s, radio offered numerous medical history dramas and educational programs underwritten by corporate sponsors. Many of these programs were dramatic adaptations of Hollywood movies, but some were documentaries, radio talks by experts, or reenactments. Most shows usually appeared within a series, such as *Cavalcade of America,* sponsored by the DuPont Company, and *Lux Radio Theater,* sponsored by Lever Brothers, each of which featured radio plays. In at least one case, the entire series was composed of medical history. During the early 1930s, the Eastman Kodak company sponsored weekly radio talks by Howard W. Haggard, an M.D. and a physiology professor at Yale. The lectures were based on his book *Devils, Drugs, and Doctors,* the title of which was used as the title for the radio series. These talks were carried coast to coast every Sunday evening over Columbia Broadcasting System. An indication that the program had a substantial following is that listeners were invited to write in for free printed copies of the talks. Lectures covered such topics as hydrophobia, pharmacy, and dentistry and such scientists as William Harvey, Antoine Laurent Lavoisier, and Rene Laennec.[1]

Revere Copper and Brass, Inc., sponsored weekly broadcasts of *The Human Adventure,* a series carried by about 120 stations across the country on Wednesday evenings in the 1940s. These broadcasts were prepared by Encyclopaedia Britannica, in cooperation with the faculty of the University of Chicago, to dramatize "the achievements of scholars and scientists working in the great universities of the world." Subjects other than medical history were included; the broadcast about

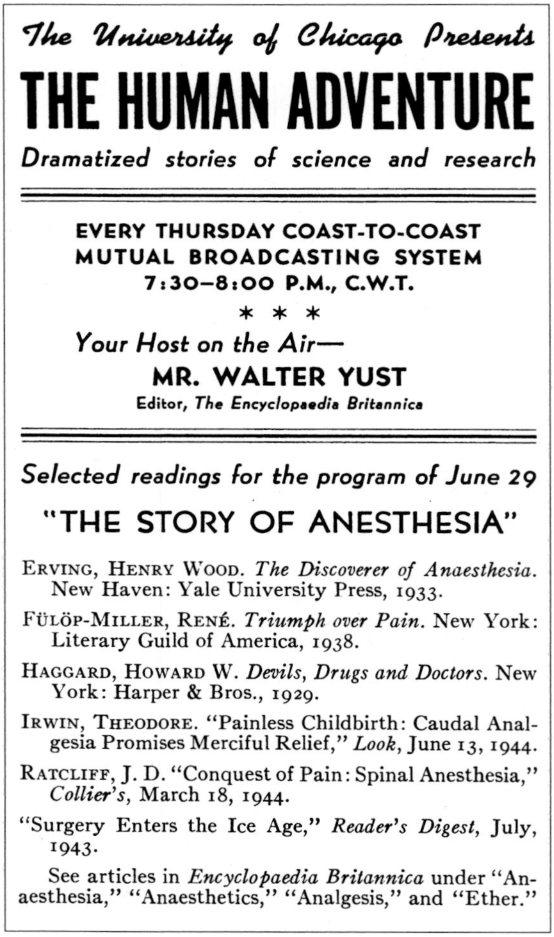

The University of Chicago Presents

THE HUMAN ADVENTURE

Dramatized stories of science and research

**EVERY THURSDAY COAST-TO-COAST
MUTUAL BROADCASTING SYSTEM
7:30–8:00 P.M., C.W.T.**

★ ★ ★

Your Host on the Air—
MR. WALTER YUST
Editor, The Encyclopaedia Britannica

Selected readings for the program of June 29

"THE STORY OF ANESTHESIA"

ERVING, HENRY WOOD. *The Discoverer of Anaesthesia.*
New Haven: Yale University Press, 1933.

FÜLÖP-MILLER, RENÉ. *Triumph over Pain.* New York:
Literary Guild of America, 1938.

HAGGARD, HOWARD W. *Devils, Drugs and Doctors.* New
York: Harper & Bros., 1929.

IRWIN, THEODORE. "Painless Childbirth: Caudal Anal-
gesia Promises Merciful Relief," *Look*, June 13, 1944.

RATCLIFF, J. D. "Conquest of Pain: Spinal Anesthesia,"
Collier's, March 18, 1944.

"Surgery Enters the Ice Age," *Reader's Digest*, July,
1943.

　　See articles in *Encyclopaedia Britannica* under "Anaesthesia," "Anaesthetics," "Analgesis," and "Ether."

FIG. 59. Postcard from *The Human Adventure: Dramatized Stories of Science and Research.* The card—postmarked on July 7, 1944, a week after the radio broadcast of June 29—was obviously mailed in response
to the listener's request for a list of relevant readings.
Author's collection.

smallpox vaccination, for example, was followed by shows on Leonardo da Vinci
and Columbus. Listeners to the smallpox program heard the simulated voice of the
eighteenth-century minister Cotton Mather defending inoculation, took in a conversation between Edward Jenner and "the great Dr. John Hunter," and (after a mu-
sical transition) listened to an exchange between Jenner and two children whom he
was vaccinating. The sponsor reinforced people's engagement with the programs by
inviting listeners to request a list of readings on a postcard (fig. 59). Additionally,
by paying one dollar, subscribers could receive nicely printed booklets for thirteen
weeks, each with a script of one week's *Human Adventure*.[2]

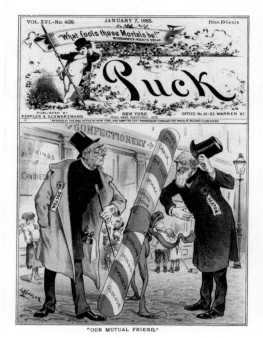

"OUR MUTUAL FRIEND."

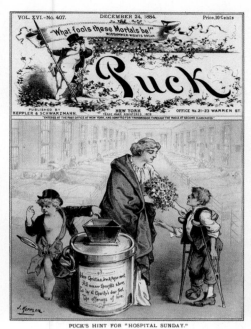

PUCK'S HINT FOR "HOSPITAL SUNDAY."

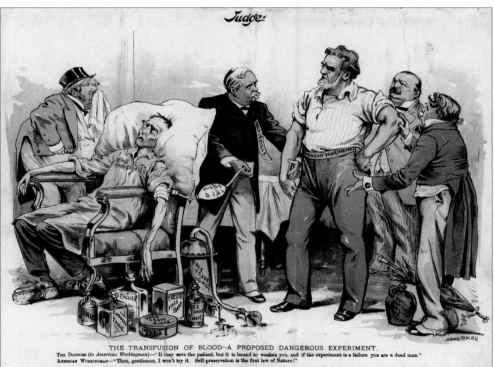

THE TRANSFUSION OF BLOOD—A PROPOSED DANGEROUS EXPERIMENT.

THE DOCTORS (to American Workingman)—"It may save the patient, but it is bound to weaken you, and if the experiment is a failure you are a dead man."
AMERICAN WORKINGMAN—"Then, gentlemen, I won't try it. Self-preservation is the first law of Nature!"

Top left: **COLOR PLATE 1.** "Our Mutual Friend," *Puck* 16:409 (January 7, 1885), cover (289). Chromolithograph by Joseph Keppler. Author's collection. *Top right:* **COLOR PLATE 2.** "Puck's Hint for 'Hospital Sunday.'" *Puck* 16:407 (December 24, 1884), cover (257). Chromolithograph by Joseph Keppler. Author's collection. *Bottom:* **COLOR PLATE 3.** "The Transfusion of Blood—A Proposed Dangerous Experiment," *Judge* 14:350 (June 30, 1888), back cover (196). Chromolithograph by Grant Hamilton. Author's collection.

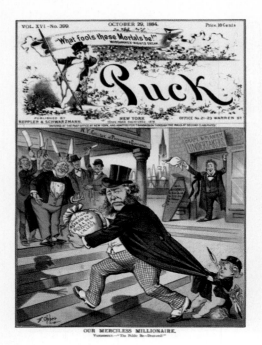

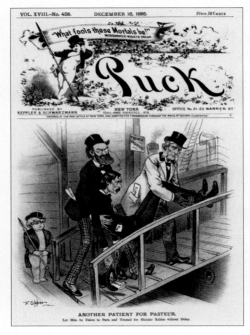

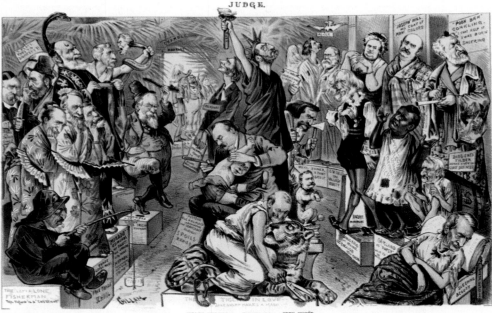

Top left: **COLOR PLATE 4.** "Our Merciless Millionaire. Vanderbilt:—'The Public Be—Doctored!'" *Puck* 16:399 (October 29, 1884), cover (129). Full-page chromolithograph by Frederick Opper. Author's collection. *Top right:* **COLOR PLATE 5.** "Another Patient for Pasteur. Let Him be Taken to Paris and Treated for Blainiac Rabies without Delay," *Puck* 18:458 (December 16, 1885), cover (241). Full-page chromolithograph by Frederick Opper. Author's collection. *Bottom:* **COLOR PLATE 6.** "Judge's Wax Works—The Political Eden Musée," *Judge* 9:227 (February 20, 1886), 8–9. Double-page chromolithograph by T. Bernhard Gillam. The middle section of this two-page spread shows "Pasteur Cleveland Inoculating the Democracy [i.e., the Democratic party] Against Spoils Rabies." Author's collection.

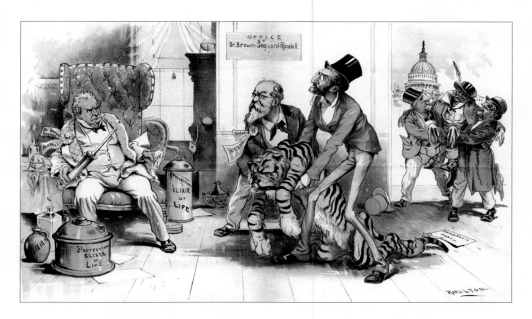

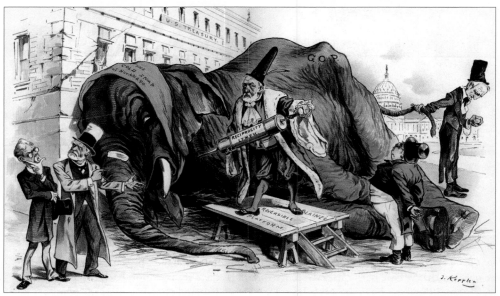

Top: **COLOR PLATE 7.** "Hopeless Cases," *Judge* 16:411 (August 31, 1889), center spread (336–337). Chromolithograph by Grant Hamilton. Author's collection. *Bottom:* **COLOR PLATE 8.** "A Bad Case of Consumption—Reciprocity Lymph," *Puck* 28:718 (December 10, 1890), center spread (276–277). Chromolithograph by Joseph Keppler. Author's collection.

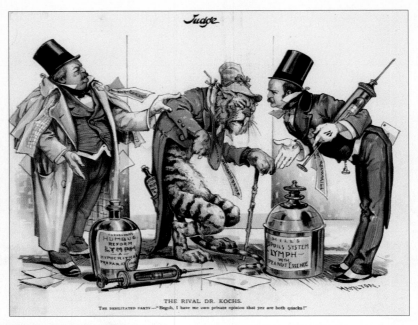

THE RIVAL DR. KOCHS.
THE DEBILITATED PARTY—"Begob, I have me own private opinion that yez are both quacks!"

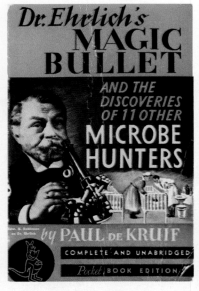

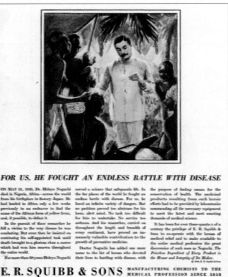

FOR US, HE FOUGHT AN ENDLESS BATTLE WITH DISEASE

E. R. SQUIBB & SONS   MANUFACTURING CHEMISTS TO THE MEDICAL PROFESSION SINCE 1858

*Top: **COLOR PLATE 9.*** "The Rival Doctor Kochs. The Debilitated Party—'Begob, I have me own private opinion that yez are both quacks!'" *Judge* 19:478 (December 13, 1890), back cover (198). Full-page chromolithograph by Grant Hamilton. Dr. Koch-Cleveland's bottle is marked "Humbug Reform Lymph—A Hypocritical Preparation," and Dr. Koch-Hill's reads "Hill's Spoils System Lymph with Peanut Essence." Author's collection. *Bottom left: **COLOR PLATE 10.*** Cover of a paperback edition of *Microbe Hunters* by Paul de Kruif (Pocket Books, 1940), employing as a tease the film title "Dr. Ehrlich's Magic Bullet" along with an image of actor Edward G. Robinson in the role of Paul Ehrlich. De Kruif successfully demanded that this cover be replaced. All rights reserved. Author's collection. *Bottom right: **COLOR PLATE 11.*** E. R. Squibb & Sons, "For Us, He Fought an Endless Battle with Disease," *Woman's Home Companion,* April 1929, 52 (full page). The same ad ran in other magazines that year including *American Magazine* and *Literary Digest.* © 1929 E. R. Squibb & Sons. All rights reserved. Reprinted courtesy of Bristol Myers Squibb. Author's collection.

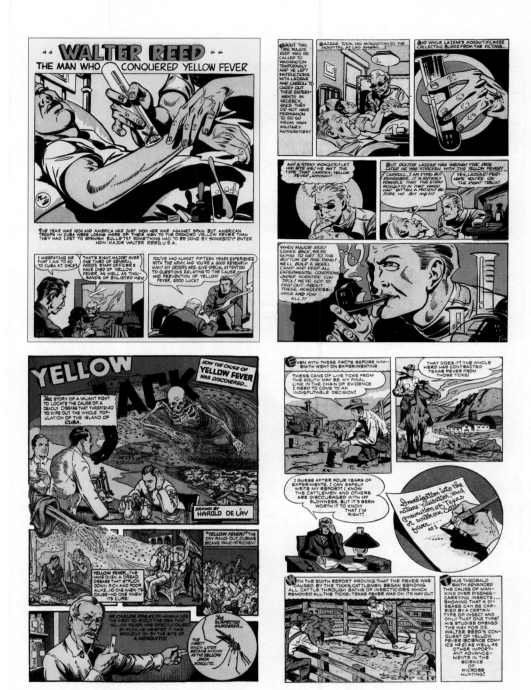

*Top left: **COLOR PLATE 12.*** Splash page of Rudy Palais, "Walter Reed," *Science Comics* 2 (March 1946), 26. © 1946 Humor Publications Inc. All rights reserved. Author's collection. *Top right:* ***COLOR PLATE 13.*** "Lazear took his mosquitoes to the hospital," full page in Rudy Palais, "Walter Reed," *Science Comics* 2 (March 1946), 29. © 1946 Humor Publications Inc. All rights reserved. Author's collection. *Bottom left: **COLOR PLATE 14.*** Splash page of Harold Delay, "Yellow Jack: How the Cause of Yellow Fever Was Discovered," *True Comics* 1 (April 1941), 37. © 1941 The Parents' Institute Inc. All rights reserved. Used with permission. Author's collection. *Bottom right: **COLOR PLATE 15.*** "Even with these facts," full page in "Theobald Smith and Texas Fever," *Science Comics* 5 (September 1946), 23. © 1946 Humor Publications Inc. All rights reserved. Author's collection.

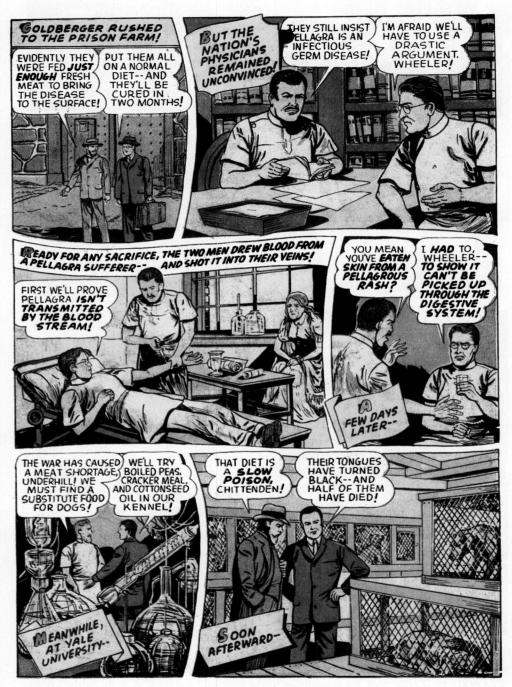

COLOR PLATE 16. "Goldberger Rushed to the Prison Farm," full page from "Famine Fighter," *Real Life Comics* 12 (July 1943), 21. © 1943 Nedor Publishing Company. All rights reserved. Author's collection.

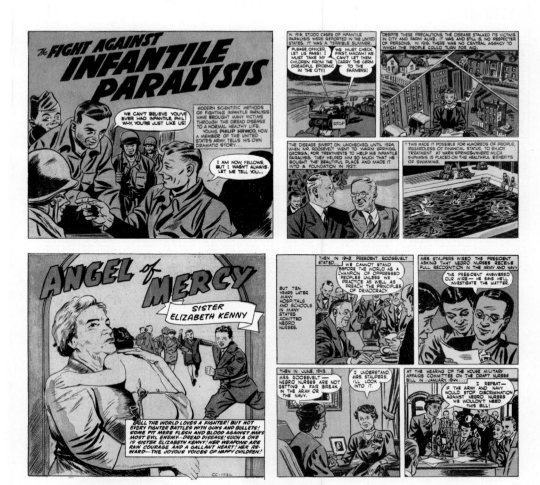

Top left: **COLOR PLATE 17.** Splash panel of "The Fight against Infantile Paralysis," *True Comics* 32 (February 1944), 26. © 1943 True Comics, Inc., a subsidiary of the Publishers of Parents' Magazine. Used with permission. All rights reserved. Author's collection. *Top right:* **COLOR PLATE 18.** "Please, officer," four panels of "The Fight against Infantile Paralysis," *True Comics* 32 (February 1944), 27. © 1943 True Comics, Inc., a subsidiary of the Publishers of Parents' Magazine. Used with permission. All rights reserved. Author's collection. *Bottom left:* **COLOR PLATE 19.** Splash panel of "Angel of Mercy: Sister Kenny," *It Really Happened* 8 (April 1947), 14. © 1947 Visual Editions, Inc. All rights reserved. Author's collection. This image is closely modeled on a photograph in *Life* magazine (September 28, 1942, 73); compare figure 95. *Bottom right:* **COLOR PLATE 20.** "But ten years later," four panels from "Dynamic Fighter: Mabel K. Staupers," *Negro Heroes* 2 (Summer 1948), 28. © 1948 National Urban League. Used with permission. All rights reserved. Author's collection.

BACILLUS

	TUBERCULOSIS	DIPHTHERIA	TETANUS	BOTULISM	GAS GANGRENE	DYSENTERY	ANTHRAX	TYPHOID PARATYPHOID	CHOLERA	PLAGUE	WHOOPING COUGH	TULAREMIA
LOCATION OF INFECTION												
CHEMICAL CONTROL — PREVENTION												
CHEMICAL CONTROL — TREATMENT												
BIOLOGICAL CONTROL — PREVENTION												
BIOLOGICAL CONTROL — TREATMENT												
STATUS OF BIOLOGICAL CONTROL	Best control, BCG vaccine, is still experimental. Streptomycin, new drug, is promising.	Toxoid and antitoxin are "effective," i.e., control disease in all but very few cases.	Toxoid is 100% effective in prevention if inoculations are repeated periodically.	Antitoxin is effective if it is administered during the earliest stages of poisoning.	Penicillin, sulfa, antitoxin good in treating. Toxoid is promising in prevention.	Sulfa drugs, used for prevention and treatment, replaced antibacterial serum.	Sulfa drugs and antibacterial serum are both effective if used in early stages.	Vaccine is effective in prevention. Streptomycin reported effective in treatment.	Vaccine is reported by some medical men to be effective in prevention of disease.	Vaccine is reported effective in prevention. Sulfa drugs now used in treatment.	Immune serum effective in treatment and prevention. Vaccine helps in prevention.	Disease often transmitted by rabbits, tularemia has no prevention or treatment.

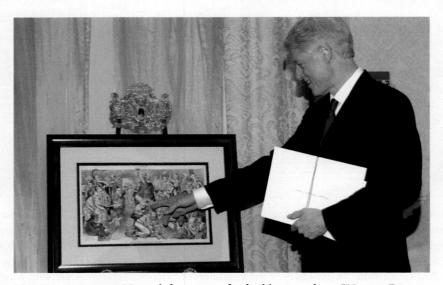

Top: **COLOR PLATE 21.** Upper left quarter of a double-page chart, "Human Diseases Caused by Germs and How They May Be Controlled," designed by Jerry Muscott, in "Germs," *Life*, November 5, 1945, 66. Page © 1945 Life Inc. Reprinted with permission. All rights reserved. Author's collection. *Bottom:* **COLOR PLATE 22.** Former president William J. Clinton with a framed print of "*Judge*'s Wax Works—The Political Eden Musée," at the Pasteur Foundation Gala on April 19, 2005. Photograph by Joe Vericker/Photobureau © 2005 Pasteur Foundation. Used with permission. All rights reserved.

The *Human Adventure,* like the earlier series by Haggard, was clearly a commercially sponsored educational program, though not without entertainment values.[3] Other radio shows about the history of medicine shifted that balance, putting more emphasis on entertainment. These were the "radio plays" common in the era. For many of these plays, *Microbe Hunters* was a handy source. For example, "Leeuwenhoek, First of the Microbe Hunters" was broadcast by WABC and WCBS in 1938. The script was adapted from de Kruif's book, and the play was produced by the Radio Division of the Federal Theater of the Works Progress Administration.[4] The same division was responsible for a 1938 broadcast of "Louis Pasteur" on WNYC.[5]

More commonly, the radio dramas of the 1930s and 1940s were closely based on film scripts, such as the productions in the *Lux Radio Theater,* broadcast from 1934 to 1955 and hosted by Cecil B. DeMille from 1936 to 1945. These were hour-long versions of major films, expensive productions with popular actors, an orchestra, and a live studio audience; the lead performers were often those cast in the original film. The high frequency of famous artists in these shows confirms that they were directed to a large audience and not to a specialized circle of history buffs. Medical history episodes sponsored by Lux included "The Story of Louis Pasteur," with Paul Muni, on November 23, 1936 (about a year after the film's release), and "Arrowsmith," with Spencer Tracy and Fay Wray, on October 25, 1937. Two years later, on February 3, 1939, *Campbell Playhouse* broadcast a radio version of "Arrowsmith" that had been dramatized by Orson Welles. Helen Hayes portrayed Leora Tozer Arrowsmith, as she had in the film. Hayes later played this role on radio again at least two more times, for the *Helen Hayes Theater of the Air* in the early 1940s and for *Electric Theater* in the late 1940s. Such broadcasts, of course, did not introduce new material to the public, but they did reinforce notions of laboratory-based medical progress and they ensured that the public was familiar with the main historical exemplars from the silver screen, not only Louis Pasteur and "Martin Arrowsmith" but also the other leading medical heroes of the popular imagination: Walter Reed, Florence Nightingale, Marie Curie, Samuel Mudd, and William T. G. Morton.

In the late 1940s, other programs continued to recycle the main medical history figures. *Academy Award Theater* broadcast a drama called "The Life of Louis Pasteur" on April 13, 1946. Then *Encore Theatre* broadcast several more medical titles in the summer of 1946, including "The Life of Louis Pasteur," "Yellowjack," "The White Angel," "Dr. Ehrlich's Magic Bullet," "Prisoner of Shark Island," and "Nurse Edith Cavell." Late in the 1940s, a perky radio show, *This Is the Story,* presented whole dramas in just five minutes, including one on Louis Pasteur's rabies work.[6] But in these dramas, a far greater number of medical heroes make an appearance than the half dozen big names. Radio writers and producers searching for material in the 1930s and 1940s found many figures who were never celebrated in a Hollywood feature film and who were not yet familiar to the general public.

In the *Cavalcade of America,* sponsored by the DuPont Company, medical history was especially prominent. These thirty-minute dramas were broadcast across the country for nearly eighteen years, from October 1935 to March 1953, first on CBS and then on NBC. The *Cavalcade of America* featured, of course, only figures from U.S. history. Yet over nearly twenty years, the shows provided a remarkable range of episodes that sampled three centuries of medical history, including both scientific developments and the social history of medicine. And these accounts were not fictional but true stories (allowing for dramatic liberties) of a historical past running right up to the present. These expensive shows offered prestige, often starring such leading performers as Tyrone Power, Loretta Young, and Myrna Loy.

Perhaps because the long-term sponsor of the series was DuPont, promising "better things for better living through chemistry," the programs featured many heroes of science and technology among its subjects, including doctors and nurses. "Heroism in Medical Science" on December 4, 1935, seems to have been the earliest medical history show in the series. It was divided between two subjects: Crawford Long's role in the discovery of surgical anesthesia in the mid-nineteenth century and William Crawford Gorgas's fight against yellow fever in the early twentieth century. Even though neither discovery took place in wartime and neither man took serious personal risks in his efforts to advance medicine, "heroism" was the word being applied in the 1930s to such work. "Hero" was the common word of the era for people who made medical history, perhaps drawing on the imagery of the combat with microbes or the battles against ignorance and intellectual inertia.

Prominent among the familiar lives celebrated in this series were Walter Reed, "Martin Arrowsmith," Clara Barton, William Gorgas, Sister Elizabeth Kenny, and Samuel Mudd. Other dramas in this series brought many less-familiar historical characters into people's homes. Yet, even within this second group, only a few of them did not already have some presence in popular media, appearing at least in magazines and comic books, if not on the big screen. Quite a number of them were women, even years prior to the wartime propaganda encouraging women to join the workforce. Individual women heroes included Elizabeth Blackwell (the first female M.D. in the United States, with shows in 1937 and 1944, the second starring Loretta Young), Marie Zakrzewska (pioneer in female medical education and hospitals for women and children), Mary Walker (Union Army surgeon captured during the Civil War), Mary Putnam Jacobi (clinician and scientist), S. Josephine Baker (public-health doctor), Clara Maass (army nurse who died fighting yellow fever), and Annie Warburton Goodrich (advocate for professional standards in nursing). A program on the Frontier Nursing Service starred Myrna Loy.

At least three *Cavalcade* programs dramatized the U.S. role in medicine's triumph over smallpox, starting with the introduction of inoculation by Cotton Mather and Zabdiel Boylston in Boston in the 1720s. Other broadcasts brought to life Thomas Jefferson's being vaccinated by Benjamin Waterhouse and then, in "Experiment at Monticello," Jefferson vaccinating his family, servants, and slaves. Among nineteenth-century American heroes, this series highlighted J. Marion Sims, "Sir Galahad in Manhattan," for founding the first women's hospital in the United States. The twentieth century was represented by Harvey Cushing, pioneer of brain surgery, and Norman Bethune (though a Canadian), inventor of the mobile blood bank that was so important in World War II. The struggle to explain mysterious diseases was explored through the work of Theobald Smith puzzling out the origin of Texas fever, Joseph Goldberger proving pellagra was a vitamin-deficiency disease, and Public Health Service scientists wrestling with Rocky Mountain spotted fever. Recent drug discoveries brought the series right to the present with a 1943 broadcast about sulfa drugs, a 1944 drama about Fleming and Florey's work on penicillin, and a 1944 show about American chemists' effort to synthesize quinine, which war had made scarce.[7] (See the appendix for a detailed list of the medical history stories in the *Cavalcade* series with titles, broadcast dates, identification of subjects, and some notes on casting.)

EARLY COMMERCIAL USES OF MEDICAL HISTORY

Many readers may recall seeing the widely distributed full-color prints of history paintings sponsored by the pharmaceutical company Parke, Davis & Company (later Parke-Davis). But although these images are the most familiar examples of the genre today, the use of medical history for corporate gain did not start with these paintings of "Great Moments in Pharmacy" (1951–1957) and "Great Moments in Medicine" (1957–1964).[8] Rather, the Parke-Davis "Great Moments" project was the climax of a long development that began modestly in the nineteenth century and then expanded greatly in the 1920s.

In the latter decades of the nineteenth century, pictorial trade cards commonly advertised stores, services, and manufactured products. Even for health-related products, these cards seldom used images of physicians; far more typical were testimonials by celebrities or pictures of the fashionable or the notorious. Popular trade-card images included opera singers, sideshow performers, suffragists, presidents, stage performers, writers (such as Oscar Wilde), and even one presidential assassin (Charles Guiteau). For most products, there was great value in creating a celebrity association or having an endorsement, but doctors were not yet credible enough to sell products. In advertising directed to the public, physicians rarely made appearances, except in the case of proprietary medicines. When a doctor did appear in a print ad before the 1920s, it was usually in medical journals or in corporate gifts for physicians, such as calendars, daybooks, office decorations, or sets of souvenir photographs.

Some late-nineteenth-century products borrowed without authorization the names of the first generation of medical heroes, including Pasteurine, Pasteur Bitters, Kochine, and Listerine.[9] But before the 1920s (and thus prior to de Kruif and his imitators), historical figures in medicine were not yet widely remembered and did not yet carry much cachet. In 1927, when *Time* reported on the centenary of Joseph Lister's birth, the magazine commented on the public's historical amnesia:

Many men have forgotten Joseph Lister's work in antisepsis. Few now know the meaning of "to listerize" and of "listerism," words brought into the language as a tribute to him. Were it not for the Lambert Pharmaceutical Co.'s broadcasting of *Listerine* (aromatic antiseptic), his name would have disappeared altogether from the colloquial tongue.[10]

Beginning in 1928, however, two major pharmaceutical companies (E. R. Squibb & Sons and Parke, Davis & Company) both embarked on extensive magazine-advertising campaigns centered on vignettes of medical history for the general public. These ads were corporate-image ads rather than direct-to-consumer product ads. Their goal was to build respect for the company, its scientific ethos, and its contributions to society's well-being.[11] Squibb's series used no overall title; Parke-Davis labeled its eighteen stories "Building the Fortresses of Health." These widely distributed efforts were soon followed by other medical-heroes campaigns created by pharmaceutical firms, by the Coca-Cola Company, and by the Metropolitan Life Insurance Company. The "Fortresses" campaign of Parke-Davis set a style and tone that was closely imitated by many others, with an influence extending over several decades and culminating in its own "Great Moments" series in the 1950s and 1960s.[12]

On occasion, Squibb's ads pictured people and events with a direct tie to its own products, allowing the company to boast, for example, about the benchmark-setting standards of purity that Dr. E. R. Squibb had established in the remedies and reagents he offered for sale. An ad entitled "The Conquest of Pain" featured the portraits and achievements of ether pioneers William Thomas Green Morton and Crawford Long, but it again took the opportunity to highlight the dependably high purity of the ether produced by Dr. Squibb.[13] Less self-referentially, Hideyo Noguchi was portrayed in a Squibb ad captioned "For us, he fought an endless battle with disease." The text explained that Noguchi died in Nigeria of yellow fever while seeking a cure for that disease (see color plate 11).[14] This Squibb series also highlighted the achievements of Louis Pasteur, Robert Koch, and others. A few years later, in January 1935, Squibb published a double-page ad showing a group of "Medical Heroes," each in the garb of his or her era, against a monumental architectural background styled like a mural in a neoclassical government building. This group introduced a new medical hero, William H. Welch, the eminent medical statesman from Johns Hopkins who had died less than a year before. From left to right, the group included Welch, Nightingale, Long, Morton, Lister, Koch, Pasteur, Ehrlich, Semmelweis, Jenner, and Claude Bernard. The caption proclaimed, "They shall serve mankind forever. These are the mighty dead who gave man victory over death."[15] These ads repeated the same increasingly familiar names. Their goal was not originality but the reassuring association of a company with the greats of history.

In Parke-Davis's "Fortresses" series, each of the full-page ads identified itself as "one of a series of messages of Parke, Davis and Company, telling how the worker in medical science, your physician, and the maker of medicines are surrounding you with stronger health defenses year by year." The ads appeared in *Collier's, Hygeia, Literary Digest, National Geographic,* and the *Saturday Evening Post.*[16] Typical ads in this series showed soldiers receiving typhoid shots, the seventeen-year-old William Henry Perkin discovering the first aniline dye, made in 1856 from coal tar, and a pith-helmeted white physician in Africa instructing a local chief to move his village away from the shores of Lake Victoria because of tsetse flies infected with sleeping sickness. Other ads touched on childbed fever, diphtheria, lockjaw, scurvy, and yellow fever.

One "Fortresses" ad reached back to the first medical breakthrough in the United States and revived the human-interest stories that had grabbed the public's attention in the 1880s.[17] Appearing first in early September 1928, a full page was headlined "3,000 Miles to Save Four Young Lives." The text helped older readers recall the Newark boys' trip to Paris while telling the story anew for younger ones. "Was there time to save these four boys? When their doctors cabled for hope, Pasteur replied: 'Envoyez les enfants toute de suite'—(send the children at once). And so Patsy and Eddie and Austin and Willy sailed for the Old World." This ad also informed readers that "today preventive treatment against hydrophobia can be given without delay by any qualified physician right in the patient's own home."[18] Under a wash drawing of four boys on the deck of the ship was a public plea: "If any of these four—the first Americans to be saved from hydrophobia by the Pasteur treatment—should see this, we would be very glad to have a letter from him."

Shortly, the company heard from one of the boys, then a man in his fifties. Parke-Davis even paid the man's way to Chicago to participate in the dedication ceremony for a new statue of Pasteur in October 1928.[19] When William Lane, the former messenger boy, spoke about Louis Pasteur's personal kindness to him and recounted his adventures in the dime museums, his sponsored appearance gave new life to an old medical breakthrough thanks to the company's ad and its outreach to him. Lane's story became news again, renewing popular interest in the origin of rabies shots. In Chicago, the *Tribune* and the *Daily Journal* ran long stories on this dedication ceremony, with several photographs.[20] The event was also covered nationally in a *New York Times* article that reminded readers of the public attention accorded Pasteur's patients, quoting from Lane's speech: "We received a great welcome [on our return to New York]. We were swamped by theatrical offers. Dr. Billings told us he wanted us to become doctors and he did not want us to accept any of these offers. But I guess our mothers wanted the money, because we went to the old Globe Theatre in New York for six weeks. We would stand up, show our scars and a man would explain how Pasteur cured us."[21] When the report described the innocent and nervous child, the altruistic scientist, the celebrity welcome back in the United States, and the public's awareness of the successful treatment, it showed that the press's focus on a human-interest story had changed little over the decades. And it was this same popular preference for richly detailed stories about people's lives that had given de Kruif's approach such appeal.

The advertisers, too, knew how to exploit this appeal and how to combine it with readers' empathic connection to the characters in the ads. In May 1931, Parke-Davis for a second time revived the public's curiosity about the boys whom Pasteur saved from death many years before.[22] It ran a modified version of the earlier ad, announcing this time that "this picture reunited two comrades saved by Pasteur in 1885": Willy and Austin. "Neither had seen the other for 40 years. They thought each other dead." The copy also noted that in just a single year, 1930, "probably 90,000 Americans were inoculated against hydrophobia" (fig. 60). A few years later, in 1936, when Warner Brothers was promoting *The Story of Louis Pasteur,* the company's agents found William Lane again to set up a newspaper interview with him about his treatment at Pasteur's laboratory in 1885. For a staged publicity stunt, the company then invited Lane to New York to join its representative to greet the ship and welcome Joseph Meister, Pasteur's first rabies patient, to the United States.[23]

THE POPULAR HEALTH HEROES OF METLIFE

In 1925, the Metropolitan Life Insurance Company (MetLife) began producing a series of booklets about historical figures under the rubric "Health Heroes." The company had become particularly well known for the large volume of informative booklets it created for its policyholders, apparently on the theory that educating customers would result in lower morbidity and mortality rates and thereby increase profits for the company.[24] These materials also served as a form of image advertising to foster the company's reputation as a caring corporation that provided health and disease information that was intelligent, attractive, calmly rational, and useful. In variety and richness, these leaflets went far beyond platitudes and simple admonitions to swat flies, eat right, and sleep with the window open. They promoted, of course, smallpox vaccination, diphtheria's Schick tests, and the prevention of outbreaks by use of toxin-antitoxin injections. But they also touched on more delicate topics, with a pamphlet on syphilis as "the great imitator," and they even used the commonly censored word "syphilis" in a print ad as early as 1928.[25] All these efforts were overseen by the company's Welfare Division, established in 1909 (later renamed Health and Welfare Division). Given the size of the company's customer base, these endeavors touched the lives of many millions of Americans. The first publication, an eight-page pamphlet on tuberculosis called "A War upon Consumption," was printed in 3.5 million copies in ten languages, and that was just the first edition. Between 1909 and 1945, the Welfare Division distributed over 1.3 billion health education booklets. A single magazine ad might yield one hundred thousand requests for a booklet. As moving pictures gained in popularity and inexpensive projectors came into use, the company produced slide shows and movies of health information. Cumulative attendance at showings of these movies by 1945 totaled 134 million viewers.[26] Many of the company's campaigns had measurable success. For example, an intensive effort to prevent diphtheria in upstate New York was credited for a remarkable drop in the number of deaths from this cause. Between 1926 and 1941, annual diphtheria deaths there fell from 738 to 6.[27]

This picture reunited two comrades saved by Pasteur in 1885

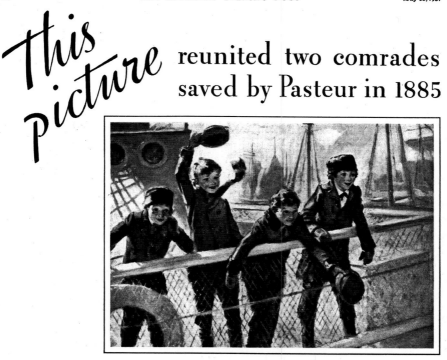

SOME months ago, a Parke-Davis advertisement, illustrated by the above picture, told how four children who had been bitten by a mad dog —the first Americans to be inoculated against hydrophobia by Louis Pasteur, in 1885—were saved from almost certain death and returned to their homes none the worse for their 6,000-mile journey to Paris and back.

The sequel to this story happened when Willy and Austin, two of that original quartet, read the advertisement and replied to it. Neither had seen the other for 40 years. They thought each other dead. Their reunion was an event in their lives.

In Pasteur's day the public was slow to grasp the significance of his great gift to medical science. On the morning the four youngsters were due to arrive home, a great New York newspaper ridiculed Pasteur's treatment in its leading editorial. It used these words: "The return of the children sent from Newark to Paris to be inoculated for hydrophobia ought to mark the close of a particularly foolish and mischievous sensation."

Of course, the past 45 years have conclusively proved the great life-saving value of Pasteur's treatment. It is estimated that in 1930 probably 90,000 Americans were inoculated against hydrophobia (also known as rabies) by their own physicians.

Why take needless risks?

Medical science has not only improved Pasteur's original vaccine, but it has also greatly simplified the method of inoculation. If ever your child is bitten by a dog, don't take any risks. Any qualified physician can, in your own home, protect your child against the possibility of rabies, safely and simply.

For three generations Parke, Davis & Company has been privileged to supply dependable drugs and medicines to the medical profession. Today the Parke-Davis label is your doctor's assurance of the purity and strength not only of antirabic vaccine, but of the many other medicinal products he uses to safeguard your family's health.

❖

The same exacting care that marks the manufacture of Parke-Davis medicines controls the preparation of the following products for your daily use at home— Parke-Davis Milk of Magnesia, Parke-Davis Standardized Cod-liver Oil, Parke-Davis Hydrogen Peroxide, Parke-Davis Shaving Cream, and Parke-Davis Neko (the original germicidal soap). Ask for them at your drug store.

BUILDING THE FORTRESSES OF HEALTH

One of a series of messages telling how the worker in medical science, the physician, and the maker of medicines are surrounding you with stronger health defenses year by year. Parke, Davis & Company, Detroit, Michigan; Walkerville, Ontario.

PARKE, DAVIS & CO.

THE WORLD'S LARGEST MAKERS OF PHARMACEUTICAL AND BIOLOGICAL PRODUCTS

FIG. 60. Parke, Davis & Company, "This Picture Reunited Two Comrades Saved by Pasteur in 1885," *Saturday Evening Post,* May 23, 1931, 104 (full page). © 1931 Parke, Davis & Company. Used with permission. All rights reserved. Author's collection.

Quite a number of the company's publications targeted children, with coloring books, nursery rhymes, games, and puzzles. The famous Health Heroes series offered illustrated biographies for school-age children, featuring Marie Curie, Edward Jenner, Robert Koch, Florence Nightingale, Louis Pasteur, Walter Reed, and Edward Livingston Trudeau.[28] The series name was explicitly chosen to "appeal to children, and to appeal to their sense of romance."[29] MetLife, through its agents and in its advertisements, offered these pamphlets to customers and schoolteachers.[30] Of the seven "heroes" in the series, six were commonly celebrated medical figures. Trudeau was less famous, but he was important, like Reed, for placing American heroes alongside the Europeans and because much of MetLife's effort was devoted to reducing the incidence of tuberculosis. The Health Heroes pamphlets were issued for several decades, with new covers that reflected changing fashions in graphic design (fig. 61). Besides the pamphlets, the company produced 35 mm filmstrips for community groups and schoolteachers. At first, the films were silent, requiring the teacher to read the narration from a printed script; later, an LP recording provided a "sound track."[31] There were also versions of the Health Heroes in 16 mm sound film as early as 1932. But since filmstrip projectors seem to have been more popular than movie projectors in the schools until after World War II, the older and simpler technology persisted along with the newer one.[32]

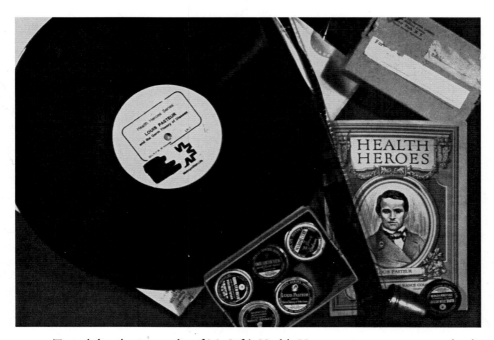

FIG. 61. Typical distribution media of MetLife's Health Heroes series, 1920s to 1950s: booklets in various editions, filmstrips with storage cans, a mailing box for filmstrips, a teacher's guide for *Marie Curie,* and a long-playing record that provided a soundtrack that was coordinated to the frames in the filmstrip for *Louis Pasteur.* Author's collection. Photograph © 2009 Bert Hansen.

The seven "health heroes" experienced an enormous circulation in booklets and in other media, both in homes and in classrooms. After the initial flood of copies to introduce a new title, the maintenance level of reprints was about one hundred thousand copies of each booklet per year. The company presumed that one copy of a booklet would serve five to ten students. By 1941, customers, teachers, and students had received from MetLife over three million copies of *Louis Pasteur*, the initial health hero booklet.[33]

DIVERSE USES OF MEDICAL HISTORY IN CORPORATE ADVERTISING

After medical history images had been introduced into mass-media advertising by Squibb, Parke-Davis, and MetLife, many other companies followed their lead in campaigns both sensible and silly. In 1932, the Coca-Cola Company introduced an image campaign called "Famous Doctors," linking the purity of its soda-fountain drinks to that of modern medicines in a series of six posters designed for countertop display. These water-color-style portraits featured Hippocrates, Harvey, Lister, Pasteur, Reed, and Roentgen.

Though not a doctor, Pasteur was a very popular figure in medical history advertising, perhaps the most popular of all. In 1936, the same year that Paul Muni was on theater screens playing Louis Pasteur, the Anheuser-Busch company ran a full-page ad in *Collier's* with a portrait of Pasteur at the center: "Pasteur learned from studying brewing methods how doctors could keep people healthier. The Home of Budweiser pioneered another important discovery by the great French scientist—pasteurization."[34] Although Pasteur had applied the technique to wine and beer, not milk, Americans in general came to associate him with that process after pasteurized milk became common in the 1920s. For example, a double-page ad in *Good Housekeeping* of June 1937 proclaims, "He made life Safer for Children," and then explains at length how "today—this great work of making life safer is carried on by the Sealtest System of Laboratory Protection" for milk, ice cream, and other dairy products.[35] In a National Dairy Products ad in *Life* magazine in late 1943 appears a painting of Pasteur at his microscope; he faces worried businessmen who ask, "Why does our wine turn sour, M. Pasteur?" The text explains Pasteur's discoveries about microbes and fermentation as the scientific basis for pasteurization and milk safety.[36]

Starting in 1939, the pharmaceutical company Wyeth began acquiring a series of six paintings, "Pioneers of American Medicine," commissioned from the well-established illustrator and muralist Dean Cornwell.[37] He produced just one painting a year owing, it was said, to his need for extensive research. Wyeth first turned the paintings into posters and magazine ads and then collected them into a small booklet under the same title in 1945. The six paintings illustrated Ephraim McDowell performing abdominal surgery; William Proctor establishing American pharmacy; Oliver Wendell Holmes combating puerperal fever; army doctors Walter Reed, Jesse Lazear, and James Carroll fighting yellow fever; army surgeon William Beaumont with his famous patient, Alexis St. Martin, making discoveries in digestive physiology; and William Osler teaching at Old Blockley. How such medico-historical figures were becoming both familiar and popular well beyond professional circles is confirmed by an article in *Coronet* magazine in 1945, which reproduced five of the paintings in color.[38]

From 1942 through 1944, Bayer Aspirin ran a series of eighteen ads in daily newspapers, each of which presented the story (in text and image) of an important medical discovery dated to a specific year and compared it with the 1898 discovery of aspirin. Evocative words such as "discovery," "triumph," "miracle," "marvel," and even "blessing" were used to characterize medical progress. The illustrations were high-quality drawings, and the large ads (a full page in a Sunday magazine or about two-thirds of a broadsheet page of a daily) were well designed with strong leads, such as "1796—Why did milkmaids never get smallpox?"; "1785—a Doctor picks a magic flower"; "1921—The Wag of a Tail"; "1882—a doctor, who dreamed of tiger hunts, bags a MAN KILLER in a bottle!"; and "1885—a MAD DOG and a fighting Frenchman!" The final entry in the series brought history right up to the present when it saluted "Penicillin, Golden Drug of the Battlefront, Blessing for Mankind."[39]

In the early 1940s, another new pharmaceutical advertising series used medical history, adopting a military angle in keeping with the mobilization for war. Ciba, the Swiss-owned pharmaceutical firm with headquarters in New Jersey, took full-page ads in U.S. magazines for a series on "Medical Heroes of the Army and Navy," later broadened as "Heroes of the United States Medical Services." One full-page ad featured "Fighter with Foods," Dr. Joseph Goldberger of the U.S. Public Health Service (fig. 62).[40]

The explosive success of penicillin during the early 1940s prompted new ads capitalizing on the favorable publicity surrounding this revolutionary breakthrough. Long before pharmaceutical companies such as Merck advertised penicillin as their product, other kinds of manufacturers picked up on images linking old breakthroughs and new ones, especially if they could bask in penicillin's aura. On a full page of the *Saturday Evening Post* in November 1944, the Crane Company of Chicago, a manufacturer of plumbing supplies, boasted about its valves and fittings with an illustration of a sanitary production facility for penicillin, "birthplace of the new wonder drug."[41] Shell Oil sought the same association with medical progress in a striking ad, whose painted illustration presents a handsome soldier walking safely out a smoldering ruin with abandoned crutches behind him: "A Prayer Is Answered. Shell research opens the way to great increases in production of the miracle drug."[42]

In the 1940s, the R. J. Reynolds Company used doctors in quite a number of Camel cigarette ads, claiming, for example, that Camels soothe a smoker's throat or that "more doctors smoke Camels than any other cigarette."[43] The copy and the

Heroes of the United States Medical Services

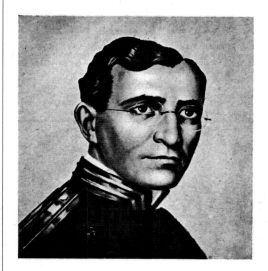

DR. JOSEPH GOLDBERGER
(1874-1929) *U. S. Public Health Service*

CLIMAXING years of outstanding research in yellow fever and other diseases, Dr. Goldberger probed one of the most baffling medical mysteries of the early Twentieth Century . . . pellagra . . . and not only discovered its dietary origin, but identified a new pellagra-preventive vitamin factor. But Dr. Goldberger gave the world more than a new vitamin . . . he gave it a greater appreciation of the importance of nutrition to health . . . an appreciation that is reflected today in the thought and care which goes into the modern scientific feeding of children and adults in government stations, private institutions, and millions of American homes.

Ciba Pharmaceutical Products, Inc. salutes the men in the Medical Services of the United States as well as those in civilian forces responsible for health "behind the lines."

Fighter with Foods

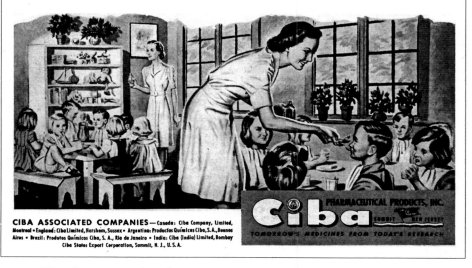

CIBA ASSOCIATED COMPANIES — Canada: Ciba Company, Limited, Montreal • England: Ciba Limited, Horsham, Sussex • Argentina: Productos Químicos Ciba, S.A., Buenos Aires • Brazil: Produtos Químicos Ciba, S. A., Rio de Janeiro • India: Ciba (India) Limited, Bombay Ciba States Export Corporation, Summit, N. J., U. S. A.

Ciba PHARMACEUTICAL PRODUCTS, INC.
SUMMIT — NEW JERSEY
TOMORROW'S MEDICINES FROM TODAY'S RESEARCH

FIG. 62. Ciba Pharmaceutical Products, Inc., "Heroes of the United States Medical Services: Fighter with Foods [Joseph Goldberger]," *Time,* Air Express Edition, May 15, 1944, 29 (full page). This entire issue was printed in black and white. In other magazines, this ad's images were in color. © 1944 Ciba Pharmaceutical Products, Inc. Used with permission of Novartis Pharmaceuticals Corporation. All rights reserved. Author's collection.

graphics in these ads frequently center on medical history heroes. For example, the painting in one Camel ad of 1947 portrays doctors with a microscope in a jungle hut, and the caption echoes the title of de Kruif's book, calling them "Big Game Hunters" in pursuit of "the biggest game of all . . . the microscopic and mysterious enemies of mankind."[44] Famous medical pioneers appear in a series of Camel ads under the slogan "Experience Is the Best Teacher." In this series could be found Claude Bernard (glycogen research), C.-E. Brown-Séquard (glycogen neurology), Paul Ehrlich (chemotherapy), Robert Koch (bacteriology), Theobald Smith (allergy), and many others. These full-page ads share a common design. Adjacent to an old-fashioned drawing of one or more physicians appears text such as, "Experience is the Best Teacher . . . Rudolf Virchow (1821–1902) proved it in pathology." Then, after a short paragraph about Virchow's work, appears the tagline "Experience is the best teacher in smoking, too!" At the bottom of the page runs the famous slogan "More doctors smoke Camels than any other cigarette."[45] Because these attractive images prompted requests from doctors for prints, the company produced an oversized booklet of them, entitled *Know Your Doctor,* which was distributed so that physicians could have it on display in their waiting rooms.[46]

Pasteur had become so famous and so useful as a general cultural hero that his image was employed to sell a wide range of products. In 1943, for example, a full-page ad in *Fortune* magazine proclaims, "Pasteur Found the Way. Now All Mankind Benefits." Along with a picture of Pasteur and a generic scientist holding a test tube, readers observed a smiling mother holding her smiling baby over this caption: "Toilet tissue is a simple essential upon which American plumbing and therefore public health depends." The advertiser was Scott Paper Company.[47]

In a 1946 ad captioned "Your Health and Victories in Medical Research," Squibb grouped two photographic views of production facilities for penicillin and influenza vaccine with a picture of a foxglove plant and a note about its role in producing a drug for certain heart conditions. But the main photograph on the page shows a cute little boy and his Boston terrier together peeking into his lunch sack. The caption invokes Pasteur's epoch-making discovery of 1885 and presents a new angle on the significance of defeating rabies: "Let no one deprive a boy of the character-building companionship of his dog" (fig. 63).

Even companies without any possible medical association invoked Pasteur's name and reputation in idiosyncratic ways. For example, Raycrest Fabrics ran a full-page ad in the Sunday magazine of the *New York Times* in late 1948. It reproduces the old engraving of Louis Pasteur watching his second patient, Jean Baptiste Jupille, receive an injection (see fig. 24 in chapter 3). How did a manufacturer of rayons and fine cottons connect its work to Pasteur? Not by a shared scientific method. No, the commonality was know-how: "Pasteur Rid the World of Hydrophobia: In Cords It's the 'Know How' that Counts." The ad explains this idea further: "When scientific brains were unable to solve complex problems, the facile 'know how' of Pasteur supplied the proper answers. . . . At the time that Pasteur was performing his great feats, the mills that make Raycrest Cords were employing their 'know how' to achieve

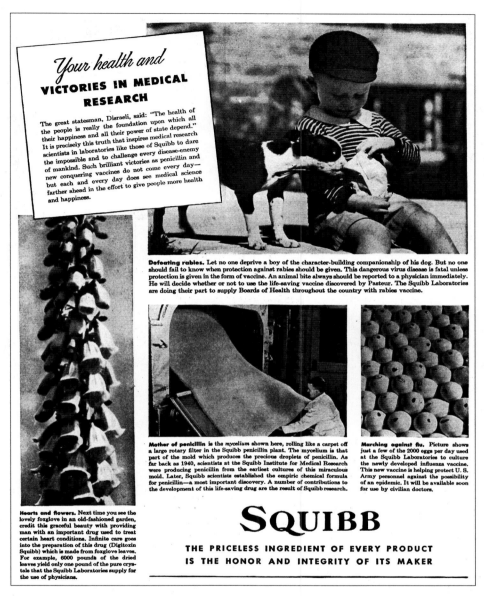

FIG. 63. Squibb, "Your Health and Victories in Medical Research," *Life*, January 28, 1946, 86 (full page). © 1946 Squibb. All rights reserved. Reprinted courtesy of Bristol Myers Squibb. Author's collection.

startling developments in corded fabrics."[48] In 1953, Dr. West's Miracle Tuft Tooth Brushes adopted the familiar image of Edelfelt's famous painting of Pasteur for its purposes with the caption "So germ-free Pasteur would have passed it!" (fig. 64).[49] This claim might seem slightly strange given that the rabies virus in Pasteur's hand had no direct connection with asepsis or with germs as a cause of disease. But the

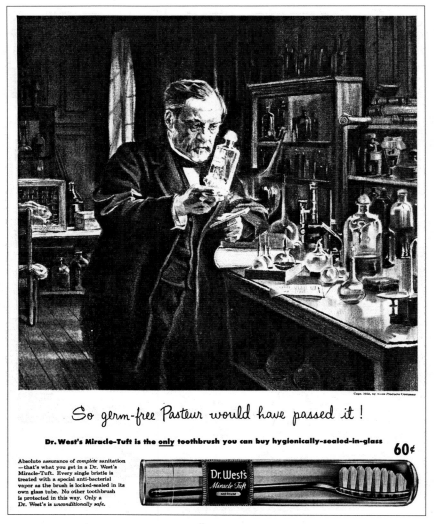

FIG. 64. Dr. West's Tooth Brushes, "So germ-free Pasteur would have passed it!" *Life* 34:19 (May 11, 1953), 151 (full page). © 1953 Weco Products Company. All rights reserved. Author's collection.

image of Pasteur looking at the rabbit spinal cord in a drying bottle had by then long ceased to signify his rabies vaccine and had come to stand in for heroic scientific discovery in general.

The graphic renderings of medical history in the advertisements of the mid-twentieth century usually recycled earlier images or imitated them. The history they evoked was one of medical progress. Through magazine advertising, successive generations of customers were continually being reintroduced to the great medical achievements of the past, and the intended effect was to honor businesses of the present as credible because they continued the legacy of a worthy past.

CHAPTER 8

POPULAR MEDICAL HISTORY IN CHILDREN'S COMIC BOOKS OF THE 1940s

TRUTH is stranger and a thousand times more
thrilling than FICTION.
    —cover tagline on *True Comics*, April 1941

THE 1940s HAVE been called a "golden age of medicine," characterized by doctors'
high social status, the profession's credibility, public confidence in miracle
cures, and an expansion of funding for medical research.[1] For the general public, it
was also a golden age of medical history in books, film, and radio. In 1941, the audience was enlarged by millions of children and adolescents when a brightly colored
genre of medical history debuted in popular comic books. Yet because the 1940s
comics with medical history stories are hard to find today, these books have been
overlooked as a source for understanding medicine in midcentury popular culture.[2]

The medical history stories in children's comic books were, however, widely disseminated, engaging, upbeat, and instructive. By placing key events of contemporary medicine within a historical tradition, they also helped to reinforce the rising
status of the medical profession in the United States during World War II and in the
postwar era. They actively promoted medical philanthropy and biological research.
The young-people's versions of the stories strongly resonated with the imagery their

parents had already encountered in film, radio, and books, but they differed by giving more attention to science and scientific method as part of their presentation of history. In the comics, the medical stories were integrated fully with the other "true adventure" stories. On one typical cover, for example, "famine fighter Dr. Joseph Goldberger" is shown with a mother and sick child threatened by the specter of Death.[3] The story of Goldberger's experimental research on pellagra jostled for space with the heroism of the Leathernecks on Guadalcanal and the military leadership of General Eisenhower (fig. 65). Also included in this book were stories about

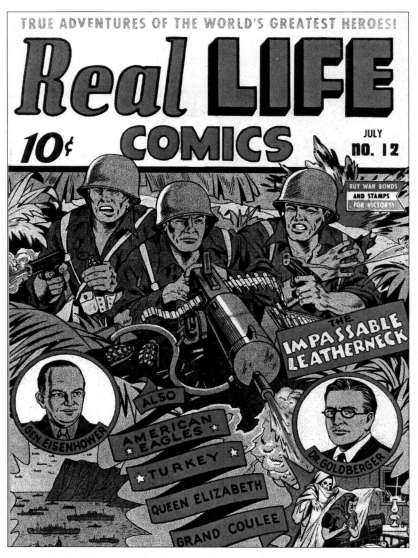

FIG. 65. Dr. Goldberger with Gen. Eisenhower and others on the cover of *Real Life Comics* 12 (July 1943). © 1943 Nedor Publishing Company. All rights reserved. Author's collection.

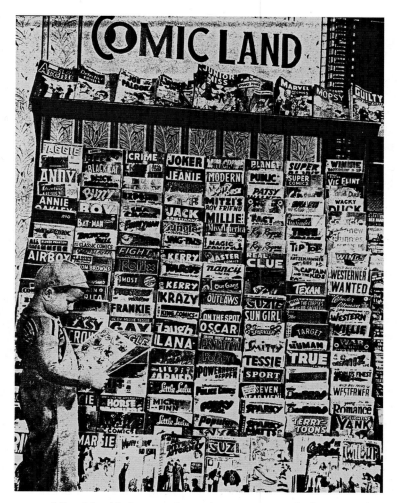

FIG. 66. "Comicland," photographer unknown, apparently first printed in *Newsdealer* magazine in 1948 and often reprinted, for example, in *Comics Buyer's Guide,* and enlarged as a poster. © 1948 Newsdealer Magazine, Inc. All rights reserved. Courtesy Maggie Thompson.

the air cadets, the history of Turkey, Queen Elizabeth I, and electrical power from Grand Coulee dam.

These books and the stories they contained were remarkably popular. Surely at no other time have medical history stories been disseminated in editions approaching one million copies. Nor is it likely that in some other era such huge numbers of young people had regular encounters with Theobald Smith, Robert Koch, or Joseph Goldberger other than in schoolbooks (and seldom even there). A newsstand photograph entitled "Comicland" (fig. 66) illustrates both the enormous popularity of comic books in the 1940s and the consumer's wide choice among the many books issued each month.[4] *True Comics, Real Heroes,* and *Real Life Comics* were on the newsstand competing with *Superman, Batman,* and many other titles. If the true-adventure books sold in smaller numbers than those of the superheroes, they still sold in the hundreds of thousands each month. But numbers are not the whole story. Comic books were ubiquitous in the lives of children and young adults from the late 1930s into the 1950s. "For at least a quarter century," according to historians Dick Lupoff and Don Thompson, "the comic book was the dominant element in the culture of American children—they read them, re-read them, collected them, traded them. During the same period, especially during World War II, when servicemen with limited off-duty time hungered for cheap and quickly readable material, it achieved great (though less publicized) popularity as reading matter for adults."[5]

THE INDUSTRY AND THE ART OF CARTOON STRIPS AND COMIC BOOKS

To understand what made these picture stories so entrancing and how they pressed their images deep into readers' minds and hearts, one needs to appreciate the visual rhetoric of comic strips, the means by which they turn the medium's constraints into opportunities and bring the stories to life. In books, magazines, and print advertising, the images are almost always subordinate to the text, and they serve only to illustrate it; meaning is carried in the verbal structure, and the illustrations are used only to catch our attention, add emotional resonance, or show things also described in the words. For example, one might get a picture of a person's face where the text mentions the person's name. Someone reading of a young scientist studying hard may be offered a picture of a boy peering into a microscope. In most print media, the images rarely carry the narrative.[6]

Action drawings do the narrative work in comic strips (also called "sequential art"), with words appearing in speech balloons as utterances or characters' thoughts and sometimes as a separate voice-over. Cartooning that depends on third-person narration is less engaging; well-designed comics closely resemble film and radio, in that skillful dramatization minimizes voice-overs, and the plot is carried as fully as possible through dialogue and sound effects. The dramatic narrative in comics has a further peculiarity in being heavily fragmented. A story in sixty panels can have as many as fifty-nine gaps in the narrative. But those gaps, hinting at action that happens "in the gutter" between frames, actually make comics particularly engaging because they force each reader to participate in imagining the story. Unlike film, which conveys predetermined auditory and visual stimuli at every moment, sequential comic art forces the reader to picture the activity in between the boxed panels and mentally to create the sounds. Comics by their nature "jump" discontinuously, for example, from a knife in a moving hand to a person lying bloody on the ground in the next panel. Silently the reader creates a picture of the stabbing and sometimes even its sound. Radio drama likewise, by virtue of the pictorial dimension it lacks, forces a listener to create mentally the complete visual scene of characters, setting, and lighting. This forced participation is what makes radio drama, radio ball games, and comic books particularly absorbing activities.[7]

Consider the initial frame, or "splash panel," of one of the Walter Reed stories (see color plate 12).[8] We do not know whose arm, what insect, why, or what will happen now. But as readers, we are likely to react by drawing our arms in closer as if to get away from the biting insect; we might also hear in our head the buzzing of a mosquito. Although the drawing is just a drawing, we do not view it as an object. We spontaneously start to imagine possible narratives, and the situation becomes "real" to us mentally even though it is just a cheaply reproduced line drawing in an exaggerated style.

How this highly syncopated form of storytelling prompts a viewer to fill the missing intervals is seen clearly in two consecutive panels from a story about penicillin (fig. 67).[9] They show a point in the narrative when penicillin was still highly experimental, of limited availability, not yet widely known, and used almost exclusively for military patients. We see only policemen cartooned with the conventional "motion lines," a few reporters, and a physician. The patient is conspicuously absent, but the two frames with their three small "speech balloons" effectively tell her story, drawing readers into picturing a definite series of actions taking place in several locales over a number of hours. It was these structural features that made comics so attractive, impressing the stories and characters deeply into children's imagination and memory.[10]

The modern comic book took shape only in the mid-1930s, even though cartoons and caricature have been around for centuries and narrative comic strips started appearing in newspapers as early as the 1890s. The first big success was *Detective Comics* in 1937, followed by even bigger ones with the introduction of a character type known generically as a superhero, such as Superman in 1938 and Batman in 1939.[11]

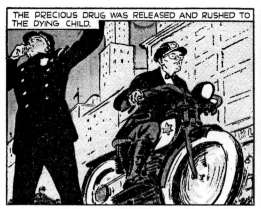
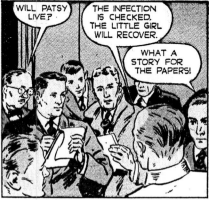

FIG. 67. "The precious drug," two panels of "Penicillin," *True Comics* 41 (December 1944), 22. © 1944 True Comics, Inc., a subsidiary of the Publishers of Parents' Magazine. Used with permission. All rights reserved. Author's collection.

Almost overnight, comic books became a major publishing phenomenon and a multimillion-dollar industry.[12] The format was quickly standardized into a booklet of soft newsprint paper, roughly eight by ten inches, printed in flat saturated colors over black line drawings (often carelessly printed with uneven registration). Each book contained several different stories. The glossy covers imitated the style of circus posters. Although the quality of actual printing was usually poor, the graphic art was sometimes excellent. If adults sometimes criticized comic books for being bad reading that hurt children's eyes, the children seem not to have noticed.[13]

Comic books became a national passion. The 60 or so titles published in 1938 rose to 108 in 1940 and swelled to 168 in 1942.[14] Average sales were two to four hundred thousand copies per issue. Single issues of *Action Comics* with a Superman story often sold about nine hundred thousand copies, and bimonthly issues of the book titled *Superman* averaged sales of 1.3 million copies.[15] Ten million comic books were being sold each month in 1940.[16] Comic books were found everywhere. They were known to everyone; and if they were read mostly by children, they were read by almost all of them. According to Nyberg, "more than 90 percent of the children in the fourth, fifth, and sixth grades reported that they read comic books regularly, averaging at least ten comics a month. . . . Readership was lower among adolescents and adults; still, 30 percent of young adults reported reading comic books."[17]

HISTORY CHALLENGES FICTION AND FANTASY

Detective fiction and superheroes in fantasy stories had such spectacular success in comic books that publishers tried other kinds of stories to tap into this huge market. Along with funny animals and funny people, "true" adventures were introduced in several new titles, jam-packed with tales of "real people" from history and the present. These books shifted attention from supermen to humans, from fantasy heroes to real people, but without abandoning heroism or the biographical narrative. These books were founded on the premise that truth could displace fantasy, and although many of the stories were gory, especially in wartime, the genre has been well characterized as "wholesome adventures."[18] In these comic books, the medical history stories appeared cheek-by-jowl with fierce battles and exotic adventures.[19] This new group of comic books tried to entertain with facts and information.[20] Although their intentions were educational, the stories were often as fresh, even raw, as the action adventures with which they competed for space and attention on the newsstands.

The true-adventure genre was inaugurated in April 1941 with *True Comics,* whose cover bore this motto: "TRUTH is stranger and a thousand times more thrilling than FICTION." The first issue featured Winston Churchill on the cover and included a story about Dr. Walter Reed's experiments on yellow-fever transmission. The intention of founder and publisher George J. Hecht was to put in children's hands a book that would "educate and stimulate them by placing before them the examples of important and courageous people." *True Comics* had been scheduled to be published every two months, but after the premier issue sold out its three hundred thousand copies, the publisher made it a monthly.[21] At times, it also appeared as a newspaper strip.[22] Before the end of the year, *True*'s publisher added two similar books to its roster: *Real Heroes* and *Calling All Girls*. The "true comics" idea was quickly copied by others, with *Real Life Comics* debuting in the summer of 1941, followed in a few years by a sister publication, *It Really Happened*. Before the end of 1941, a third publisher's magazine entered this market under the title *Trail Blazers*. After the war, publishers attempted to add further titles in the "true comics" genre, but none of them met with success. *Real Fact* was introduced in 1946 and lasted just twenty-one issues. *Science Comics* published its only five issues between January and September of 1946. In 1947, *Picture Stories from Science* folded after its second issue. *Negro Heroes* appeared only twice.

The "wholesome adventure" comics did not achieve the huge circulation numbers of fantasy books like *Batman* and *Superman,* which sometimes sold over a million copies an issue. But by April 1942, *True Comics, Real Heroes,* and *Calling All Girls* had attained a combined monthly circulation of 750,000.[23] For 1944, audited circulation figures of *True Comics* alone had risen from its 1942 monthly averages of around 325,000 up to a circulation high of 559,625.[24] But measuring the impact of comic books must also take into account that they were often reread and were regularly traded among friends. Collecting and sharing were especially popular among GIs. At military post exchanges, comic books "outsold *Life, The Reader's Digest,* and *Saturday Evening Post* combined at ten to one."[25]

Like all newsstand comics, the books in the true-adventure genre were commercial endeavors with full-page ads for bubble gum, candy, toy rifles, and other popular or faddish goods. They competed for purchasers in the mass market. *True Comics* was, however, established and owned by a different kind of publisher from other comics: Parents' Institute, Inc., the publisher of *Parents' Magazine. True Comics* listed as "junior advisory editors" such celebrities as Mickey Rooney, Shirley Temple, and Eddie Cantor's daughter, Janet, along with "senior advisory editors" such as George H. Gallup, Hendrik Willem van Loon, and two Columbia University professors. The values expressed in the medical stories in the series may be characterized as secular humanism.[26] Unfortunately, comic-book historians have given short shrift to the "wholesome adventure" comics because they were not the biggest sellers and did not contain any of the fantasy characters such as Superman or Mickey Mouse, who reappeared in successive issues and became enduring celebrities with millions of fans. Nor did the true-adventure books typically get the better artists or allow them to sign their own stories. Nonetheless, even if the true-adventure comics were smaller in circulation, in artistic stature, and in the making of devoted historians, they achieved a substantial readership for medical history among youngsters in the United States. At their best, they brilliantly combined good science with high adventure and such excellent art as that of cartoonist Rudy Palais (see color plate 13).[27]

The success of the true-adventure comics was not sustained beyond the mid-1940s. The genre disappeared along with the other publications of an era now designated "the golden age" of comic books.[28] What ended in the late 1940s was not simply the huge sales numbers and the quality of the books but youth culture's universal passion for comics and comics' commanding place in the culture at large. The prominence and centrality that comic books had held in mass culture from the late 1930s disappeared as a result of political attacks and the rise of television. Their dominance was challenged first by an anticomics crusade that included book-burnings in schoolyard bonfires in the summer of 1948[29] and then by the fierce attacks of the psychologist Fredric Wertham, culminating in his 1954 book, *Seduction of the Innocent*.[30] Even the U.S. Congress held public hearings on the dangers of comic books. The industry was seriously hurt, and it established self-censorship with an industry code of approval.[31] In the 1950s, the rise of television deeply undercut the commanding position of comic books in young people's entertainment. Still, for most of the 1940s, true-adventure comics were enormously popular, and they were peopled with the likes of Paré, Pasteur, and the penicillin scientists.

WHO WERE THE HEROES OF CHILDREN'S MEDICAL HISTORY?

Walter Reed and Louis Pasteur had the most frequent appearances in the true-adventure comic books, just as they had in the other media for popular history of medicine.[32] Each of these men had been featured in a major Hollywood film of the mid-1930s, as well as in de Kruif's writings. Reed's story was perfect for the era: he was a soldier, an American, and the man credited with solving the problem of yellow fever in the context of a government-sponsored investigation. Reed was the very first of the comic-book medical heroes; "Yellow Jack: How the Cause of Yellow Fever Was Discovered" appeared in the inaugural issue of *True Comics* (see color plate 14).[33] When "Major Walter Reed, an army doctor," was introduced to readers on the second page of the story, the drawing would have been familiar to many of them, as it replicated the portrait on a commemorative postage stamp issued a year earlier, in April 1940.

The storyline in this comic book was a familiar series of guesses, observations, hypotheses, and dangerous experiments, including the death of Dr. Jesse Lazear, "a martyr to science." The experiments were explained clearly and made visually prominent (figs. 68 and 69). As pedagogy, such pictures neatly illustrated how experimental

Opposite, top: **FIG. 68**. "Phew!" panel of Harold Delay, "Yellow Jack," *True Comics* 1 (April 1941), 42. © 1941 The Parents' Institute, Inc. Used with permission. All rights reserved. Author's collection. *Bottom:* **FIG. 69**. "One more test," four panels of Harold Delay, "Yellow Jack," *True Comics* 1 (April 1941), 43. © 1941 The Parents' Institute, Inc. Used with permission. All rights reserved. Author's collection.

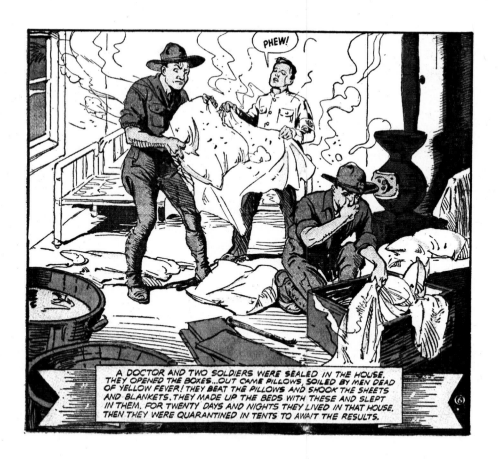

PHEW!

A DOCTOR AND TWO SOLDIERS WERE SEALED IN THE HOUSE. THEY OPENED THE BOXES...OUT CAME PILLOWS, SOILED BY MEN DEAD OF YELLOW FEVER! THEY BEAT THE PILLOWS AND SHOOK THE SHEETS AND BLANKETS. THEY MADE UP THE BEDS WITH THESE AND SLEPT IN THEM. FOR TWENTY DAYS AND NIGHTS THEY LIVED IN THAT HOUSE. THEN THEY WERE QUARANTINED IN TENTS TO AWAIT THE RESULTS. (6)

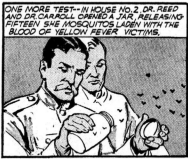

ONE MORE TEST-- IN HOUSE NO. 2, DR. REED AND DR. CARROLL OPENED A JAR, RELEASING FIFTEEN SHE MOSQUITOS LADEN WITH THE BLOOD OF YELLOW FEVER VICTIMS.

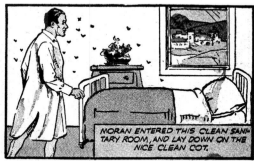

MORAN ENTERED THIS CLEAN SANITARY ROOM, AND LAY DOWN ON THE NICE CLEAN COT.

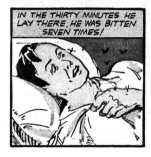

IN THE THIRTY MINUTES HE LAY THERE, HE WAS BITTEN SEVEN TIMES!

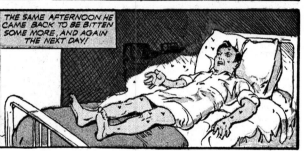

THE SAME AFTERNOON HE CAME BACK TO BE BITTEN SOME MORE, AND AGAIN THE NEXT DAY!

controls functioned in the testing of hypotheses. As scary and ugly doings, they offered the thrill of horror that suited their place in an adventure comic for a largely male, adolescent and preadolescent readership.

A second story about the yellow-fever breakthrough by Reed and his colleagues appeared in *Real Life Comics,* where Reed shared the magazine's cover with Jacob Riis and the Fighting Seabees (fig. 70). With comic strips' characteristic conciseness, four panels on the last page of this story showed the soldier Moran being carried out sick from the experiment's "clean house" as Reed announced that "a filthy house without mosquitoes can't cause yellow jack—but a clean house with one mosquito is a death trap." The next panel showed Dr. Gorgas ordering the removal of stagnant water from the streets, and the final one proclaimed, "Ninety days later—for the first time in two hundred years there was not a single case of yellow fever in Havana! Major Walter Reed and his daring associates had won another battle in the endless war against disease!"[34] Yellow-fever stories also appeared in *Science Comics* and *Picture Stories from Science.*[35]

Pasteur made his comic-book debut in the October 1942 issue of *Trail Blazers,* followed quickly the next month by a story in *Real Heroes.*[36] Whereas *Real Heroes* told only the story of "sick wine," *Trail Blazers* recounted quite a number of important episodes, which had also appeared in the 1936 film and other popular accounts: homesickness making a youthful Pasteur abandon study in Paris, his later return to study at the École Normale, a chemistry professorship at Strasbourg, spoiled wine, disease among silkworms, airborne germs and disease, the public anthrax-vaccine experiment, rabies vaccine and Pasteur's anxiety over its first use in a human being, his election to the French Academy, and the benefits we all gain from pasteurized milk. The story was sketchy, factually loose, and cliché ridden, but it conveyed a great deal of information in only forty-four frames on nine pages. Filling in the gaps may have been easy for readers, as much of the story had been presented repeatedly in books, films, and radio dramas. The story's drawings by Gary Gray (a pseudonym of the prolific cartoonist Jack Farr, whose art appeared in early *Superman* and *Batman* comics) had an unusual style for the true-adventure comics, as he gave the characters a very twentieth-century appearance or, more accurately, the appearance of modern comic-strip figures.[37] Louis Pasteur and Madame Pasteur were thin and as handsome as movie stars. Their facial features and their 1940s hairstyles could have appeared in *Blondie* or *Dick Tracy* (though without the latter's physiognomic exaggerations), two popular comics of the day.[38]

In *Real Heroes* for November 1942, an unsigned, but well-drawn story, "Pasteur and the Unseen Enemy," showed how Pasteur puzzled out the problem of good French wine that often spoiled when shipped to England. The story illustrated Pasteur's cleverness in staging the successful experiment comparing heated and unheated wines.[39] The microscope played a prominent role in this triumph, and readers learned that wines with different problems harbor different groups of microbes. The story's artwork has a distinctive style, with the highly exaggerated body language often found in comics and a successful use of worm's-eye views and bird's-eye views

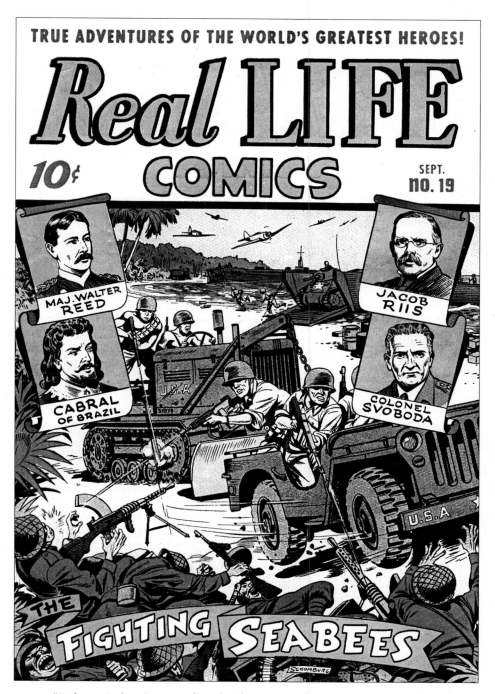

FIG. 70. "Fighting Seabees," cover of *Real Life Comics* 19 (September 1944). © 1944 Nedor Publishing Company. All rights reserved. Author's collection.

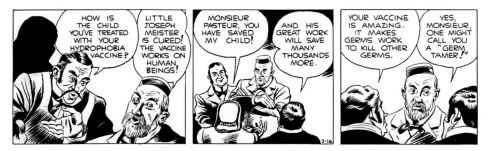

FIG. 71. [Sam Glankoff], "Louis Pasteur: Germ Tamer," first three frames in *True Comics* newspaper strip of four frames, ca. 1943, original ink drawing on Strathmore board, approximately 4 by 20 inches, marked up for the printer in blue pencil. Used with permission. Author's collection.

to add action to the scenes. No artist was given a credit line for this story, but the style is unmistakably that of Sam Glankoff, a frequent contributor to 1940s comics and a successful artist in his own right.[40] And when Pasteur made his appearance in the newspaper comic strip entitled *True Comics,* the unsigned drawings were clearly by Glankoff as well (fig. 71).[41]

Pasteur also made several appearances in an unusual series of noncartoon stories published in two comic-book titles, *Real Life Comics* and *It Really Happened.* The texts were written by Nat Schachner, a chemist, who began his career in public health and in chemical warfare. Schachner then became, in turn, a lawyer, a very successful science-fiction writer in the 1930s, and a historical biographer, with books on Burr, Hamilton, Jefferson, the founding fathers, and the American Jewish Committee.[42] Most of Schachner's comic-book stories were about Jewish heroes, and several of these men had made their mark in medicine or science, such as Waldemar Haffkine.[43] Noncartoon drawings illustrated the text and showed Haffkine speaking with Pasteur, Haffkine using a microscope (in a drawing based on a nineteenth-century image of Pasteur), and people dying of disease along a roadway in Asia. Along with the usual story of mysterious diseases overcome with laboratory discoveries fostered by cleverness and determination, readers learned as well that the Jewish Haffkine was invited by Elie Metchnikoff, a Russian microbiologist who pioneered immunology, to take a place at Mechnikoff's institute in Odessa. But this opportunity was blocked by the Russian government's anti-Semitic policies, and Haffkine moved to Paris. When Haffkine first announced his plans to conquer cholera, he was warned by all that Pasteur and his colleagues had worked on it for years without success. Undaunted, Haffkine managed to develop an inoculation for cholera, tested it on himself under Pasteur's care, and then took it to India with great success. "It should have been enough for one man. But Haffkine was not content. There was that other scourge—the bubonic plague!"[44] After years of work, he had another triumph. "In the midst of the raging plague, [he] inoculated his hundreds of thousands. Again, the plague retreated before him and fled this lonely human being who, single-handed, had fought through and won where hundreds of others had failed. Waldemar Haffkine, whom Russia had once dismissed because of his religion, had banished from earth two of the worst diseases that had ever plagued mankind!"[45] Schachner published at least three other scientific biographies in comic books: "The Magic Mold" (1946) about Dr. Ernest Chain, who shared a 1945 Nobel Prize with Alexander Fleming and Howard Florey for developing penicillin; "Master of Medicine—A True Story of Scientific Achievement" (1947) about Dr. Simon Flexner and the establishment of the Rockefeller Institute for Medical Research; and a story about the great anthropologist Franz Boas, "A Foe of Prejudice" (1946).[46] Like Haffkine, Chain, Flexner, and Boas were all Jewish.

Despite the popularity of Pasteur and Reed and the comic books' substantial and unacknowledged dependence on the writings of Paul de Kruif, the range of medical history heroes in the comics was fairly wide. Among those who had their own separate stories, Ambroise Paré was the historically earliest figure.[47] Paré also appeared in a survey, "The Story of Medicine," a cover story depicted by a scene of battlefield care of the wounded, where a prominent feature is the bag of a blood product hanging from the butt of a rifle that stands upright with its bayonet in the ground, an image that occurred often in these books (fig. 72). Both Paré stories focused on his observation that soldiers' wounds healed faster in the cases in which doctors had run out of the hot oil normally used to cauterize them. Progress came from his open-eyed observations and his willingness to reconsider tradition.

Edward Jenner's discovery of the vaccine against smallpox anchored two biographical stories about him, and it was mentioned in other accounts as well. Both biographies feature the anecdote of Napoleon's consenting to release British prisoners when he sees Jenner's name in a plea for clemency. One version carelessly puts Jenner on the list of prisoners, rather than on the list of petitioners.[48] The control of smallpox is also highlighted in a comic-book story about Catherine the Great, who, when persuaded by animal experiments that "vaccination" is safe, overrules the skeptical local physicians in favor of Dr. Dimsdale from London and has herself "vaccinated" so that she can safely minister to her people and serve as proof of the value of "vaccination." "In the weeks that followed, Russians of high and low estate flocked to Moscow to receive the magic immunization." In truth, what Catherine brought to Russia in the 1760s was the technique of inoculation, or variolation, not vaccination.[49] Another story contains the same error, applying the term "vaccination" to General George Washington's order to have his troop variolated, an event that took place during the Revolutionary War, about fifteen years before vaccination was invented.[50]

"Death Fighter" Robert Koch, with beard and microscope, is a cover figure on the third issue of *True Comics,* containing a didactic but lively eight-page story about his anthrax work.[51] The story explains cellular staining, techniques of distinguishing microbes from one another, Koch's identification of the cholera germ, his work in Asia and Egypt, and his Nobel Prize. In the closing frame, on a scroll of honored scientists with Aristotle heading the list, Koch's name is inscribed and

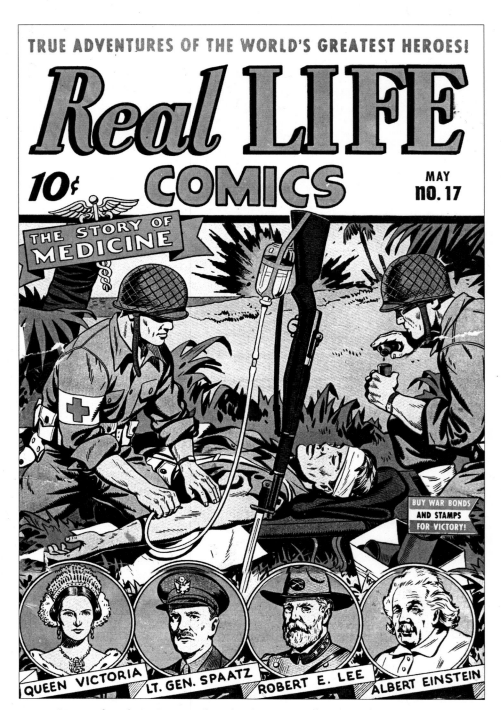

FIG. 72. "Story of Medicine," cover of *Real Life Comics* 17 (May 1944). © 1944 Nedor Publishing Company. All rights reserved. Author's collection.

he is designated as "the father of bacteriology." Koch reappeared in May 1943 as "Herr Doktor" in another lengthy and rich account, "The Conquest of Diphtheria," in which readers also encounter Emile Roux, Friedrich Loeffler, and Emil August Behring as the key figures of the 1890s.[52] This account climaxes with a magnificent American triumph: "Decades later, Dr. Park of New York achieved the final victory!" He replaced antitoxin therapy with a new injection that allowed children to build their own immunity rather than to receive it passively from horse serum. "In New York State alone, diphtheria deaths dropped from 4,500 in 1922 to less than 60 in 1940—with healthy children everywhere providing a living memorial for Loeffler, Roux, and Behring!"[53] Even during World War II, German doctors were still being honored for their exciting achievements, as was the Italian Giovanni Battista Grassi, who later that same year shared a story about malaria with the British physician Ronald Ross.[54]

Searching for a beri-beri germ is the starting point for the adventures of the Dutch physician Christian Eijkman in the East Indies, where he observes the surprising contrast between men sick and dying in a clean prison where they are fed high-quality white rice and generally healthy prisoners in the "poor, ill-kept Jangro prison . . . a miserable place."[55] He secures permission to have two groups of prisoners switch prisons and confirms from this experiment that food is more likely a cause of the illness than filth and germs. Two prisoners die in this experiment. His research continues with beri-beri induced in chickens, experiments with brown and white rice, and a failed search to isolate the key "something" in the brown casings of whole rice kernels that kept people well. This story about "The Discoverer of Hidden Hunger" ends with Eijkman's being awarded the Nobel Prize for discovering the cause and cure of beri-beri. A caption notes that "Dr. Eijkman began the work which gave us our knowledge of the vitamins we all need for good health" and promises "another vitamin story" soon.[56] The very next issue brought another vitamin triumph, this time the story of an American chemist working in the Philippines, Robert R. Williams, who devotes twenty-five years of study to rice bran. He finally succeeds in isolating Vitamin B_1 and then shows how to put it back into prepared foods.[57]

All these adventures in the laboratory did not, however, preclude attention to public health. Stephen Smith was introduced to readers as a young man appalled by urban disease, who developed a powerful "vision of a healthful city" and waged "a heroic battle that gave America her first public health laws!"[58] As a young doctor in 1858, Smith notices the high prevalence of typhoid in filthy slum settings but is rebuffed in his demand that a rich landlord keep the tenements cleaner. "A smouldering revulsion in young Stephen Smith burst into a fire of action!"[59] He compiles facts and figures, and he drafts a law for New York State, but it is blocked by sleazy politicians. He comes back again and again, with more and bigger studies, the backing of more doctors, and newspaper editorial support. In time he triumphs, when a new legislature makes history by passing his public-health law, just as cholera is approaching. In the closing panel, readers are addressed directly by a man approaching his ninety-ninth year, reading from "the proudest entry" in his journal: "I have seen my health bill, after forty-five years, become the model for such bills all over the nation."[60]

Stories of another doctor Smith, Theobald this time, engaged readers with detailed microscopic images and walked them through several controlled experiments of medical microbiology. This government bacteriologist was featured in two substantial stories in *Real Life Comics* and *Science Comics*.[61] The first of these stories declares that a "mysterious death stalked among America's teeming herds—until a young scientist sought the cause!"[62] Six pages of colorful drawings show field trials with labeled stock pens, close-up views of ticks both young and mature for egg laying, bacilli in the circle that conveys a microscope's field, and the triumphant cleansing of disease-bearing ticks from cattle in insecticidal troughs. The closing frames describe Smith's proof of an insect-borne disease as a clue that made possible both David Bruce's tracking of sleeping sickness to the African tsetse fly and Giovanni Battista Grassi's discovery of the source of malaria. The later story, "Theobald Smith and Texas Fever," has stronger cartooning but shows the same inquisitive young scientist in settings taken from cowboy movies (see color plate 15).[63] An elegant splash drawing opens the story with a herd of longhorns and a concise overview: "Fifty years ago, northern cattle shipped to graze in the south got sick and died from a mysterious disease the cattlemen called Texas fever. Southern cows shipped to the north trailed this disease with them, killing more northern cattle. To explain this riddle, Theobald Smith devoted several years of his life, experimenting in the laboratory and on the range. He was the first and greatest of all American Microbe Hunters!" As in the earlier account, his triumph is linked to further discoveries, opening "the way for Dr. Walter Reed's conquest of yellow fever . . . as well as other important advancements in the science of microbe hunting!"[64]

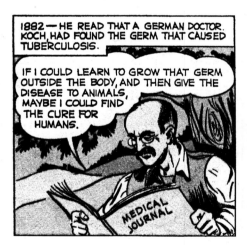

FIG. 73. "If I could learn to grow that germ," panel of "Conqueror of the White Plague," *True Comics* 19 (December 1942), 57. © The Parents' Institute, Inc. Used with permission. All rights reserved. Author's collection.

In the 1940s, the general public was already familiar with Edward Livingston Trudeau for his personal recovery from tuberculosis through a bracing outdoor life in the Adirondacks and for his opening a sanatorium at Saranac Lake to treat successfully thousands of fellow sufferers. When *True Comics* presented his biography to young readers under the title "Conqueror of the White Plague," the story transformed him from an innovative clinician into a laboratory-oriented microbe hunter. Reading in a medical journal that a German doctor Koch has found the germ that causes tuberculosis,

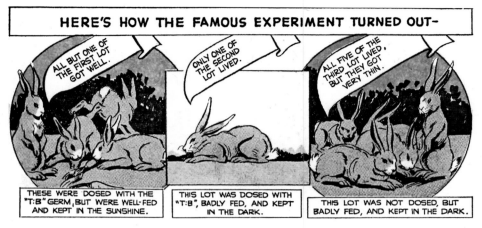

FIG. 74. "Here's how the famous experiment turned out," panel of "Conqueror of the White Plague," *True Comics* 19 (December 1942), 59. © The Parents' Institute, Inc. Used with permission. All rights reserved. Author's collection.

Trudeau muses to himself, "If I could learn to grow that germ outside the body, and then give the disease to animals, maybe I could find the cure for humans" (fig. 73). He builds himself "a small, rude laboratory with home-made equipment."[65] This account makes later events in the clinician's life and work dependent on a modest experiment he had undertaken with two groups of five rabbits, all ten injected with the newly discovered tubercle bacillus. These groups are placed in either good or bad conditions, and another five are kept as an uninfected control in bad conditions with little food (fig. 74). Preceding frames show him injecting the rabbits with a large needle and syringe; like so many of the other scientific doctors portrayed in these stories, he casually experiments on animals as if no one had ever raised an objection, and there is no attempt to protect youthful eyes from views of the sacrificed animals. Just after the frame with the groups of rabbits, which illustrates the data, Trudeau draws his conclusion for both the reader and himself: "Now I know my treatment is right! Bad living conditions alone do not cause the disease, or the third lot would have died. Fresh air and sunlight, good food and rest cured all but one of the first lot—they will cure human beings, too, in most cases of tuberculosis."[66]

A story about Joseph Goldberger delivers substantial scientific complexity and detail in only forty-six small images; readers of "Famine Fighter" discover not only a remarkable man's career in the public-health service but solid information about physiology, the experimental method, and clever detective work in science. The elements of the plot—some repulsive, some lusciously appealing—encompass a number of features that would have made it especially compelling to a preteen audience (fig. 75). The adventure starts in Goldberger's youth, with an epiphany about the exciting new frontier of medical research: a "war against disease" waged by an "army wielding scalpels and test-tubes."[67]

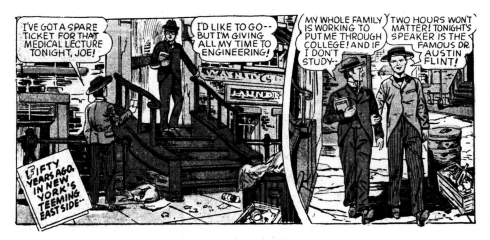

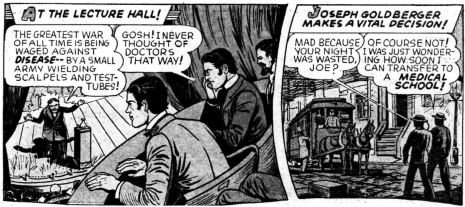

FIG. 75. "I've got a spare ticket" and "At the lecture hall," four panels from "Famine Fighter," *Real Life Comics* 12 (July 1943), 15–16. © 1943 Nedor Publishing Company. All rights reserved. Author's collection. Young Goldberger hears Dr. Austin Flint's lecture and decides on medical school.

After becoming a government scientist, Goldberger takes up the study of pellagra, a disease that was endemic across much of the United States in the early twentieth century, especially in the South. The disease was characterized by an ugly scab-forming rash, and it also caused physical weakness, mental deterioration, and death. When Goldberger begins his study in the pellagra-ridden insane asylums, his observation quickly takes in the overlooked fact that the staff did not contract the disease. This moves him to begin doubting the likelihood of finding a pellagra germ and to wonder about questions of diet. He brings a detective's eye to the matter, noticing that in an orphanage where over two-thirds of the children have pellagra, the cases are all in one age group, from six to twelve years old. This leads to questions of what protected both the very young and the adolescents from this mysterious suffering. By further sleuthing, he learns that the younger children have milk in their diet, and he discovers that hungry adolescents are stealing food at night. With a new theory that pellagra arises from a deficiency of protein, he tries an experiment in an orphanage with a diet of eggs, milk, and fresh lean meat. A year later, all but one case out of 130 recover on this diet.

In exchange for pardons, a group of prisoners agrees to an experiment in which they live on the monotonous, if common, southern diet of fatty pork and corn syrup. In a perfect fantasy for a children's story, the men are thrilled to have this rich sweet diet and as much of it as they want. After a while, they get sick and beg to stop the trial, even giving up the promised release from prison. All these observations lead Goldberger to reject a germ explanation for this widespread ailment, earning him the mockery of experts. A key experiment to demonstrate that germs are not involved required that Goldberger, his co-workers, and his wife ingest pellagra victims' scabs and inject themselves with sick people's blood (see color plate 16). Goldberger's theory that pellagra is caused by some yet unknown deficiency in a fat-rich diet finally receives experimental confirmation when, by manipulating dogs' diet, he first manages to engender pellagra in them and then restores them to health with a special diet (fig. 76). And best of all, he finds that adding minute amounts of yeast to the regular diet of millions of ordinary Americans would be enough to prevent thousands of cases of debility and death from this common disease. Goldberger was a microbe hunter with a difference. He showed that, despite the stirring successes of the germ theory, unnoticed dietary deficiency was a major cause of disease, and he established a preventive model for public-health intervention on a national scale.

A very different kind of hero and a distinctive kind of medical innovation are featured in the story of the Mayo brothers, Will and Charlie, from Minnesota. They began medical study in their father's practice before entering medical school. Out of their personal achievements, they proceeded to create a nationally recognized

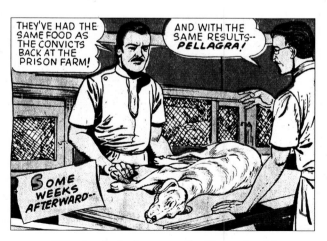

FIG. 76. "They've had the same food," panel of "Famine Fighter," *Real Life* 12 (July 1943), 22. © 1943 Nedor Publishing Company. All rights reserved. Author's collection.

institution for research, training, and patient care. They were great innovators in surgery and surgical education, and their success enabled them to become generous philanthropists.[68]

Several medical heroes risked death to help humanity. Dr. Samuel Mudd single-handedly cared for everyone in a prison when yellow fever broke out, and in 1943 children were given the same story that their parents already knew from a 1936 film and several radio dramas.[69] Dr. David Livingstone, a missionary in Africa, is portrayed in a comic book as struggling "for the betterment of thousands of savage natives."[70] The British nurse Edith Cavell served in war-torn Belgium in 1915, treating the wounded no matter what their allegiance or nationality. But she also helped Allied soldiers to escape from German-controlled areas, actions for which she was tried and then executed. The comic book that tells Cavell's story, twenty-eight years after her death and in the midst of another war, presents her noble story with better-than-average artwork, and it salutes her as "selfless, gallant, fearless."[71]

Whereas Cavell calmly faced the perils of human treachery and evil, doctor Wilfred Grenfell battled the elements of nature at its most brutal, and he survived by means of a steely courage, the loyalty of his dogs, his own clear thinking, and his ability to do what the situation demanded—no matter how painful or grotesque. Grenfell was an English missionary doctor who went to Canada in 1893. In addition to providing medical services and establishing hospitals in remote Labrador, he wrote popular outdoor-adventure books for adults and younger readers.[72] The comic-book stories focus on one particularly dramatic episode, tagged on the cover of *True Comics* as "Adrift on an Ice Pan: Dr. Wilfred Grenfell."[73] A second version of his story appeared less than a year later in *Real Life Comics*.[74] The six-page story in *True Comics* has clean, powerful graphics, with good action drawings. When making a late-winter house call, the doctor and his sled dogs lose contact with land when the ice sheet in an inlet breaks into pieces. Grenfell urges his dogs to swim to a larger chunk of ice and, holding their traces, he is pulled through the icy water to safety, having lost his coat and gloves. "In order to keep from freezing to death, the doctor had to kill three of his dogs. He laced the dog skins into a rug and piled up the bodies for a windbreak." He wraps himself in dog skins, "snuggling against his biggest dog" to keep warm. When that pan of ice begins to drift out to sea, he ties dog bones together to make a flagstaff in case a boat might find him. One does, and he is saved. Then, despite frozen feet, he hurries to take care of the sick boy who is now in the hospital. The closing frame, which in other comic-book stories often memorializes the heroic doctor, shows a bronze tablet reading, "To the Memory of three noble dogs—Moody, Watch, and Spy—whose lives were given for mine on the ice, April 21, 1908, Wilfred Grenfell."[75] It is not hard to see how young children were both repelled and attracted by a story of devoted, noble dogs, in which their skinned carcasses and bloody bones are fully depicted.

Far across the continent some years later, a sled dog named Balto became an international medical hero by facing tremendous dangers to save a town from diphtheria. In early 1925, Balto led a team over the last segment of a six-hundred-mile run to bring antitoxin to Nome, Alaska, in order to stop a diphtheria epidemic when planes could not fly in the antitoxin. The suspense of whether Balto and his team would make it in time to save these lives made headlines for weeks all across the nation.[76] The event was so famous that when leaders of the "No More Diphtheria" campaign in New York State wanted a publicity stunt, they restaged the race in the streets of Syracuse with an Alaskan musher taking his dog sled right to City Hall.[77] Balto himself later became a showpiece on the vaudeville circuit, but after his fortunes declined, he was displayed for a while in a dime-museum freak show in Los Angeles. A Cleveland businessman, who found him there, raised funds to buy him and placed him in the Cleveland zoo. On Balto's first day in Cleveland, fifteen thousand people came to see him. When he finished his days there, he was mounted by a taxidermist and placed on exhibit at the Cleveland Museum of Natural History.[78] Balto was celebrated in stories, books, pamphlets, and even a statue in Central Park. His medical heroism made appearances in *Heroic Comics* and *Real Heroes,* both in 1946.[79]

Several heroes and heroines were featured for making some founding contribution to health care, if not as creators of new scientific knowledge. It was not accidental that the category of "firsts" was dominated by women, who had generally been excluded from professional positions in medicine and faced high barriers to participation in science.

The earliest of these firsts to get a story-length profile in comic books was the seventeenth-century heroine Jeanne Mance, "Canada's pioneer nurse, whose courage inspired the founding of the city of Montreal and its famous hospital, Hotel Dieu." As striking as a starlet, she is first seen holding a baby and a gun (fig. 77). Arriving from France in 1642, she refuses to stay in the established settlement at Quebec and pushes further into new territory. In a frontier fort, Mance cares for sick and hungry children and maintains everyone's courage while besieged by "savage Iroquois, [who] harassed the settlers."[80] The Mance story illustrates how the comics borrowed heavily from cinema's visual style. Many visual resemblances to movies (body language, viewpoints or camera angles, abrupt cuts between scenes) served the comics well and deepened readers' engagement by helping to bring movement and personality to the cartooned figures.[81]

The nineteenth century furnished the comic books with several role models of women in both nursing and medicine. Florence Nightingale, the famous "Lady with the Lamp," was the initial presentation when the premier issue of *Wonder Woman* in 1942 inaugurated a regular feature called "Wonder Women of History."[82] The story of how Nightingale talked her way into war-front service in the Crimean War and proved her mettle and the value of her trained nurses, winning all to her cause, was already familiar from books, pamphlets, and a Hollywood film. The "Wonder Women of History" feature injected true-adventure stories into a comic book that was otherwise entirely fantasy. A few issues later, another installment in this series profiled Lillian Wald as "The Mother of New York's East Side." The story recounts her nursing training, her public-health work, her creation of school nursing, "her

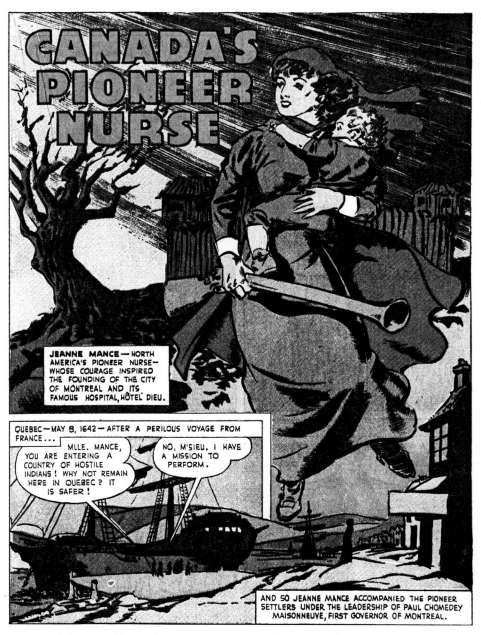

FIG. 77. Splash page of "Canada's Pioneer Nurse," *True Comics* 24 (May-June 1943), 15. © 1943 The Parents' Institute, Inc. Used with permission. All rights reserved. Author's collection.

inspiring idea of a federal children's bureau," her leadership in nursing during World War I, and her heroic service during a wartime epidemic, probably influenza, though the comic book calls it typhoid.[83]

The story of Clara Barton illustrated not only the help her nursing care brought to the Civil War wounded but also the feminist struggle she fought even to be allowed to serve on the front. Also mentioned was her later work to establish the American Red Cross.[84] A stress on wartime heroism in the early 1940s shaped the account of Dr. Mary Walker. In other contexts, Walker's late career as eccentric feminist in top hat and trousers tended to be the focus of attention, but in her comic-book story the focus is her youth and service in the Civil War; she is celebrated as "First Lady of the Army Medical Corps." She had chosen her calling early: "I don't want to do girls' work. I want to be doctor like my daddy." Despite her medical degree, Walker is restricted in the Civil War to nursing duties at first, even though she is better skilled than some of the doctors under whom she is serving. In time, her skills are recognized. Her dress-reform interests are noted without being sensationalized, and her efforts on behalf of women's struggles for voting and entry to the professions are mentioned. She is shown receiving the Congressional Medal of Honor for her wartime service and looking back with satisfaction at what women had achieved by the end of her life.[85] In a presentation of Elizabeth Blackwell's pioneering entry into the medical profession, three of the four pages are devoted to her attempts to enter medical school, with only one more frame each to show women patients who regard her medical work as improper for a lady, her opening of a dispensary staffed by women, and her establishing the first women's medical college.[86]

CONTEMPORARY MEDICINE CAME TO BE PORTRAYED AS HISTORY

True-adventure comic books, like the other media of the 1930s and 1940s, seamlessly integrated the tradition of Pasteur, Koch, and Reed with the present, placing new discoveries such as penicillin into the canon of medical history, associating contemporary researchers with greats of the ages, and bestowing on present-day medicine a golden aura of the past. The most substantial examples of contemporary medical celebrities in the comics are Alexander Fleming, as the main star of the penicillin discovery, and Sister Elizabeth Kenny, as the most visible practitioner in the polio field before Jonas Salk came to the fore in the 1950s.

Penicillin began receiving significant newspaper and magazine coverage only in 1943, as the scale-up to industrial production was making headway. By late 1944, the story of its discovery and use was being explained in the comic books in the same manner as discoveries from earlier times. It appeared first in *True Comics* 41 (December 1944) and then in *Science Comics* 1 (January 1946). Both comic books mentioned the story on the cover. Penicillin's development could not be recounted

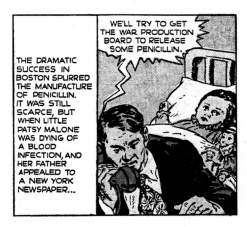

FIG. 78. "We'll try," panel of "Penicillin," *True Comics* 41 (December 1944), 21. © 1944 True Comics, Inc., a subsidiary of the Publishers of Parents' Magazine. Used with permission. All rights reserved. Author's collection.

strictly as a biography because the narrative had to include several teams in different institutional settings. First, there was Fleming's discovery in England, which had no effect until it was later reconfirmed by Ernest Chain and Howard Florey; this work was followed by the animal and human tests using only the limited amounts of penicillin that could be cultivated in the laboratory. Under the pressure of war in Europe, the project moved to the United States, where government and industry worked together to produce it successfully in the quantities demanded by the war.[87] *True Comics* included a recent event from just the prior year, when a little girl's special treatment made the news in daily papers in August 1943. The father of Patsy Malone, who was dying of a blood infection, appealed to friends at a New York newspaper after he read about the use of penicillin in treating victims of a nightclub fire in Boston (fig. 78). When little Patsy was treated and survived (fig. 67), the medical miracle generated further press coverage, with a happy child at the center of touching human-interest stories.[88] Patsy's story was retold some months later, with her photo, in the *Time* magazine edition that featured Fleming as the cover story.[89] *Time*'s photo of Patsy in bed with a doll at her side was probably the model for her image in *True Comics*. Not surprisingly, *Science Comics* gave less attention to the human-interest side of penicillin's history than *True Comics* did, while devoting more attention to the laboratory work: molds, bacteria, the difficulties of industrial production, and the need to develop strains that would grow submerged instead of just on the surface of the nutrient medium.[90]

Even a decade before Jonas Salk and the March of Dimes gave the world a polio vaccine, stories about the children's disease were remarkably upbeat. In the comics, efforts to deal with polio were turned into success stories. Not surprisingly, President Roosevelt's overcoming his disability and various efforts of the National Foundation for Infantile Paralysis were included in these naturalistic cartoons. The polio victim as a hero is portrayed by a hardy young soldier, Philip Hawco.[91] The story is artificial, with little plot, but the device of a soldier chatting with buddies conveys a fair amount of information in a limited number of frames by getting the readers to imagine for themselves each situation that is suggested by a snapshot image with short dialogues or voice-over texts. Phil tells his army buddies all about "The Fight against Infantile Paralysis" when prompted by the exclamation "We can't believe you've ever had infantile, Phil! Why, you're just like us!" (see color plate 17).[92]

Phil describes the loneliness he had experienced as a cripple at home until he was sent to a special hospital for free treatments, through which he recovered completely. He then tells his buddies about the 1916 epidemic, in which people felt helpless and small-town residents feared catching the disease from fleeing city dwellers. He mentions the absence at that time of any central agency from which to get help. His buddies then learn about Warm Springs, Georgia, and a new foundation established to support treatment there (see color plate 18).[93] Other panels illustrate the founding of the National Foundation in 1938, the leadership that FDR's former law partner Basil O'Connor brings to the foundation, the therapy of Sister Kenny, and the participation of celebrity performers in fund-raising (fig. 79). Phil even explains just how funds are distributed by the National Foundation, and he asserts the patriotic need for all Americans to pull together to continue what "hard work and generosity have accomplished."[94] A remarkably rich and coherent account of three decades of polio's history is achieved in only eighteen panels on four pages.

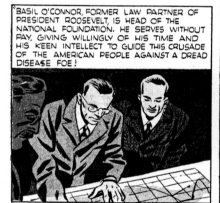
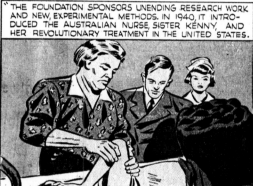

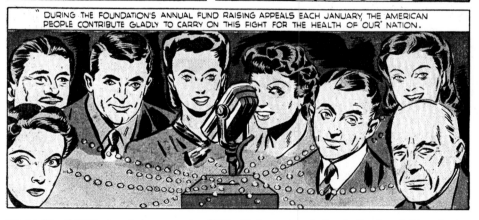

FIG. 79. "Basil O'Connor," three panels of "The Fight against Infantile Paralysis," *True Comics* 32 (February 1944), 28. © 1943 True Comics, Inc., a subsidiary of the Publishers of Parents' *Magazine*. All rights reserved. Used with permission. Author's collection.

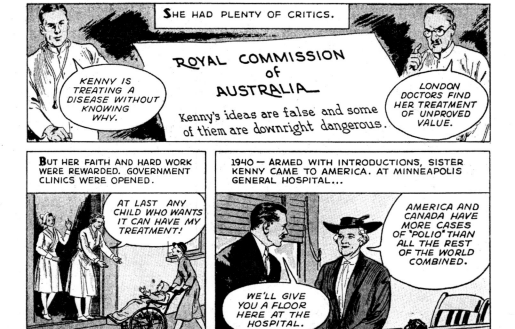

FIG. 80. "Kenny is treating," three panels of "Australian Bush Nurse," *Real Heroes* 5 (July 1942), 26. © 1942 The Parents' Institute, Inc. Used with permission. All rights reserved. Author's collection.

Sister Kenny's contributions to therapy are acknowledged in just one frame of soldier Phil's narrative. But in three other comic books, Kenny earned stories of her own (see color plate 19).[95] Her biography, when recounted at length, was molded to resemble that of a de Kruifian hero, moving from an obscure background to a passion for discovery, often facing ridicule from men in authority, and finally achieving therapeutic success and public acclaim (fig. 80). Several factors account for the substantial number of pages Kenny was given: the public's familiarity with infantile paralysis, the attention her work had received in the news media, the large role that children play in her story, and the fact that her approach to therapy was an active regimen of massage, exercise, and hot packs—more emotionally appealing than the competing immobilization technique.[96] Two of the stories close with the image of a ceremony in Australia dedicating a park in her honor, at which one of the participants is an old man whose polio had been cured by the treatments she applied when he was a boy. Continuing recognition of the individual pioneering patients echoes the attention given to the grown-up Newark boys, who had been the first Americans to receive Pasteur's injections for rabies.

In early 1943, Dr. Margaret Chung, another contemporary figure given a history in the comics, was featured in *Real Heroes* as "Mom Chung and Her 509 'Fair-

Haired Foster Sons.'"[97] In 1916, Chung had become the first U.S.-born Chinese woman to earn a medical degree in the United States. The cartoons illustrate the struggles faced by a woman becoming a doctor but also the pride Chung took in her success. Besides her medical practice, she devoted much energy, after the Japanese invasion of China in the 1930s, to gathering financial and political support in the United States for China's efforts to defend itself. She received media stories at many points in her long career, becoming more famous for her political and social activism than for her medicine. It was her work with airmen whom she informally adopted that prompted the title of the comic-book story about her: "Fair-Haired Foster Sons"; in adult magazines, the boys whom this unmarried woman looked after were usually called her "bastards."[98]

Mabel Keaton Staupers, a contemporary of Dr. Chung, also combined health care with activism. She had been one of the first African American nurses to earn an advanced degree. Working in Harlem, she rose to become a national leader in the nursing profession, and she used her position to advance the integration of African American women and men in the armed forces during and after World War II. The comic-book story conveys Staupers's status and achievements by showing her in meetings with first lady Eleanor Roosevelt and President Franklin Delano Roosevelt (see color plate 20).[99]

PATTERNS IN THE COMICS' PICTURE OF MEDICAL PROGRESS

Despite the diversity of historical figures and the medical challenges they faced, these dozens of stories shared a consistent picture of medical progress, and it seems likely that the young readership absorbed the beliefs and values they expressed. That the stories were often formulaic, uncritical, and sometimes erroneous is beside the point. Popular attitudes are less clearly embedded in an era's fine art or high literature than in what has been called its "formula literature."[100] As active commemorations of medicine's past, these stories established a canonical group of familiar heroes, and the list gained an apparent objectivity by the reappearance of the same figures within this genre and across genres.

Comic-book history of medicine cultivated an appreciation for medicine just as art history does for fine art. Given the young audience, it would be surprising if the comic-book stories did not have some effect on career aspirations as well. In these stories, even the most unusual people are portrayed as potential role models, and ordinary children are helped to identify with them because the narratives often begin with the heroes' humble origins and show how these individuals became devoted to science or medicine in their youth (as in fig. 75). The modeling of career roles is made explicit in a reader's letter from Harold Copeland of The Bronx, New York, published in *True Comics*. Harold was a thirteen-year-old who wanted to become a doctor and wrote to thank the company for a story about the Red Cross in an early issue. The editors asked whether he also liked their recent story about Dr. Grenfell and promised that more like it would be coming soon.[101]

These comic books directly encouraged public support for science, not only by making doctors' actions heroic but also by depicting the social benefits of scientific progress and by illustrating the necessity of funding of research. Cattle ranchers and wine merchants invited laboratory workers to solve practical problems. Parents and doctors fretted over dreaded ailments incurable without new knowledge. When the Mayo brothers become wealthy, they funded a large research center. And even two nonmedical stories about the financier and statesman Bernard Baruch both emphasized the importance of providing funds for medical progress. In the first of these stories, readers learned that "in 1944, he provided $1,100,000 for medical research." One scientist tells another, "With Baruch's money we can do research that will help returning veterans." The next panel's caption explains that "he also spends thousands of dollars on private investigations." Baruch gives instructions to a colleague: "I want a thorough report on the methods of making artificial limbs for veterans."[102] In a second story the following year, Baruch was credited with building a hospital after World War I and then with supporting research after World War II. The seventy-six-year-old visitor asks a hospitalized veteran, "How are you coming along? That arm any better?" The bandaged patient replies, "Yes, Sir! We vets sure appreciate the medical research you're sponsoring, Mr. Baruch!"[103] Similarly, the penicillin and polio stories in the comic books strongly emphasize the good things that come when substantial resources are devoted to research and development.

Among the medical heroes, the number of American women is significant, despite the dominance of European and American men. Given the dearth of attention to minority-group doctors and nurses in any writings of that era, one cannot be surprised that these books may have had only a single example each of an African American health hero and an Asian American one. That the limited presence of black medical heroes derived more from historiography than from any editorial or audience prejudice is confirmed by the numerous stories of many other black notables in the true-adventure comics, such as Mary McLeod Bethune, George Washington Carver, Frederick Douglass, Paul Robeson, Jackie Robinson, and Harriet Tubman. And even during a war against Germany and Italy, medical heroes from these countries were not ignored, although there seem to have been no stories about the well-known Japanese American medical scientist Hideyo Noguchi.

Comic strips by their very nature require dramatization. Readers saw people in action and were given striking tableaux. Even when sitting alone and still, a person in a comic frame could be undergoing a change, as in the image of Edward Livingston Trudeau reading about Robert Koch's discovery (see fig. 73). Youthful readers saw men actively taking the steps to observe phenomena for themselves, to invent new concepts, and then to test them out. Though these stories are less didactic than science textbooks, many of the concepts are explained rather well in a compact form. In these wholesome little stories, comic-book art turns didacticism into dramatic situations that neatly convey both scientific information and moral inspiration. Attentive readers would easily have learned a fair amount of basic science that was worked into the historical narratives. These graphic stories automatically emphasize the concrete physical realities of the situation, including experimental conditions. Facts and evidence are paramount.

Although scientific theories are generally less visible than facts in the comics, there are two major exceptions: the ubiquitous germ theory of disease and a basic theory of scientific method. If readers learned rather little about how cells or germs live and die, how immunity or vaccination works, just how vitamins are essential to physiological processes, they repeatedly discovered that evidence, properly interpreted, was the only foundation for knowledge or cure. Hunches and intuition, guesses and lucky breaks all played a part, but these always needed to be verified by experiments. Again and again, comic-book readers were taken through the steps of a controlled experiment. This popularization of a highly simplified version of the experimental method of doing science was an important cultural achievement, however much scholars observe that actual scientific research rarely proceeds in accord with the simple model. The attempt to cultivate the rationality and materialism characteristic of the natural sciences was exactly what George J. Hecht, the originator and publisher of *True Comics*, had in mind.[104]

Many of the experiments depicted in the comic books also brought children face to face with suffering, death, and vivisection. The stories of yellow-fever research, for example, spotlight the experiments using human beings. And even children are shown dying in the diphtheria story (fig. 81). Some of the experiments to understand tuberculosis and pellagra are illustrated with sick or dying animals (in fig. 76, for example). The optimistic march of progress that pervades these stories stepped unhesitatingly over the dead patients, the sacrificed animals, and even the men who died from experimentally induced yellow fever, with a frank acceptance

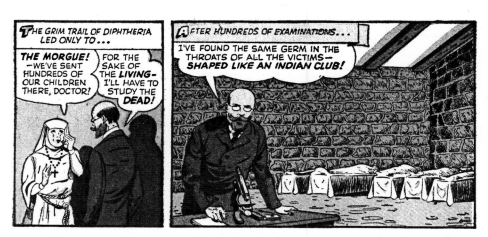

FIG. 81. "The morgue!" two panels of "The Conquest of Diphtheria," *Real Life Comics* 11 (May 1943), 31. © 1943 Nedor Publishing Company. All rights reserved. Author's collection.

of risk and death that was permissible in children's book in wartime. The prominence of visible suffering is explained partly by the demands of the graphic medium and partly by the violence that was being depicted routinely in the battle stories during the war.[105]

Probably the most detailed display of vivisection is in a remarkable story about Russian experiments with a mechanical heart-lung device published in the first issue of *Marvels of Science* in March 1946, "Dog Dead or Alive?"[106] This three-page story was clearly based on a film, *Experiments in the Revival of Organisms,* made in Moscow in 1940 and circulated in the United States.[107] The panels showed young readers such procedures as the draining of all a dog's blood, followed by observations of the inert animal ("his bloodless cadaver"). Then after the dog's being dead for fifteen minutes, the blood was pumped in again from the device serving as heart and lungs. "Twelve hours later the dog sat up, and, back on his feet again, ran barking to a friend he recognized!"[108] In two other frames, a device called the "autojector" maintains life in a dissected set of dog lungs, and a dog's dissected heart is kept beating regularly from the artificial supply of oxygenated blood. Four images show how the device supposedly kept a dog's severed head alive for many hours (fig. 82). Three frames illustrate tests confirming that the head is alive and functioning: its eyes blink in response to a bright light, it salivates when citric acid is applied to its lips, and its ears cock at the noise of a pistol firing blanks.[109] The comic-book images, which match the film closely, were probably based directly on a 1943 article in *Life* magazine, in which twenty-one frame enlargements from the movie were reproduced.[110]

This graphic display of scientific naturalism, unsuppressed in children's comics and in a family magazine, was remarkably different from the kinds of experimental procedures that could be shown in Hollywood movies of the era. The film industry's production code largely prevented the display of any images of vivisection or even of the actual injections of vaccines and therapies.[111] In schools, by contrast, vivisection was not yet taboo—even if sex was. A special "text edition" of *Microbe Hunters* published in 1948 for use in schools retained "Massacre the Guinea Pigs" as the uncensored title of the chapter on diphtheria research while silently cutting the entire chapter about Paul Ehrlich's work on a magic bullet to cure syphilis.[112]

But if the unavoidable presence of death and vivisection in the 1940s true-adventure comic books may be surprising to some twenty-first-century readers, something that might have been expected was not found in these books, namely, the evil doctor and the mad scientist. This anticipated figure is missing because the true-adventure comics drew their heroes from historical and contemporary reality, and such devilish figures had simply never existed outside the imagination of Mary Shelley and her many heirs. Furthermore, the naturalistic ideology of secular humanism that seems to have shaped the overall enterprise of the true-adventure comic books set itself in opposition to the fantastic stories in the superhero comic books, and perhaps implicitly against science fiction and horror films as well. The motto "truth is . . . more thrilling than fiction" was not just a promotional slogan; it expressed the values of

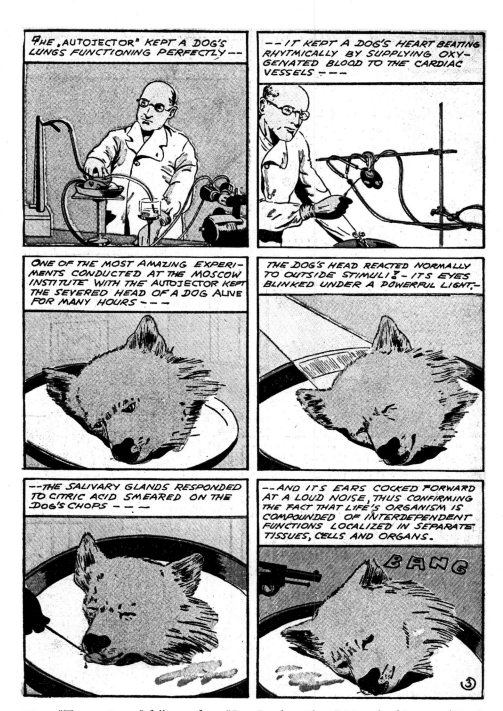

FIG. 82. "The autojector," full page from "Dog Dead or Alive?" *Marvels of Science* 1 (March 1946), 48. © 1946 Charlton Publications, Inc. All rights reserved. Author's collection.

the enterprise. In many of these stories, of course, laymen's superstition, ignorance, and obscurantism challenge a scientific doctor, and occasionally benighted physicians try to hold back the march of progress. But these traditionalists have nothing in common with the diabolical monsters who made appearances in the Superman and Batman comics and in Hollywood's horror films of the same era.

The humane, edifying stories in the true-adventure comics present an important corrective to a commonplace notion that scientists have been universally represented in twentieth-century popular culture as goofy nerds, at best, and more commonly as deeply vicious madmen. Such figures have often been in the center of scholarship on the popular imagery of the scientist.[113] This skewed portrait may have arisen by scholars' paying undue attention to creative works of literature, film, and fantasy comics without looking sufficiently at comic books such as these or at this genre's important nonfiction predecessors: biopics, radio dramas, and a substantial body of popular writing about medical history.

Did these colorful little history stories have any effects on children's thinking and feeling about medicine? Did stories about the past shape attitudes toward the present and the future? For several reasons, it seems likely that they did. First was the powerful consistency of the image across all the stories. Second, by mixing the historical heroes with contemporaries, these colorful books helped to aggrandize medical research and the medical profession for the wartime and postwar United States. Third, the image in the comic books resonated strongly with that exhibited in radio shows, films, books, and magazines. Further, these popular incarnations of medical history were widely dispersed in the popular culture.

The triumphalism observed in medical history stories across the full range of popular media in the 1930s and 1940s helped create a widely shared social optimism about medical science. Historian George Basalla, in his groundbreaking study of what he called "pop science," postulated a relationship between the image of science in popular culture and "public willingness to support scientific education and research."[114] In my view, these popular images and values were what helped raise funds for the March of Dimes and its research projects for nearly twenty years, before its successful vaccine emerged. They were the attitudes that conditioned reactions to the polio-vaccine trials in the 1950s. They were the same values that a few years later helped to mold responses to the heart transplants and the trials of the first artificial hearts, as journalists and readers at the time of those breakthroughs had been children or teens during the heyday of comic books filled with "real" medical heroes. Although it would be claiming too much to attribute new postwar funding for biomedical research, especially the great expansion of the National Institutes of Health in the later 1940s, to the optimistic image of medical progress found in children's magazines, the powerful reinforcement of common themes in mass culture should not be discounted. In the comics, as in the wider culture, this was medicine's golden age.

As an assessment of the impact of such stories in the comic books and in the other mass media, the depiction of medicine that they offered probably had more social power than it could have had in another era, just because the popular culture of the 1940s was so consistent and ubiquitous. Although it would be wrong to exaggerate consensus for politics or intellectual life in that era, the visual imagery seen in comic books and in *Life* magazine thoroughly pervaded the culture, and it provided a unifying complex of shared impressions. In that era, when popular culture was more unified and people more frequently sat together near a "common hearth" to consume en masse the iconic photographs in *Life* magazine as a universally held image of the United States, people had more in common than they did in later years, when U.S. popular culture became more fragmented.[115]

PART IV

THE MODERN IMAGERY OF MEDICAL PROGRESS

CHAPTER 9

LIFE LOOKS AT MEDICINE

MAGAZINE PHOTOGRAPHY AND THE AMERICAN PUBLIC

The great fascination of these old magazines is the completeness with which they "date." Absorbed in the affairs of the moment, they tell one about political fashions and tendencies which are hardly mentioned in the more general history books.

—George Orwell

WHAT WAS THIS magazine that brashly took the title *Life*? Not *Boy's Life* or *Outdoor Life*, or even *American Life*, but simply and boldly *Life*—in huge white letters framed in solid red on the upper corner of the large cover photograph? *Life* magazine began in November 1936 and quickly gained a circulation in the millions. To print *Life's* large photographs with sufficient clarity, it was necessary to develop special coated paper and to reengineer printing plants. The scale was staggering: a single week's issue required seven million pounds of paper and two hundred thousand pounds of ink. After the magazine was printed in Chicago each week, enough copies were bundled in four hundred miles of wire to fill 360 railroad boxcars on their way to homes in the United States.[1] The magazine prospered from President Franklin Roosevelt's second term in the midst of the Great Depression through the countercultural 1960s until its sudden death at the end of 1972.[2] For the mid-twentieth century, *Life* magazine was perhaps the most potent single force in shaping Americans' visual images of themselves and the world at large.[3]

Life became Americans' family photo album. People returned to copies of the magazine again and again for years. Before television, only *Life* provided images that became so familiar they took on the status of icons. Although people might see cheerleaders or nurses or doctors in their own lives or in their local newspapers, it was *Life* photographers who created in the public's eye such archetypes as The Cheerleader, The Army Nurse, or The Medical Researcher. Ordinary Americans came to picture things around them as posed and framed by *Life*'s photographers and editors, who somehow made their images seem more real than reality itself. And for people and things not readily observed in everyday life, *Life*'s photos were even more powerful in creating shared images, whether of a celebrity such as Marilyn Monroe or of a promising new device such as the huge two-million-volt linear accelerator hovering over a patient and touted as "fresh hope on cancer."[4] The power of magazine photographs in establishing a uniform culture was delineated as early as 1923 by Edwin E. Slosson, founding editor of Science Service, even though he could not then have imagined the overwhelming presence that *Life* managed to achieve fifteen years later. Slosson claimed that "the seeing of the same pictures and reading the same magazines at the same time by the greater part of the one hundred million people of the United States tends toward conformity in tastes and ideas, toward the standardization of the American."[5]

THE NATURE OF LIFE

For the American public, *Life* took on many roles. *Life* liked to be the ringmaster for a circus of astonishing scenes. *Life* could also be a docent, gently and helpfully instructing readers about history, art, science, and culture. Often *Life* played the intrepid reporter, capturing scenes of political drama or monstrous disaster. At times the magazine was a muckraker, and at others a comedian. It happily flacked Hollywood films, stars, and starlets. But sometimes *Life* was the preacher, reminding readers of their duties, helping them honor their ancestors, and scolding their hypocrisies. Quite frequently it was the teenager looking for a good time. At the same time, *Life* was the adventurous explorer, taking a camera into exotic or exclusive haunts, whether that be a medical school classroom or the palatial homes of the very rich, the undersea world or an operating room—or even inside the human body itself. If its visual style was often breathless, *Life* could also be thoughtful—if seldom humble. Yet even when it chose to be caring and reflective rather than splashy, this was achieved with no sacrifice of its graphic stylishness.

Life was more than entertainment and civics, the subjects for which it is perhaps best known. It was a voice for decency and progress. It was progressive in the old sense, especially in its enthusiasm for the rationality of science and medicine. But this enthusiasm was less that of the public-relations man than that of the easygoing high school science teacher, with a cheery display of show-and-tell from the natural and physical worlds, offering photographs and diagrams of the wonders of nature and of scientists' exploration of them. *Life* was also the school nurse with calm explanations of sex and childbirth, assuring us that natural events were nothing to be embarrassed about.

In more than a thousand news articles and features, with photographs iconic and prosaic, *Life* portrayed medicine with images that sank into people's brains and remained there. Medical stories were numerous and frequent, averaging two or more each month. Among U.S. magazines, *Life* was the one most likely to be saved and re-read over months, years, and even decades, except perhaps for *National Geographic.* Family homes and barber shops and doctors' offices held on to their copies of *Life,* and people went back to those copies again and again for the delight and satisfaction they continued to find there. In an age before television, old *Life* magazines entertained many children on rainy days at home. Before the rise of broadcast television, *Life* was the United States' most consistent purveyor of visual impressions, including an imagery of the medical world, with wide-ranging effects on public awareness and consciousness.

Because of *Life*'s prominence—its very hegemony in Americans' imagery of themselves—its pictures of medicine shaped ordinary people's understandings of medicine and attitudes toward it. These pictures articulated the notions of medical progress established by the popular histories of medicine that flourished in the 1920s and 1930s. They shared themes and stories with the true-adventure comics (even providing images that were sometimes copied directly into the comic books). *Life*'s interest was more in the present than in the past, yet history of medicine had its place, serving the same function as in the comic books, namely, to show continuity of effort in medical research.

Life detailed new kinds of medical care, the latest discoveries, and active medical research. It published many memorable photos of medical figures, making some of them iconic (fig. 83). Equally important, it provided careful explanations that were intellectually engaging and sometimes of practical use; a remarkable amount of science was successfully conveyed by the magazine's pictures and diagrams. And by taking ordinary citizens into specialized medical settings such as cancer clinics and operating rooms, *Life* normalized those settings, perhaps reducing anxiety for patients and their families who might be entering them. It supported biomedical research by presenting it in interesting ways, by making clear the importance of research funding, and by cheerfully celebrating the use of animal and human experiments to generate life-saving science and technology. *Life* also offered sympathetic reporting on public-health activities, including sex education, all grounded within a sensible, humane naturalism.

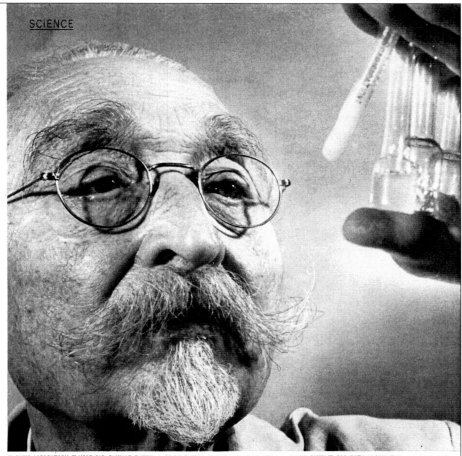

IN PARIS LABORATORY 77-YEAR-OLD CAMILLE GUERIN, A CO-DEVELOPER OF BCG, HOLDS UP DRY AND LIQUID SAMPLES FOR BOTH VACCINATION AND ORAL USE

TUBERCULOSIS VACCINE

U.S. doctors try out immunization drug after years of controversy

Snubbed by U.S. doctors for years, the only vaccine known to immunize against tuberculosis has now been accepted for a large-scale tryout in this country. The vaccine, called BCG, is already being given to test groups in eight states. In one group of 3,000 American Indians the tuberculosis mortality rate among those vaccinated was nine times lower than among the unvaccinated.

Discovered in 1908 by two French scientists, the drug is made by growing the germs of cow tuberculosis in a medium which weakens the organisms' virulence. During early tests the vaccine received a bad name when 75 German children died after being injected. These deaths were actually caused by a technician's mistake. But medical men continued to hold BCG suspect until years of tests proved that the vaccine was not only harmless but built up a high degree of immunity in persons not already infected. In Europe some 15 million children are being vaccinated. In the U.S. mass immunization may be years away, but at least BCG has won the support of many tuberculosis experts.

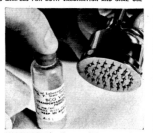

VACCINATOR has 40 prongs which puncture a drug-soaked paper, deposit vaccine in holes in patient's skin.

FIG. 83. Splash page, "Tuberculosis Vaccine," *Life,* May 2, 1949, 67. Photograph of Camille Guerin by Carl Perutz of Magnum; lower photograph by Cornell Capa. Page © 1949 Life, Inc. Reprinted with permission. All rights reserved. Author's collection.

INFORMATION THAT STICKS AND HONEST SCIENCE

Laying out the magazine's goals in an advance prospectus, *Life*'s founder, Henry R. Luce, provided a strong vision for a new kind of weekly magazine. Although coverage of science and medicine easily fit within Luce's general goals for the new magazine, these subjects were accorded special status. Luce wrote that he wanted *Life*'s readers

> to see life; to see the world; to eyewitness great events; to watch the faces of the poor and the gestures of the proud; to see strange things—machines, armies, multitudes, shadows in the jungle and on the moon; to see man's work—his paintings, towers and discoveries; to see things thousands of miles away, things hidden behind walls and within rooms, things dangerous to come to; the women that men love and many children; to see and to take pleasure in seeing; to see and be amazed; to see and be instructed.[6]

From the start, science received an exemption from constraints affecting other coverage. Luce himself made the case:

> We shall not insist that Science shall always be pictorially arresting. In fact, to Science we will give the privilege of not being pictorially arresting. We will be happy to have pictures which, if given a little time and study by the reader, will yield information which sticks. . . . The fact is that today most people—most educated people—walk through a world which has been amazingly analyzed by Science without having the least idea of what the world looks like to the eye of the Geologist, the Engineer, the Astronomer, the Biologist, the Chemist or the Bacteriologist. . . . We have . . . to put up a sign: "Honest Science Sold Here."[7]

Luce wanted honesty in science coverage, and he got it. But he got celebration as well. And that, too, was in keeping with the magazine's general approach to all its subjects. Again, in Luce's own words: "*Life* has a bias. *Life* is in favor of the human race, and is hopeful. *Life* likes life. *Life* is quicker to point with pride than to view with alarm." Luce once remarked to a colleague, "I always thought it was the business of *Time* to make enemies—and of *Life* to make friends."[8]

Such grand ambitions required a realignment of text and image in magazine layouts, giving photographs a new role. To accomplish this, Luce drew on new technology and editorial styles borrowed from Europe. Photographs had been appearing in books since the mid-nineteenth century, but they were printed separately from the text and tipped into the books. By the 1890s, the new halftone screening process allowed newspapers and magazines for the first time to print images and text together. But until the late 1920s, the photographs in magazines and newspapers usually served just to illustrate the text. They did not carry the meaning of a story, nor did they control the layout of words and images on the page. Breaking this mold, visionary European photographers and editors developed the photoessay, which reversed the usual functions of text and image. New technologies supported pictures' rise in status: the smaller and lighter—hence candid—Leica camera (1924) and the flashbulb (1925). The pioneers in this new magazine genre were *Vu* in Paris (1928) and the *Berliner Illustrirte Zeitung* (founded in 1890 but transformed in 1929 by introduction of the photoessay). *Life* in the United States (1936) was quickly followed by *Picture Post* in England (1938).[9]

Life magazine was primarily a picture show. Aiming high, it secured outstanding camera work. The originality of the photographs and the imaginative editing made *Life*'s medical coverage far more influential than similar stories in its competitors, *Look,* the *Saturday Evening Post,* and weekend newspaper supplements. As in museum exhibits, arrangement and aesthetics were just as crucial as the images selected. The goal in *Life*'s photoessays—and even in many of its single photos as well—was to have the pictures tell the story. As *Life*'s first science editor later recalled, "Pictures showed what was happening. In truth, the words underneath the picture were the illustration; the story was carried by the picture. What you did with the caption was answer the questions excited by the picture."[10] This approach was, of course, the same one used in comic strips.

Medical stories were handled by the magazine's science editor, and the coverage conformed to the principles of honesty and significance. Although foolishness and anger were excluded, this did not mean that humor was absent from the medical stories or that the stories lacked a firm point of view. In the medical photographs, the visual aesthetic often adopted one or more of three common modes: celebration or veneration, strong internal composition, or eccentricity. All three approaches strongly shaped the image and the viewer's reaction to it—within, of course, Luce's bounds of honesty and optimism. Individual heroes of medical discovery were usually honored with a photo portrait. Often the camera moved in close to shoot from a low position so that viewers looked up at the figure, like worshipers gazing at a statue in a church. With the surroundings reduced to a minimum, one larger-than-life figure usually dominated the composition.

Life photographers used many compositional structures, but one that the editors seem to have held in great favor was the generation of rhythmic patterns achieved through repetition of elements, often similar figures in groups or massed as a crowd in which no single person or object dominates. But the overall harmony, often embodying a strong feeling of geometric symmetry, caught a reader's eye. Alfred Eisenstaedt repeatedly employed this technique to great effect, as in an early photoessay on nursing students (figs. 84 and 85).

Opposite, top: **FIG. 84**. Cover, "Student Nurses," *Life,* January 31, 1938. Photograph by Alfred Eisenstaedt. Cover © 1938 Life, Inc. Reprinted with permission. All rights reserved. Author's collection. *Bottom:* **FIG. 85**. Splash pages, "The Student Nurse Prepares for an Arduous but Noble Profession," *Life,* January 31, 1938, 40–41. Photographs by Alfred Eisenstaedt. Pages © 1938 Life, Inc. Reprinted with permission. All rights reserved. Author's collection.

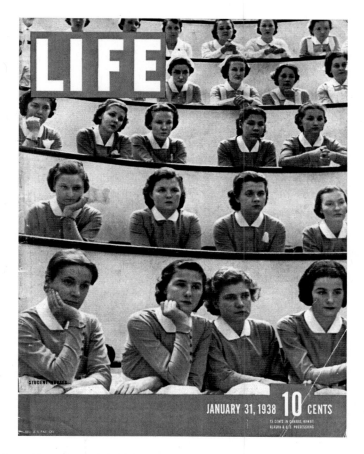

LIFE

STUDENT NURSES

JANUARY 31, 1938 **10** CENTS

15 CENTS IN CANADA, HAWAII
ALASKA & U.S. POSSESSIONS

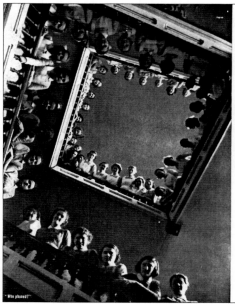

"Who phoned?"

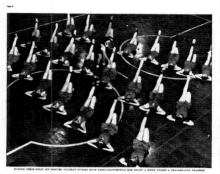

DURING THEIR FIRST SIX MONTHS STUDENT NURSES MUST TAKE CALISTHENICS ONE NIGHT A WEEK UNDER A TRAINED GYM TEACHER

THE STUDENT NURSE PREPARES FOR AN ARDUOUS BUT NOBLE PROFESSION

At Roosevelt Hospital School of Nursing she studies, has fun, cares for the sick

Most of the 49 nurses peering into the door will at left have no caps. This means that they are novices. Fresh from their high schools, they entered the Roosevelt Hospital School of Nursing in New York last Sept. 15 to train for a difficult but noble profession. By now the few months have been climacteric. March 11 will be the first important day in their new careers. For then, with solemn ceremony, they will be "capped" by the school director. The caps they will don their probationary status and officially become analysts in a great sisterhood of healers. Two and a half years later they will again line up for an important ceremony, this time to receive the golden pin that qualifies them finally for the worthy title of graduate nurse.

In the meantime they will have studied hard at microbiology, hygiene, materia medica and the science of nursing, will have spent hours of vigil in wards, will have had classes in nutrition and psychology. But not all of a nurse's life, as these pictures by Alfred Eisenstaedt show, is hard work. The modern nurse plays hard, swims, dances, keeps herself fit, leads a healthy social life. For she well knows that nursing today requires more than knowledge. It calls for patience, devotion, tact and the reassuring charm that comes only from a fine balance of physical health and adjusted personality.

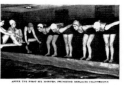

AFTER THE FIRST SIX MONTHS, SWIMMING REPLACES CALISTHENICS

CONTINUED ON NEXT PAGE

Eccentric images, even of science, could be justified under Luce's guidelines: "to see and to take pleasure in seeing; to see and be amazed; to see and be instructed." An article about the science museum in Cologne opened with a shot of a technician preparing the exhibit; but readers saw only his torso and legs, as his head and neck disappeared into the gaping mouth of a giant plaster head.[11] Twins offered both quirkiness and repetition when used to illustrate a story on heredity.[12] In the 1930s, blood transfusion was still a new procedure and a big advance, so *Life* returned to it again and again. One such story in 1938 covered a veterinary convention at which was announced success in establishing blood types for horses. Since the doctors could now perform safe transfusions in horses, they were photographed performing one in the hotel ballroom.[13] To celebrate a devoted donor who had given 871 pints of blood, *Life* used a startling upward shot of this vaudeville strongman towering over the viewer.[14] When doctors reported trials of powerful new drugs that restored the spark to lethargic tuberculosis patients, *Life* showed the patients dancing.[15] But sometimes *Life* simply captured the mundane from an unusual perspective, as when microphotography brought viewers inside an egg or into the body's interior.

Four "visual hallmarks" of *Life*'s photography have been delineated by Philip Gefter, a picture editor at the *New York Times,* as "clear subject matter, strong composition, bold graphic effect and at times even a touch of wit."[16] For me, *Life*'s striking photographs operated as they were intended: to amaze and instruct at the same time. But not everyone agreed. Marshall McLuhan, a well-known critic, denigrated *Life*'s "penny-arcade vision" as "nursery entertainment" for "homo boobiens," writing in 1948 that its "pictures and ads produce an aura of sentimental awe for the sub-rational reception of rapid-fire prose."[17]

Medical stories appearing in *Life* fell into one of three main types. A few dozen were long, artistic photoessays by such leading photographers as Alfred Eisenstaedt, Fritz Goro, Hansel Mieth, and W. Eugene Smith. Images from these essays are remembered decades later and have sometimes been reprinted. Far more numerous were the hundreds of news stories, including reports on the development of penicillin, the experimental trials of cortisone, the discovery of antihistamines, the testing of the polio vaccine, and the achievement of the first heart transplants. Feature stories, which did not require an immediate news hook, illustrated such subjects as surgical novelties, new instruments, war injuries and rehabilitation, and Sister Kenny's polio therapy, as well as sad conditions in mental hospitals and new reforms sparked by the exposure of institutional deficiency.

Life's dramatic images from all three kinds of stories remained vivid long after the reader turned the page. *Life*'s most forceful photographs of medical progress — blood banking, heredity, the X-ray campaign against tuberculosis, the use of animals in medical research, Salk's polio vaccine — persisted in people's minds. *Life* achieved this effect primarily by means of artistry within the images and the innovative layout of the pages. The power of these iconic photographs, their sheer attractiveness, helps explain why readers continued to page through long-out-of-date issues.

MEDICINE IN LIFE: *THE FIRST YEAR*

Right from the outset, *Life's* attention to medical subjects received accolades from readers. In the second issue, dated November 30, 1936, *Life* introduced an enduring and popular feature, "Speaking of Pictures." The initial installment carried an intentionally understated title, "This Is a Brain Operation." But the novelty of close-up photos of surgery on the human brain, as well as other insider images that followed them, grabbed the attention of laypeople and professionals alike. Appreciation by physicians and medical societies was recorded not only in the magazine's letters column but also in *Life's* advertising and in commentary by other magazines.

Within a few months, *Life* introduced its first science cover story by crowding its cover with "274 Laboratory Mice." The photograph's design abandoned internal composition in favor of uninterrupted repetition, a common aesthetic device in *Life,* offering a semiabstract composition in shades of black, white, and gray (fig. 86). The picture stimulated curiosity since the purpose of the mice was not stated on the cover. These mice were, however, more than just a cute pictorial tease; they were essential participants in the story of research. "U.S. Science Wars against an Unknown Enemy: Cancer," a seven-page story with thirty-nine images, presented the clinical picture, the nature of the research, the coordinated medical efforts, and the best remedies then known, with rubrics that sustained the title's military metaphor.

The large splash-page photograph was captioned "Biggest Gun in the War against Cancer Is Crocker Laboratory's 1,250,000-volt X-Ray Machine." The following page opened with the caption "Here Is the Enemy: Living Cancer" and a microphotograph of a dividing cancer cell. "Some Captains in the Cancer War" used ten photo portraits, with names that almost sound like royal titles: Andervont of Harvard, Ewing of Memorial, and so on. This style presumes that the public will—or should —recognize the names and the institutions. "Mice Replace Men on the Cancer Battlefield" showed living mice with various tumors alongside microphotographs comparing healthy and cancerous mouse mammary tissue. Jackson Memorial Laboratory was described as the "biggest source for cancer mice in the U.S.," supplying 150,000 each year for research, about one-third of those for cancer work. The laboratory head, Dr. Clarence Cook Little, "has made valuable discoveries which tend to substantiate the theory that susceptibility to cancer is inherited."[18] The section "Doctors Can Find and Cure Early Cancer" opened with a large photograph of an "aspirational biopsy," showing the needle entering a breast, "whose retracted nipple and 'orange-peel' skin indicate cancer." "Metastasis: Cancer on the Move" presented photos of dissected cancerous organs: lymph glands, heart, brain, and uterus (fig. 87). "Only the Surgeon's Knife or Radiation Can Cure Cancer" was illustrated by photos of lead-shielded devices, a radium handler in protective gear, high-voltage radiation generators, and two photos showing a man's face before treatment and then after his "dreadful skin cancer" was cured with two years of therapy.

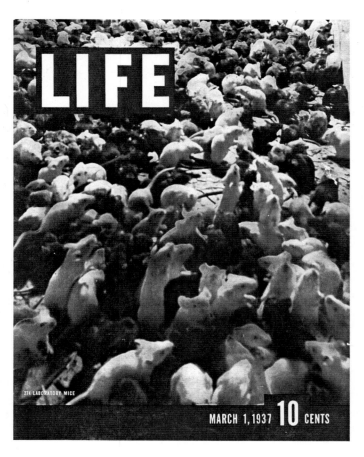

274 LABORATORY MICE

MARCH 1, 1937   10 CENTS

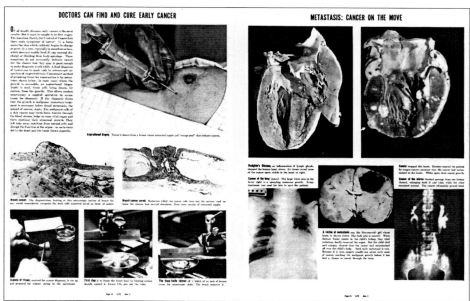

DOCTORS CAN FIND AND CURE EARLY CANCER

METASTASIS: CANCER ON THE MOVE

Although the presentation is livelier than a medical textbook and far less detailed, it stands as a remarkably rich examination of the subject, not bowdlerizing its gruesome features or exaggerating either fear or promise. *Life's* engagement with cancer in early 1937 formed part of a wide wave of agitation and publicity about the disease. In Congress, three different bills on cancer were introduced, with a compromise worked out during the summer, and the National Cancer Institute Act was signed into law by President Roosevelt in August.[19] *Life's* photoessay presented cancer as a natural phenomenon but did not dissociate the tissues and tumors from the patients who were receiving treatment. At a time when, it has been said, cancer was a word rarely to be spoken and a stigma as much as a diagnosis, the calm clarity of this extensive presentation offered its message in a loud and forthright voice, businesslike in tone, neither sensationalized nor sanitized. The frankness of its showing a syringe's needle penetrating human flesh challenged some cultural assumptions of respectability. The article prompted numerous commendation letters from doctors, medical societies, and members of the general public, but some readers also criticized the article for its disturbing pictures and for the fear it might cause.[20]

A single issue with four different medical stories offers a special opportunity to observe the variety of *Life's* subjects and its styles of coverage. "American Medical Association and the U.S. Public Health Service Join in Syphilis War with Movie" was a full-page news item with nine photos taken from a film shown at the AMA meeting in Atlantic City. Screenings were for physicians only. The unnamed film was intended to help physicians "look for, recognize, and follow up syphilitics," and it was a parallel effort to a campaign by Surgeon General Parran "to help laymen prevent the spread of syphilis." This kind of publicity among the general public seems intended to make it easier for physicians to bring up the delicate subject with patients; and it might also have created an incentive for patients to raise it themselves. *Life* observed that "while the taboo surrounding the word 'syphilis' has been somewhat dispelled, most people do not realize that early, persistent treatment will cure the majority of cases."[21]

In the same issue, readers could enjoy a lyrical photoessay about the work of the Frontier Nursing Service in Kentucky, with large, sweeping photos of the countryside alternating with close-ups of the nurses working with their impoverished, backwoods patients distant from hospitals and doctors' offices. "The Frontier Nurse" saluted the nurses' accomplishments, their devotion, and the dignity of the people they served.[22] Captions from two of the eleven images convey the article's

Opposite, top: **FIG. 86**. Cover, "274 Laboratory Mice," *Life*, March 1, 1937. Photograph by Henry M. Lester. Cover treatment © 1937 Life, Inc. Image © Henry M. Lester. Page reprinted with permission. All rights reserved. Author's collection. *Bottom:* **FIG. 87**. Interior opening, "Doctors Can Find and Cure Early Cancer" and "Metastasis," in "U.S. Science Wars against an Unknown Enemy: Cancer," *Life*, March 1, 1937, 14–15. Photographs by Henry M. Lester and William F. Payne. Pages © 1937 Life, Inc. Reprinted with permission. All rights reserved. Author's collection.

tone: "Midwives, old and new, chat by a Kentucky cabin. The modern Frontier Nurse must be a good horsewoman, a registered nurse, a tactful friend, quick to spur ahead when she hears outside her cabin the hoarse shout, 'Come on, ma'am. My woman's punishing turrible.'" "Prenatal visits during which the blood pressure is taken are a part of the routine for the busy Kentucky Frontier Nurses. Note the primitive plainness of this Kentucky mountaineer's well scrubbed home, the sturdy well-bred features of its hard-working mistress." These sympathetic images of working folks closely resembled other popular photographs of Depression-era families.[23]

Also appearing in the same issue were a news report with two whimsical photographs of gigantic models of an eyeball and an ear in a hygiene exhibit in Vienna, Austria, and a human-interest story about a young American who had been struck by infantile paralysis while abroad. He was being brought home from China in an iron lung at the cost of fifty thousand dollars.[24] This newly famous polio victim, Fred Snite, remained a popular media subject (*Life* itself did a follow-up a month later), and events in his life were photographed and reported in several newsmagazines over many years.[25]

Life soon established its credentials as a respected producer of unusual and captivating images of natural phenomena, even when the nature in question involved delicate subjects such as sex and reproduction. For example, in October 1937, still within the inaugural year, *Life*'s readers were invited to look inside a fertilized egg with twelve images in a developmental series, snapshots of a chick embryo from day one to day twenty-one. This story presented two pages of full-color photographs, very uncommon at this date.[26] There was no particular discovery here, just the rarity of the photographs. Although the story was titled "A Camera Looks inside the Egg" and it was placed in the Science and Industry section of the magazine, the primary effect was aesthetic, not practical. It is an early example of *Life*'s many articles celebrating the wonders of nature. The images were beautiful, even awesome, in an era when color photography was often crude, and embryology for the public was unprecedented. Of course, this sort of image became more familiar over time, partly through *Life*'s accomplishments. But even thirty years later, Lennart Nilsson's color photographs of human embryos and fetuses, which appeared in *Life* in 1965, would attract wide attention.[27] If this was teacherly show-and-tell, it rose to a sublime level.

Life chose to play the role of a friendly instructor, providing an invitation for many readers to explore a natural science they had not learned in school, given that only a small portion of Americans in the late 1930s had attended college and that fewer than half of them had attended high school. Even for those in school or college, no textbook of that era could afford to publish the kinds of illustrations that *Life* delivered weekly to American homes. *Life*'s curiosity included both natural phenomena and the scientific and technological manipulation of them in the laboratory. For example, the same issue that carried viewers inside the egg took them also into the realm of Erlenmeyer flasks, incubators, and microscopes in a story about the New Deal's Civilian Conservation Corps, "300,000 CCC Boys Get Pneumonia

Vaccine." Men receiving injections were in the lead photograph, but the other nine illustrations offered various laboratory scenes explaining the production process for the vaccine.[28]

MEDICAL COVERAGE KEPT GROWING

The week after *Life*'s first-anniversary issue, which had a year-old baby on its cover, the magazine published two articles that blended medical history with present-day news. "Tuberculosis: A Menace and a Mystery" was an eight-page photoessay with its most important pictures taken by Alfred Eisenstaedt.[29] Images marked by strong black-and-white contrasts and rhythmic patterns illustrated scientific research on tuberculosis, public-health activities, and patient care in rich detail. A half century of patients' experience and laboratory science at the Trudeau Sanatorium at Saranac Lake was included. The same issue reported a news story about a measles break-through: "Woman Researcher Identifies Measles Virus."[30] In time, the test developed by Jean Broadhurst, a bacteriologist at Teachers College of Columbia University, enabled doctors to identify highly contagious measles cases several days before the characteristic rash appeared, allowing the infected children to be isolated earlier and thereby reducing the spread of the disease.[31]

A few weeks later, *Life* published a major photoessay on therapeutic progress for pneumonia, an article almost as long as the cancer and tuberculosis stories. Although a decade later antibiotics would be used to control pneumonia, the best treatment in the 1930s was a complicated sequence of procedures, with individualized laboratory work required for each patient. The identification of a specific bacterial strain, followed by prompt treatment with serum of the same type, saved thousands of lives. This extinct therapy is now largely forgotten, but for nearly half a century it was one of the most prominent examples of a modern cure created in the laboratory.[32] This photoessay was given a news headline: "Pneumonia Morality May Be Cut in Half by Use of New Serums: Photographs for *Life* by Hansel Mieth."[33] The splash page was dominated by a huge, high-contrast close-up of something fleshy in a beaker of liquid, held up by a gigantic hand with darkness behind it and no further context. In a move that *Life* would use again and again, the reader was drawn into puzzling out the image before turning, already engaged by curiosity, to the text (fig. 88). The calm, ordinary prose that opened the article heightened the dramatic tease of the photograph, and its understated tone stressed the tragedy of the numerous victims: "In the glass above are two pieces of guinea pig lung. The one floating on top of the water is a healthy, air-filled specimen. The other sank to the bottom of the glass because it was solid from pneumonia. Any infected part of the 400,000 human lungs which are annually attacked by pneumococcus in this country would behave the same way if dropped into water." The article carefully explained to its readers that fighting pneumonia was complicated because of the many strains: four types known

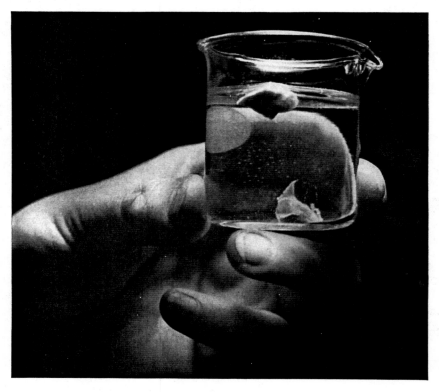

LIFE

VOL. 3, No. 25

DECEMBER 20, 1937

PNEUMONIA MORTALITY MAY BE CUT IN HALF BY USE OF NEW SERUMS

Photographs for LIFE *by Hansel Mieth*

In the glass above are two pieces of guinea pig lung. The one floating on top of the water is a healthy, air-filled specimen. The other sank to the bottom of the glass because it was solid from pneumonia. Any infected part of the 400,000 human lungs which are annually attacked by pneumococci in this country would behave the same way if dropped into water.

In the past, all sorts of treatments have been used to combat pneumonia which takes a toll of 100,000 lives in the U. S. every year. None has had any dependable effect. The principal reason was that the malady, though produced by a family of germs that looked alike and caused similar symptoms, actually consisted of 32 different types, which required different methods of attack. In 1913 three different types of pneumococci were definitely classified as I, II, and III and all the others summarily lumped under Group IV. The late Georgia Cooper in 1932 completed classification of all 32 types. Next month specific serums for all these types, covering 95% of all pneumonias, will be made available through Lederle Labora-

tories, Inc., following pioneer work done by the Rockefeller Institute of Medical Research. Even more important, a serum for the dreaded Type III, which kills half its victims, will go on the market. Thus the oft-repeated phrase " pneumonia control " may finally become more than a phrase. For, though the spread of pneumonia cannot yet be halted, the mortality rate may be reduced by more than 50% through use of serums.

In the next four months of cold weather, about 200,000 persons will contract pneumonia. Public health authorities point out that unless obstacles to the distribution of serums are overcome, some 25% of this group will perish. Because serums are at present expensive (from $35 to $150 for a case), philanthropic and public health funds will be required to aid their distribution. And because it is impossible to administer a specific serum until the specific cause of the pneumonia has been definitely typed, the primary need is for more typing stations throughout the country and the active co-operation of the general practitioner.

FIG. 88. Splash page, "Pneumonia Mortality," *Life*, December 20, 1937, 9. Photograph by Hansel Mieth. Page © 1937 Life, Inc. Reprinted with permission. All rights reserved. Author's collection.

in 1913 and thirty-two by 1937. But the report was optimistic: "next month specific serums for all these types, covering 95% of all pneumonias, will be made available through Lederle Laboratories, Inc., following pioneer work done by the Rockefeller Institute for Medical Research." Because the serums were expensive, philanthropic and public funds were required for an effort to halve the two hundred thousand cases likely to occur in coming months. This story might have been prompted by a national pneumonia campaign organized by Surgeon General Thomas Parran, or it might have already been in the works when Parran convened a national committee in November 1937 to raise pneumonia's status as a threat comparable to tuberculosis and venereal disease. A few years earlier, Parran had started a similar public-health program in New York State before taking the federal post.[34]

Additional text and photos illustrated pneumonia research, including the mice used to test the serum, the horses used to produce it, and the happily recovered John Forrest, a postal clerk treated for pneumonia at Harlem Hospital. Several narrative and visual elements in this story dated back to the first rabies shots: an ordinary citizen placed in the national spotlight when saved by a breakthrough, therapeutic materials extracted from animals, diligent laboratory investigations employing numerous workers, and the sacrifice of numberless animals. But what was different now was the power of the photoessay form and its presence in a single publication with a huge distribution. In earlier times, people across the country all encountered roughly the same story—American boys getting rabies shots in Paris, for example—but different people in different places saw it in different newspapers and magazines with variations in the verbal and visual presentations of it. Here, millions of Americans in the same week were all being introduced—through precisely the same images—to Mr. Forrest and the doctors who saved his life.

With the pneumonia story, *Life* succeeded in creating wide public awareness of the very latest developments coming out of East Coast medical centers. The magazine received and printed letters of acknowledgment and gratitude for its medical reporting. One Virginia physician thanked the magazine for making the public "conscious of the rapid strides in medicine," for doing it "in such a fine, simple and really understandable way," and for helping patients "know serum is a first resort and not a last resort." A Pennsylvania physician, proud to be a charter subscriber to *Life* magazine, applauded the "scientific, terse, and complete presentation of the pneumonia problem and its recent advances."[35] More significant, the article itself was even credited with saving a man's life in Florida, where the newest sera were not yet available. Just a week after the article was published, a Florida physician identified a patient's illness as "Type Three lobar pneumonia, the most deadly of all of the thirty-two known types of this dreaded disease." He contacted the patient's son in Pennsylvania, who "had seen the *Life* article and realized at once the seriousness of his father's condition." The son reached New York early the next morning and secured "all the available serum they had from the laboratory," taking it on an afternoon flight to Florida and delivering it to his father's bedside by 11:30 P.M. that night. His father recovered, and a long letter recounted the story in *Life*.

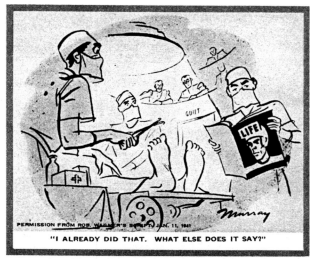

"I ALREADY DID THAT. WHAT ELSE DOES IT SAY?"

MEDICAL STORIES describing doctors' and surgeons' work have brought widespread praise from both the profession and readers, but LIFE never received quite the recognition suggested in this 1941 cartoon, drawn by Murray.

FIG. 89. "I Already Did That. What Else Does It Say?" cartoon signed by "Murray," first published in *Rob Wagner's Script*, January 11, 1941, as reprinted in *Life*, November 25, 1946, 6. Cartoon © 1941 Wagner Publishing Company. Caption © 1946 Life, Inc. Reprinted with permission. All rights reserved. Author's collection.

Accompanying the account was an editor's note: "Within a week Lederle Laboratories expect to begin distributing the serum for Type III pneumonia to their branch offices throughout the U.S."[36]

This youthful and ambitious magazine with a burgeoning circulation and a balance sheet still in the red recognized the double value of strong medical coverage: it engaged the general public while also garnering approval from professional elites. The editors singled out their medical coverage in a self-promoting page that ran in the same issue as the long letter about a man's life being saved by *Life*'s pneumonia story. This ad sampled the dozens of commendatory letters the editors had received from doctors and from medical associations, largely prompted by the photographic essay on cancer in the magazine's fifteenth issue. Headlined "The Doctor Looks at *Life*," this ad explained that "from hundreds of readers have come letters urging *Life* to go on using pictures to inform men and women about mankind's unending fight against disease and death." From the letters, both lay and professional, the "editors draw a deep encouragement, and reprint them here that *Life*'s readers may see that *Life* uses pictures not only to inform, but to inform responsibly and *accurately*."[37] As *Life*'s reputation for medical close-ups grew and as it continued to brag about the praise it received from doctors, the subject even prompted cartoons in other magazines (fig. 89).[38]

Despite *Life*'s significant attention to doctors and medical scientists inside the magazine, the only medical cover among the early issues showed that mess of mice. Even with many hundreds of medical stories, *Life* did not use a physician in a cover photograph until the late 1950s.[39] On the other hand, young nurses were quickly recognized as photogenic enough to catch readers' eyes on the newsstand. *Life*'s first nurse cover announced a photoessay by Alfred Eisenstaedt, "The Student Nurse: Her Work and Play at Roosevelt Hospital" (see figs. 84 and 85). In this article—an elegant photoessay with the story carried almost entirely by the images —Eisenstaedt and the editors gave free rein to the use of repetition and geometry in the compositional structure of the photographs. This stylistic technique heightened interest without distracting from content, at the same time that it made the essay more recognizable and memorable. In a group of two images, one photo showed three rows of students practicing calisthenics, and the other showed a row of swimmers poised to dive into a pool. For two operating-room views, the photographer composed the scenes with strong bilateral symmetry. The article was more than cheesecake and artistically patterned photographs; readers viewed the young women rising early, studying hard, working long shifts, and practicing a variety of skills. Over the following five years, five more *Life* covers featured nurses or nursing aides, with none after that.[40] Of the six stories, five focused on wartime health care services. Two major *Life* stories on the work of individual nurses, Elizabeth Kenny (in 1942) and Maude Callen (in 1951), were not cover stories.[41] Nor were any of several human-interest photoessays on medical subjects by W. Eugene Smith, a leading *Life* photographer.[42]

Life's commitment to honest science encouraged a naturalistic outlook even for such controversial subjects as venereal disease, the biology of childbirth, and the use of animals in medical research. While restraining themselves from direct advocacy or editorializing on contentious subjects, the editors tried to achieve Luce's original goal: "*Life* can open many eyes." In numerous articles, some of them unconventionally frank, the pages of *Life* showed its readers "what the world looks like to the eye of . . . the Biologist." For example, in 1938, when *Life* reported on Senate hearings for a controversial new campaign against venereal disease, the magazine eschewed moralizing and made its naturalistic sympathies clear in both the story and its photographs.[43] Two months later, in a story that featured forty-eight close-up stills of a birth sequence, *Life*'s editors opened many Americans' eyes with a candid public-health approach to reducing maternal and infant mortality. The photographs were taken from a nationally released educational film, *The Birth of a Baby,* and the article reported on the film's sponsors and its goals.[44] But seeing photographs of a baby's delivery was entirely new to most Americans and pushed the bounds of propriety. Contemplating the public's reaction, the magazine mailed a warning letter to all subscribers a week before publication, explaining that the center-spread pages of birth photos could be easily removed by parents who might feel a need to keep them from children's eyes.[45] Not surprisingly, the alert mostly seemed to generate excited anticipation. Few parents, it seems, removed the pages, and many wrote in to say how interesting all this was to their children. But photos of a naked infant and a draped pelvis seemed obscene to some police officers, who gave *Life* extra publicity by confiscating the issue at newsstands.[46] The *New Yorker* magazine immediately parodied the story in an extended cartoon sequence, "The Birth of an Adult."[47] The magazine's approach to pictures of childbirth was at once progressive, naturalistic, obscene in the eyes of some people, and slightly opportunistic. Eight years later, the editors referred to this article as "the most controversial story *Life* ever ran."[48]

LABORATORY ANIMALS

Life devoted a long, richly illustrated article in 1938 to the pros and cons of vivisection, asking in the title, "Animal Experimentation: Is It Essential to the Progress of Medicine?"[49] The opening statement from two famous female entertainers (former dancer Irene Castle McLaughlin and popular actress Marion Davies) presented the negative answer on one page. Then any pretense of a balanced debate immediately disappeared, as the facing page offered portraits and quotations from six famous men (intellectuals, scientists, and religious leaders) in support of the affirmative position: Surgeon General Thomas Parran; Dr. Alexis Carrel, co-inventor of the artificial heart with Col. Charles A. Lindbergh; Dr. Karl T. Compton, president of the Massachusetts Institute of Technology; Clifford Morehouse, editor of *The Living Church*; Archbishop John J. Cantwell of Los Angeles; and Ray Lyman Wilbur, president of Stanford University. The next seven pages supported vivisection with a series of twelve affecting images. Even if the presentation was one-sided, the celebrities were not unusual choices, as the caption explained: "No. 1 anti-vivisectionist is the plumed former dancer Irene Castle McLaughlin who now keeps a home for stray dogs. . . . Actress Marion Davies is the most powerful anti-vivisectionist through publisher-friend William Randolph Hearst." Castle, a friend of Hearst and of his mistress, Davies, was a popular spokesperson and lecturer for the cause; and Hearst's newspapers and magazines regularly published aggressive attacks and sensationalized articles about animal experimentation.[50] Hearst's media empire competed, of course, with *Time* and *Life*.[51]

Life's photoessay paired photographer Hansel Mieth's moving images of clinical and experimental settings with brief factual statements. Perhaps as a way to deflect some potential criticism from animal lovers, the editors specifically highlighted the personal experience of the photographer herself. "Miss Mieth, who spent three full days at [the Harvard Medical School], has specialized in scientific photographs, her most recent story being the sex-hormone experiments on chicks in last week's *Life*. She followed the Harvard experiments with more than professional interest since she owns a dog and several cats herself."[52]

A large photograph showing nurses in starched white uniforms carried a firmly factual caption: "Twenty-four cats proved iron lung could save children" (fig. 90).

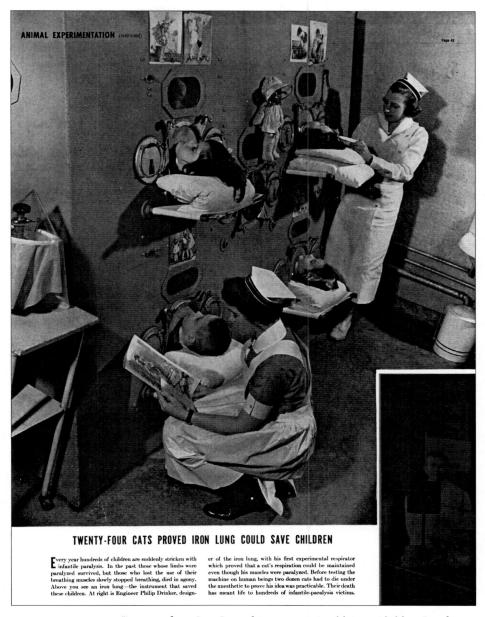

ANIMAL EXPERIMENTATION (continued)

Page 48

TWENTY-FOUR CATS PROVED IRON LUNG COULD SAVE CHILDREN

Every year hundreds of children are suddenly stricken with infantile paralysis. In the past those whose limbs were paralyzed survived, but those who lost the use of their breathing muscles slowly stopped breathing, died in agony. Above you see an iron lung—the instrument that saved these children. At right is Engineer Philip Drinker, design-er of the iron lung, with his first experimental respirator which proved that a cat's respiration could be maintained even though his muscles were paralyzed. Before testing the machine on human beings two dozen cats had to die under the anesthetic to prove his idea was practicable. Their death has meant life to hundreds of infantile-paralysis victims.

FIG. 90. Interior page, "Twenty-four Cats Proved Iron Lung Could Save Children," *Life,* October 24, 1938, 48. Photograph by Hansel Mieth. Page © 1938 Life, Inc. Reprinted with permission. All rights reserved. Author's collection.

The facing page had another photograph of nurses with patients, labeled "Giant Respirator Breathes for Paralysis Victims." The text explained that the experimental respirator invented by engineer Philip Drinker "proved that a cat's respiration could be maintained even though his muscles were paralyzed. Before testing the machine on human beings, two dozen cats had to die under the anesthetic to prove his idea was practicable. Their death has meant life to hundreds of infantile-paralysis victims."[53]

The next opening included a drawing of a seventeenth-century anatomical theater and antique portraits of Sir William Harvey, Louis Pasteur, and Lord Joseph Lister, matched with photographs showing that "dogs teach the students at Harvard Medical School to be good surgeons."[54] Photographs included close-ups of surgeons learning to tie knots on blood vessels and a dog being injected with an anesthetic. The final opening, headlined "Horse Serums, Tested on Rabbits, Save Thousands of Children's Lives Each Year," had a small image of a rabbit being held down for an injection ("diphtheria anti-toxin is tested on rabbits"), setting off two huge matching close-ups. Dominating the left-hand page was a horse's head and neck with a tube and needle placed in a vein to draw off the healing serum. And on the right was seen an angelic child's head and arm closely encircled by the arm of a nurse in a surgical mask while a male figure (only head and hands visible) held a syringe and needle from which he was injecting antitoxin into her arm.[55] The text masterfully combined the specific tale of one particular horse with grand observations about medical progress in general:

> Two gallons of blood are being drawn . . . from Patches, a horse given to the Massachusetts Antitoxin and Vaccine Laboratories. . . . Because the horse was inoculated with diphtheria germs, treated so as not to harm it, the blood will serve to produce diphtheria anti-toxin. [The] only way of testing the potency of the product is to inject it into a rabbit. . . . Anyone who has seen a diphtheritic infant suffocating, clutching at his neck as if to tear out the disease, pleading with eyes filled with terror, twisting his puffy fevered face, knows the value of anti-toxin. In modern times there is no need for children to suffer and die by the thousands from diphtheria, smallpox, or meningitis—for Patches and hundreds of other horses on U.S. laboratory farms spend their old age munching grass and producing the substances which prevent and help cure these scourges.

The article concluded solemnly, "The 20th Century has been prolific in important medical discoveries. These have cut deeply into the ravages of cholera, yellow fever, typhoid fever, encephalitis, and syphilis. Pernicious anemia can be controlled. From experimenting on dogs, Sir Frederick Banting produced insulin, the substance which keeps millions of diabetics alive. Critics of vivisection forget these facts."[56]

Life mustered all its graphic and rhetorical tools to make the case for animal experimentation, melding historical discoveries and contemporary achievements into one strong argument.[57] A growing list of well-known medical advances such as insulin and the iron lung supported the defense against antivivisectionists. The argument was clearly strengthened by the public's renewed familiarity with the historical cases such as vaccination, rabies shots, and the antitoxins—stories regularly seen and heard on the screen, on the airwaves, and in the comic books, as well as in *Life* itself. By the late 1930s, the general public's awareness of medical history as a history of triumphs made vivisection defensible in a way that had not been possible during prior antivivisection controversies of the nineteenth and early twentieth centuries.

The magazine's enthusiasm for the medical use of animals and the graphic images used in this article and elsewhere provoked no serious discomfort for Americans. Popular sensibilities on this issue, at least through the 1940s, were still being shaped, it seems to me, by most people's firsthand experience of the use and killing of lower animals.[58] Two *Life* stories from 1943 and 1944, for example, showed children themselves casually, even proudly, involved in the slaughter of animals, even in urban settings. In an article in 1943, children were encouraged to breed rabbits to cope with wartime food shortages: "Rabbits, Raising Them for Meat Is Now a Helpful Patriotic Hobby."[59] A second illustrated article the following year profiled a seven-year-old boy who killed rats for the three-cents-a-piece bounty, improving both the city environment and his own finances: "U.S. Children Help Wage Big War on Rats."[60]

A few years later, children were again in the forefront of a vivisection story in *Life*. A five-page report on the surgical breakthrough for "blue babies" opened with a huge photo of a child hugging a dog: "Michael Schirmer, 9, Meets Anna, the Dog That Saved His Life" (fig. 91). The headline explained further: "Blue Baby Research: Anna, Now 7 and Pensioned, Is One of the Canine Heroes in the Long Campaign That Has Saved Hundreds of Children."[61] This "dog hero" imagery was not unique. It appeared in newspaper articles too, and it was specifically promoted by medical research organizations.[62] The article's ten other photos diagramed the operation, showed that the animal surgery used the same antisepsis and anesthesia as human surgery, and gave readers close-ups into a surgical field dominated by a tangle of hemostats.

HEALTH POLICY ISSUES IN LIFE

Life's willingness to take on controversial subjects such as vivisection and sex education did not encompass American medicine's widest public quarrel, a political conflict over proposals for some form of national health insurance, an idea often characterized by opponents as threatening to establish "socialized medicine." The Depression had exposed the plight of millions of Americans who could not afford health care, just when medicine was gaining new powers in breakthrough after breakthrough. President Franklin Delano Roosevelt's plans for what became Social Security initially included some medical benefits for the elderly, but that component was dropped in fear that opposition from the American Medical Association

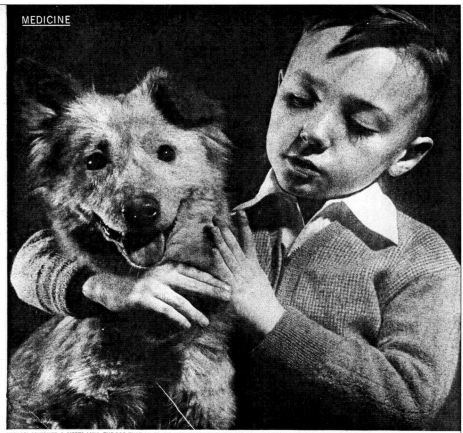

MEDICINE

MICHAEL SCHIRMER, 9, MEETS ANNA, THE DOG THAT SAVED HIS LIFE BY SERVING AS A SUBJECT ON WHICH SURGEONS PERFECTED THEIR "BLUE BABY" OPERATION

BLUE BABY RESEARCH

Anna, now 7 and pensioned, is one of the canine heroes in the long campaign that has saved hundreds of children

The affectionate meeting above took place recently at The Johns Hopkins Hospital, where Michael Schirmer, an ex-blue baby, still goes occasionally for checkups. There, on this visit, he met Anna, one of the dogs who made it possible for him to be alive and healthy today.

As a baby Michael spent most of his time in bed. His lips and fingernails were always blue, and if he tried to move around too much his whole body turned bluish. He could not even walk across a room without huffing and puffing; he had to be carried up and down stairs and wheeled in a buggy on the street. He had a heart defect that kept his body from getting enough oxygen, and he seemed destined to be a cripple until a premature death.

About that time, however, Dr. Alfred Blalock and Dr. Helen Taussig of Johns Hopkins were using Anna and 75 other dogs in a long experiment designed for children like Michael. Their surgical techniques were too dangerous to risk on human babies; so Anna and her colleagues became the first subjects. The operation (*pp. 106, 107*) was a success—and gradually Dr. Blalock perfected his techniques until they could be used with relative safety on a human being. Since then at least 2,000 blue baby operations have been performed in the U.S., with a better than 80% record of success. Anna, now a middle-aged 7 but still hearty, is a pensioner in the Johns Hopkins kennels, the heroine of one of medicine's most spectacular triumphs.

FIG. 91. Splash page, "Blue Baby Research," *Life*, March 14, 1949, 105. "Michael Schirmer, 9, meets Anna, the dog that saved his life by serving as a subject on which surgeons perfected their 'blue baby' operation." Photograph by F. W. Goro. Page © 1949 Life, Inc. Reprinted with permission. All rights reserved. Author's collection.

(AMA) might prevent any change at all. From 1937 to 1939, many magazines ran stories about ideas for health care insurance animated by New Deal politics in general and stimulated by specific calls for reform from the New York County Medical Society, a group that did not share the AMA's conservative agenda. *Life* acknowledged this dispute only in a short June 1937 report on the AMA convention and in a few letters to the editor late the following year.[63] In contrast, *Look,* a biweekly competitor, published a substantial illustrated critique of the AMA's position entitled "An Open Letter to American Doctors." A rebuttal by AMA spokesman Dr. Morris Fishbein appeared in the following issue, "An Open Letter to the American People."[64] Luce's other magazines, *Time* and *Fortune,* gave the topic more attention. Fishbein was *Time*'s cover feature on June 21, 1937 (the same date as *Life*'s brief report on policy debates at the AMA). Then eighteen months later, *Time* placed on its cover a prominent supporter of socialized medicine, Dr. Henry E. Sigerist, director of the Institute of the History of Medicine at Johns Hopkins, just when *Look*'s articles were being published in January 1939. *Fortune* had run a long story about the AMA, featuring Fishbein prominently, in November 1938.[65] In a second wave of public controversy over a proposed national health-insurance plan in the late 1940s, *Life* published only a short editorial, "Health by Compulsion: The President Proposes Much That Is Good, but There Are Better Ways to Achieve His Goals."[66]

Life's humane naturalism, conveyed through its characteristic aesthetics, gave shape and substance to a nine-page photoessay on mental illness published in March 1938: "The Shadow of Insanity: What the U.S. Is Doing about It."[67] The marginless splash page was covered edge to edge with a deceptively plain Eisenstaedt photograph of part of the wall of a brick building with windows—no people, no ground, no doorway, no sky, just a wall half-covered by a triangular shadow. In a box placed over a small part of this photo, the opening text intoned,

> In U.S. hospitals, behind walls like the one shown here, are currently 500,000 men, women and children whose minds have broken in the conflict of life. About the same number, or more, who have lost their mental equilibrium, are at large. Their doctors say they have mental diseases. Their lawyers call them insane. Mentally-balanced people shun and fear the insane. The general public refuses to face the terrific problem of what should be done for them. Today, though their condition has been much improved, they are still the most neglected, unfortunate group in the world. On [the] following six pages are various pictures showing the dark world of the insane and what scientists are doing to lead them back to the light of reason.[68]

Half the article's photographs (by Alfred Eisenstaedt) portrayed patients, posed for their privacy with their faces turned away. Other photographs (by Hansel Mieth) illustrated doctors administering new therapies (including insulin shock for schizophrenia and fever therapy for paresis). One man, cured by an insulin coma, was photographed and identified by name. Like so many of *Life*'s medical stories, this one was clearly intended to heighten concern and engagement by reducing people's distance from pathology—naturalizing or normalizing it—and to commend scientific research as the main source of progress.

> Insanity is a disease. It is as destructive to the mind as cancer is to the body. As such, mental illness should receive as much care and treatment as physical ailments. This is not the case. Until recently asylums were practically jails where the mentally afflicted were sequestered for life. Today asylums are becoming hospitals equipped and staffed to cure these patients. Today it is being recognized that the majority recover under good treatment, and that it costs less to cure them than to feed and house them for life.[69]

Although such editorial remarks framed the article, the real story was in the photographs: of people who were different from the readers, but, at the same time, just like them too; people having a hard time, but not people so desperate that readers wanted to shun them and turn the pages quickly. Though this was not a light or pleasant subject, these portraits were visually and emotionally engaging, perhaps even as much as the pictures of parties, polo, and picnics that *Life* liked to run.

EVER BIGGER BREAKTHROUGHS

During the 1940s, *Life* published frequent stories of medical news, often carrying the same themes that the magazine had articulated in the 1930s: valuable and intellectually interesting experiments, innovations in therapy and prevention, the dignity of the health professions, and the growth of medical progress from its nineteenth-century origins. Early in the decade, just before war news came to dominate, *Life* featured the newly opened National Cancer Institute (NCI), a prototype for large-scale, government-funded research, which grew rapidly at the National Institutes of Health (NIH) after the war. The point of the story was not the specific people or research projects mentioned but the expanding institutionalization of support for biomedical research. Beneath a dramatically shaded photograph of a dozen white-coated scientists at a conference table in a darkened room with a tissue specimen projected on a screen behind them, the story was headlined "Cancer: Exploration of Its Nature and Cause Will Be Organized in National Research Center" (fig. 92). The following page saluted Dr. Clarence Cook Little of the Jackson Memorial Laboratory at Bar Harbor, whose million "mice have proved heredity is a factor in cause of cancer." Following that, as an illustration of how the NCI would coordinate independent researchers across the country, readers were introduced to two researchers at John Hopkins, who "take movies of cancer cells."

The United States' entry into the war opened new frontiers for news photographers, and *Life* took a lead in bringing battlefield photography to readers on the home front. Newsreels in the movie theaters took up the dramatic subject too, but the black-and-white stills in *Life* took root more deeply in people's consciousness

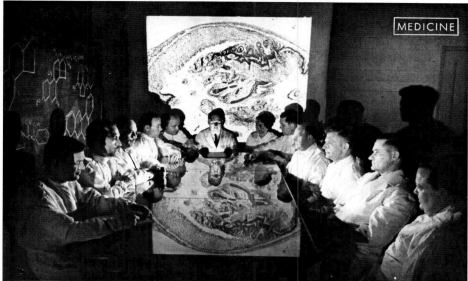

WITH MANY TIMES MAGNIFIED CANCER SPECIMEN PROJECTED ON A SCREEN, RESEARCH STAFF OF NATIONAL CANCER INSTITUTE MEETS FOR REGULAR WEEKLY DISCUSSION

CANCER
EXPLORATION OF ITS NATURE AND CAUSE WILL BE ORGANIZED IN NATIONAL RESEARCH CENTER

Cancer is the biological counterpart of social revolution. For reasons yet unknown, a group of normal tissue cells becomes disengaged from the integrated functioning of the living body. Reproducing quickly and growing vigorously, they set up their own riotous tempo. From the first center of upheaval they break loose in small clumps to invade the rest of the body or thread out in long columns into surrounding tissue. Cancer cells starve and smother neighboring tissue by foraging on its nutrition system. Once lodged in a vital organ, cancer disrupts its normal operation, brings death to the entire organism.

Though thousands of cancers are cured by early treatment, 150,000 people in the U. S. still die of this disease every year—a death rate second only to heart failure. To stem the steadily increasing number of deaths the U. S. Government has launched a major research offensive to determine the nature and cause of cancer. Headquarters is the U. S. Public Health Service National Cancer Institute at Bethesda, Md., where recently a staff of 87 scientists and helpers set up their equipment. On a Congressional appropriation of $570,000 a year, the Institute will support its own and other research projects and

bring cancer researchers all over the country into collaboration on their single problem.

In the Institute laboratories all related branches of science are represented. Cancer has been induced by innumerable agents from sunlight to sex hormones, with more than 100 different chemicals included. Some established causes of cancer, like the radiation of X-rays and radium, are also standard treatment. The mystery deepens with the discovery that certain chemicals can check chemically induced cancers, that male sex hormones will retard cancers caused by female sex hormones. In a germ-free laboratory in the Institute (*left*) one project is devoted to converting normal cells into cancer cells outside the body where the cultures cannot be contaminated.

To supplement its work the Institute plans to establish co-ordination with privately endowed laboratories. Among the first to make such a connection is Geneticist Clarence Cook Little, long a leader in cancer research and managing director of the American Society for the Control of Cancer. His 10-year-old Jackson Memorial Laboratory at Bar Harbor, Me. with its 60,000 pedigreed mice is the leading genetics laboratory engaged in cancer research.

CONTINUED ON NEXT PAGE

In sterile laboratory scientists try to induce cancer in normal cells where bacteria cannot invade and choke them off.

Effect of radiation (*below*) on normal cell division clarifies X-ray effect on cancer. Specimen at right reproduces nor-

mally into two, four and eight. Under radiation, specimen at left is first inhibited, then divides suddenly into three.

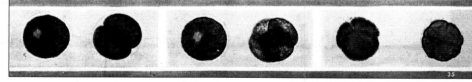

35

FIG. 92. Splash page, "Cancer: Exploration of Its Nature and Cause Will Be Organized in National Research Center," *Life*, June 17, 1940, 35. Photographs by Herbert Gehr. Photomicrographs by courtesy of Dr. Paul S. Henshaw. Page © 1940 Life, Inc. Reprinted with permission. All rights reserved. Author's collection.

because readers could pause over them and return to them more than once. The war generated heartwarming medical stories in *Life*: battlefield care, expansion of health care personnel, GIs struggling with their injuries, surgical innovations, and advances in rehabilitation. Predictably, the magazine gave an optimistic cast to many of these stories, but without suppressing the painful elements, and the narratives merged medical progress with human-interest details in such titles as "A Wounded Veteran Gets a New Face: Sgt. Charles Wise, Badly Hurt in Battle, Gets New Features, a College Education and a New Start in Life" and "Teaching the Crippled to Walk: Rehabilitation Institute in New York Shows Its Patients How to Make the Most of What Little They Have."[70]

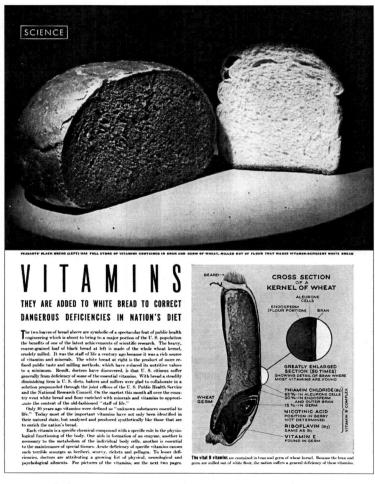

FIG. 93. Splash page, "Vitamins," *Life,* April 21, 1941, 65. Page © 1941 Life, Inc. Reprinted with permission. Photograph © 1941 Hansel Mieth, used with permission of Center for Creative Photography, University of Arizona. All rights reserved. Author's collection.

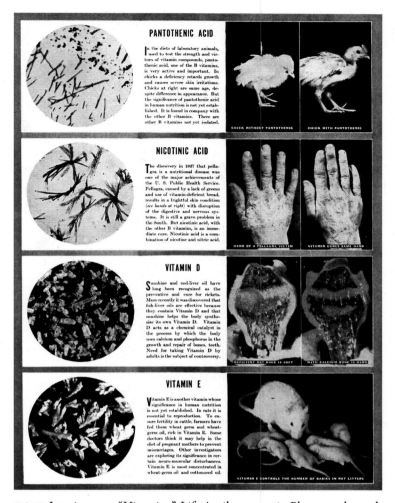

FIG. 94. Interior page, "Vitamins," *Life,* April 21, 1941, 67. Photographs credited to Merck, Squibb, and other biomedical laboratories. Page © 1941 Life, Inc. Reprinted with permission. All rights reserved. Author's collection.

But even with the deluge of war coverage, presentations of scientific advance and science education continued the pattern established in *Life*'s first few years. For example, a dramatic composition of two loaves of bread, shot by Hansel Mieth, opened a feature on vitamins: "Peasant's Black Bread (left) Has Full Store of Vitamins Contained in Bran and Germ of Wheat, Milled Out of Flour That Makes Vitamin-Deficient White Bread" (fig. 93). If the message seems prosaic and familiar today, it was more novel in the early 1940s, and it has never been more elegantly illustrated. The following pages examined eight vitamins, with a photo of crystalline forms alongside paired specimens of animals or body parts showing the effects of vitamin deficiency (fig. 94).

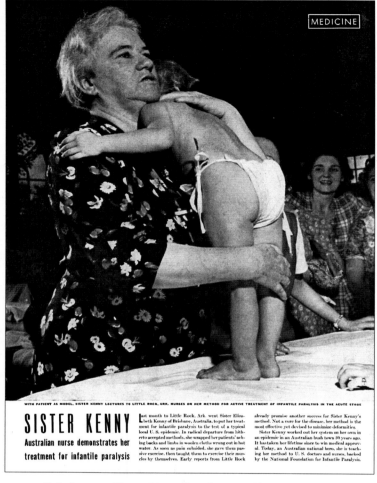

WITH PATIENT AS MODEL, SISTER KENNY LECTURES TO LITTLE ROCK, ARK. NURSES ON HER METHOD FOR ACTIVE TREATMENT OF INFANTILE PARALYSIS IN THE ACUTE STAGE

SISTER KENNY

Australian nurse demonstrates her treatment for infantile paralysis

Last month to Little Rock, Ark. went Sister Elizabeth Kenny of Brisbane, Australia, to put her treatment for infantile paralysis to the test of a typical local U. S. epidemic. In radical departure from hitherto accepted methods, she wrapped her patients' aching backs and limbs in woolen cloths wrung out in hot water. As soon as pain subsided, she gave them passive exercise, then taught them to exercise their muscles by themselves. Early reports from Little Rock already promise another success for Sister Kenny's method. Not a cure for the disease, her method is the most effective yet devised to minimize deformities.

Sister Kenny worked out her system on her own in an epidemic in an Australian bush town 30 years ago. It has taken her lifetime since to win medical approval. Today, an Australian national hero, she is teaching her method to U. S. doctors and nurses, backed by the National Foundation for Infantile Paralysis.

FIG. 95. Splash page, "Sister Kenny," *Life,* September 28, 1942, 73. Photograph credited to Ed Clark and the *Nashville Tennessean.* Page © 1942 Life, Inc. Reprinted with permission. All rights reserved. Author's collection.

A clinical advance in polio treatment was given new publicity in September 1942, with *Life* portraying Elizabeth Kenny's mode of polio therapy as a successful breakthrough.[71] Sister Kenny's active treatment of acute paralysis was depicted as a celebrated departure from received wisdom, although, in fact, by 1942 Kenny had been practicing her method for years, garnering a mix of condemnation and approbation in medical circles.[72] She was already a popular medical heroine, well known to the American public.[73] The timing of the September 1942 article was probably prompted by an earlier story in the *Saturday Evening Post.*[74] *Life*'s feature opened with a grand photo of Sister Kenny in a print dress, helping a diapered child stand against her shoulder, as she was presenting to an audience the case for her treatment method (fig. 95; see also color plate 19). Although Kenny was a nurse, *Life* covered her therapeutic method as a medical advance and treated her as it treated doctors, without bringing in her personal life, as it typically did in the magazine's articles about nurses.

In 1943, penicillin started making its way into the news after many years of unsuccessful laboratory efforts that achieved nothing substantial enough to merit publicity. *Life*'s initial penicillin story in May 1943 could do little more than proclaim its promise and depict the laboratory where it was being produced artisanally in hundreds of individual flasks (fig. 96).[75] Fourteen months later, the magazine could celebrate successful realization of factory-scale production and a record of clinical successes. *Life*'s photoessay, "Penicillin: Mass Production of Drug Replaces Slow

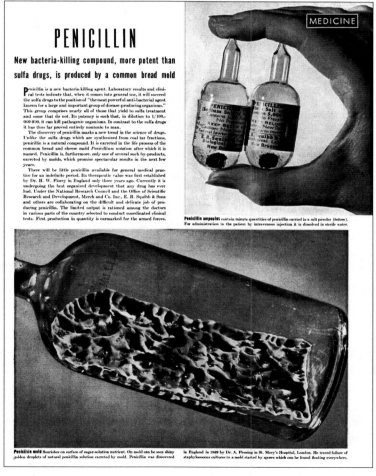

FIG. 96. Splash page, "Penicillin, New Bacteria-Killing Compound," *Life*, May 24, 1943, 53. Photographs by F. W. Goro. Page © 1943 Life, Inc. Reprinted with permission. All rights reserved. Author's collection.

Laboratory Methods to Meet Military Needs and Provide a Limited Civilian Supply," used the kind of rhythmically elegiac industrial pictures that the editors loved to publish (fig. 97). *Life* also gave readers close-ups of mold colonies in petri dishes, tubes of "weirdly beautiful mold cultures," and drawings of the life cycle of penicillium notatum. Two of the pages were in full color, and they did elegant justice to the subtle colors of mold growing on bread and fruit.

Penicillin was not the only huge therapeutic success in 1944. American scientists created synthetic quinine to overcome both wartime interruption of natural supplies and the greater need for this drug due to U.S. military presence in malarial regions.

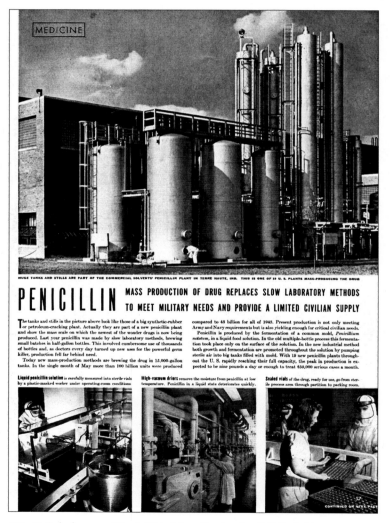

FIG. 97. Splash page, "Penicillin, Mass Production," *Life,* July 17, 1944, 57. Photographs by F. W. Goro. Page © 1944 Life, Inc. Reprinted with permission. All rights reserved. Author's collection.

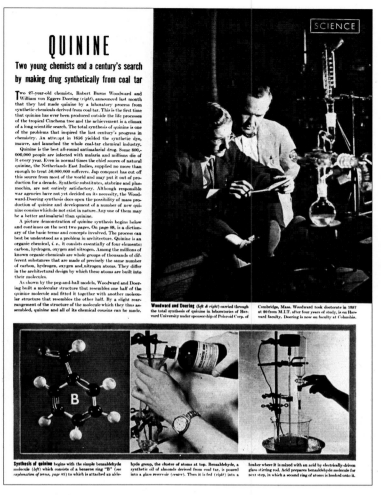

FIG. 98. Splash page, "Quinine: Two Young Chemists," *Life,* June 5, 1944, 85. Photographs by F. W. Goro. Page © 1944 Life, Inc. Reprinted with permission. All rights reserved. Author's collection.

The breakthrough was covered in "Quinine: Two Young Chemists End a Century's Search by Making Drug Synthetically from Coal Tar," a photoessay by Fritz Goro, who specialized in scientific subjects (fig. 98).[76] Besides dramatic images of men at work in the lab, the story included many photos of three-dimensional models of the molecules, explaining the seven steps in a synthesis, starting with benzaldehyde. One page illustrated molecular models in general, explaining how atoms bond into molecules with precise structures, how structures can be changed, and how certain groups of atoms (such as ethyl and methyl groups) can replace single atoms to create more elaborate structures. This rather substantial introduction to structural organic chemistry in a general-interest magazine confirmed that *Life* took intellectual issues seriously and was willing to stretch its readers' minds.

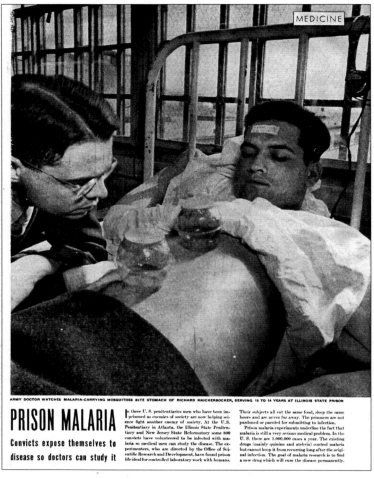

MEDICINE

ARMY DOCTOR WATCHES MALARIA-CARRYING MOSQUITOES BITE STOMACH OF RICHARD KNICKERBOCKER, SERVING 10 TO 14 YEARS AT ILLINOIS STATE PRISON

PRISON MALARIA

Convicts expose themselves to
disease so doctors can study it

In three U. S. penitentiaries men who have been imprisoned as enemies of society are now helping science fight another enemy of society. At the U.S. Penitentiary in Atlanta, the Illinois State Penitentiary and New Jersey State Reformatory some 800 convicts have volunteered to be infected with malaria so medical men can study the disease. The experimenters, who are directed by the Office of Scientific Research and Development, have found prison life ideal for controlled laboratory work with humans.

Their subjects all eat the same food, sleep the same hours and are never far away. The prisoners are not pardoned or paroled for submitting to infection.

Prison malaria experiments underline the fact that malaria is still a very serious medical problem. In the U. S. there are 1,000,000 cases a year. The existing drugs (mainly quinine and atebrin) control malaria but cannot keep it from recurring long after the original infection. The goal of malaria research is to find a new drug which will cure the disease permanently.

FIG. 99. Splash page, "Prison Malaria," *Life,* June 4, 1945, 43. Photograph by Myron Davis. Page © 1945 Life, Inc. Reprinted with permission. All rights reserved. Author's collection.

A different kind of scientific effort to improve control over malaria was described a year later in a report on the use of prisoners as experimental subjects, "Prison Malaria: Convicts Expose Themselves to Disease So Doctors Can Study It."[77] As usual, the photography was top-notch and the tone was naturalistic. The splash photo echoed popular illustrations of yellow-fever studies, with bottled mosquitoes being applied to the skin: "Army doctor watches malaria-carrying mosquitoes bite stomach of Richard Knickerbocker, serving 10 to 14 years at Illinois State Prison" (fig. 99). And at that time, prior to the emergence of ethical concerns raised by the Nuremberg Tribunal's revelations about Nazi medical experiments on humans, the article betrayed no hesitation about the use of human subjects or any questions about whether prisoners could freely consent to their participation.[78]

Two substantial articles, on tropical diseases in May 1944 and on germs in November 1945, provided expansive overviews of their subjects by combining the individuality of strong photography with the comprehensiveness of tables and charts to present a large compilation of information in a form that was both memorable and intelligible. "Tropical Diseases: They Include Appalling Human Afflictions" opened with close-ups of a louse, an anopheles mosquito, and a helminth worm at the top of the page (fig. 100). At the bottom ran photos showing victims of elephantiasis,

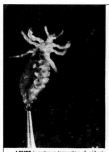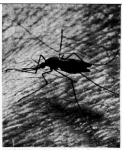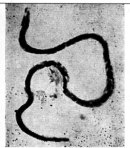

LOUSE is vector or transmitter of epidemic typhus from man to man. Delousing of persons and clothing is a primary typhus preventive.

ANOPHELES mosquito transmits malaria. The *Aëdes aegypti* mosquito transmits yellow and dengue fevers. The members of these two types, native to the U. S., are potential carriers.

HELMINTHS is name for worms which cause, among other afflictions, elephantiasis (*below*). Above is much-enlarged larva of *Loa loa* helminth which infests the subskin tissues.

TROPICAL DISEASES
THEY INCLUDE APPALLING HUMAN AFFLICTIONS

Tropical diseases, before the war, were the exotic specialty of medical missionaries and of medical officers in the Army, Navy and U. S. Public Health Service. Today with thousands of U. S. troops exposed to tropical diseases, they have become an immediate concern of the whole medical profession, not only for doctors in uniform but for doctors at home, who must now be on the alert for them in domestic practice.

The term "tropical diseases" embraces broadly those diseases that occur commonly in warm countries. Their distribution is, however, not limited by warmth of climate. More direct factors are the low standards of nutrition and sanitation prevailing in the tropics. Most of the diseases can and do exist in the temperate zones. They are, in fact, rare only where people are protected by modern medical technology.

Tropical diseases include some of the most loathsome and appalling of all human afflictions. Scientifically they are impressive in the variety of their infecting and infesting agents—submicroscopic viruses and Rickettsiae, single-celled Protozoa and bacteria of all kinds and the multicelled helminths (*above right*).

A map in color on the following spread of this issue shows the major tropical diseases in their general distribution around the planet. The pink area of the map, defining the region in which malaria is prevalent, defines roughly the geographical province of tropical medicine as a whole. At the bottom of the map each of the diseases is keyed to a symbol by which its distribution may be found. Most of the symbols represent the insects and vermin which have been specifically convicted as active vectors or passive reservoirs for each of the diseases. Not keyed on the map are the dysentery (*i.e.*, intestinal) diseases which prevail throughout and beyond the malarial regions. Together with malaria they afflict continuously at least half the population of the tropics.

For actual treatment of the diseases doctors of our armed forces are equipped with an increasing number of medical weapons produced by collaboration between clinicians in the field and the laboratories at home. Against some infections, U. S. troops are protected by their long series of immunizing inoculations. To guard them from new infections, medical units, like one shown opposite in New Guinea jungles, make continual surveys of native health in occupied areas. But the best protection is the discipline of sanitation and personal hygiene maintained among our troops. The fact that most of the tropical diseases can be so effectively controlled by preventive medicine is assurance that, though they may be imported, they will not become established in continental U. S.

ELEPHANTIASIS is late symptom of filariasis, helminthic infection of the lymphatics. Blocked lymph circulation causes swelling.

SLEEPING SICKNESS, African variety, is caused by protozoan invasion of central nervous system, ends in stupor and mania. Natives have chained this victim to heavy log.

LEPROSY is a bacterial infection which attacks skin and nervous system. The victims may live for years, becoming progressively disfigured by the rotting parts and skin ulcers.

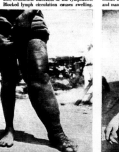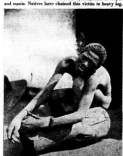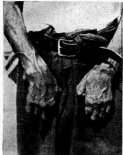

FIG. 100. Splash page, "Tropical Diseases," *Life,* May 1, 1944, 60. Photographs, left to right, upper then lower, by A. T. Hull Jr., Andreas Feininger, U.S. Public Health Service; Dr. Eugene Kellersberger (2), Dr. Douglas R. Collier. Page © 1944 Life, Inc. Reprinted with permission. All rights reserved. Author's collection.

sleeping sickness, and leprosy. The facing page, in full color, captured scenes of medical researchers working in grass huts in New Guinea. The following opening was
a huge double-page chart (twenty by fourteen inches), "World Map of the Major
Tropical Diseases." Symbols for fourteen diseases were placed on the map in the
regions where they were found. On the lower part of the pages, each symbol was
explained in four or five sentences. Pages like this could be read at various levels of
detail. An overall first impression would suggest the magnitude and the complexity
of the problem. Successive closer readings could proceed either from a region to a
symbol to a disease description or, alternatively, from a disease back to the map to
find its locations. In many ways, this design was like that of a good science textbook,
except that textbooks in the 1940s never had pages this large and they seldom had
color printing or graphic design of this quality. The fact that learning from charts
such as these required time and patience was not an obstacle to the engagement of
readers, who might otherwise be turning pages quickly in a popular magazine. The
pages displayed such interesting details that a curious person could examine them
slowly or return to them again and again, moving through the array of facts in a variety of pathways. The next four pages of the article on tropical diseases offered five
color photographs by Fritz Goro, illustrating how "living chick embryos produce
new vaccines," and black-and-white photos explaining how prevention is the "surest
of all cures."

About eighteen months later, another comprehensive medical science article ven-
tured into the realm of bacteriology, with an educator's approach and a photographer's artistry. Sinister-looking, shadowy black-and-white photomicrographs of normally invisible microbes opened the long report, "Germs: Medical Science Helps the
Body in Its Fight against Six Great Groups of Them."[79] Readers were immediately
shown the six major types: bacillus (causing fourteen diseases), coccus (five), spirochete (five), rickettsia (four), virus (seventeen), and protozoa (three). Following
these images was a double-page chart, printed in red, pink, gray, and black, which
condensed a remarkable amount of information on forty-eight different ailments in
the six groups (see color plate 21). For each condition, a body outline was marked to
indicate physical locations of the infection. Boxes below these figures revealed the
available weapons, if any, for chemical prevention, chemical treatment, biological
prevention, and biological treatment. As appropriate, these boxes contained symbols for vaccine, antibacterial serum, sulfa drugs, arsenical, penicillin, and so on.
And for each disease, there was a short verbal note on the status of its control. This
science lesson linked bacteriology with clinical conditions, therapeutics, and prevention in each vertical column. One could also read the chart horizontally to learn
which ailments could be prevented by vaccines, for example, or treated with sulfa
drugs. The large array helped readers see the patterns that underlay the myriad facts
of modern medical science. Just as in the "World Map of Tropical Diseases" published a year earlier, this chart encouraged a reader to wander in and out of various
categories. The graphic design organized the huge quantity of information in a such
a clear array that the result was intriguing, not intimidating. Fritz Goro's striking

photographs on the following three pages supplied concrete details of animals and serum injections; the section was captioned "Biologicals: Germs Are Cultivated to Make Their Own Controls" and showed the now familiar and humble rabbits and guinea pigs, as well as the always dignified and imperturbable horses being bled for serum (fig. 101).

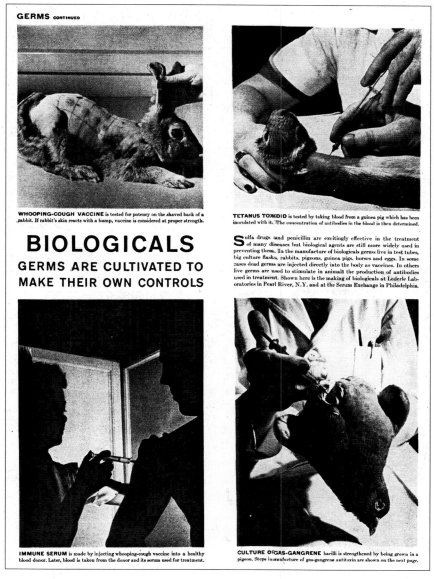

GERMS CONTINUED

WHOOPING-COUGH VACCINE is tested for potency on the shaved back of a rabbit. If rabbit's skin reacts with a bump, vaccine is considered at proper strength.

TETANUS TOXOID is tested by taking blood from a guinea pig which has been inoculated with it. The concentration of antibodies in the blood is then determined.

BIOLOGICALS
GERMS ARE CULTIVATED TO MAKE THEIR OWN CONTROLS

Sulfa drugs and penicillin are excitingly effective in the treatment of many diseases but biological agents are still more widely used in preventing them. In the manufacture of biologicals germs live in test tubes, big culture flasks, rabbits, pigeons, guinea pigs, horses and eggs. In some cases dead germs are injected directly into the body as vaccines. In others live germs are used to stimulate in animals the production of antibodies used in treatment. Shown here is the making of biologicals at Lederle Laboratories in Pearl River, N.Y. and at the Serum Exchange in Philadelphia.

IMMUNE SERUM is made by injecting whooping-cough vaccine into a healthy blood donor. Later, blood is taken from the donor and its serum used for treatment.

CULTURE OF GAS-GANGRENE bacilli is strengthened by being grown in a pigeon. Steps in manufacture of gas-gangrene antitoxin are shown on the next page.

FIG. 101. Interior opening, "Biologicals," in "Germs," *Life*, November 5, 1945, 68–69. Four photographs by F. W. Goro (in center of opening with adjacent advertising on both pages). Pages © 1945 Life, Inc. Reprinted with permission. All rights reserved. Author's collection.

In 1949, two new treatments provided *Life* with occasions to use remarkable before-and-after photos. Such juxtapositions achieved several of the magazine's aspirations: they were informative; they used rhythm and repetition to catch the eye; and their peculiarity engaged readers. When the success of cortisone ("Compound E") in liberating some patients from crippling arthritis was documented with a movie of Mayo Clinic patients' miraculous improvement with the experimental drug, *Life* included stills from the film.[80] The upper series captured a patient grimacing with arthritic pain when a doctor touched his hand and then having great difficulty walking down steps. The third frame showed how, a week after his injection, he handled the same task with aplomb (fig. 102). In a photograph on the facing page, this patient was comfortably jogging. But the caption sadly acknowledged the limits of this experimental treatment: "Patient runs with complete freedom of motion after Compound E frees him from pain, stiffness, and other distressing symptoms. He also experienced a remarkable increase in appetite and vitality. There was not enough of drug available to continue injections, however, and his symptoms returned soon after treatments were stopped."[81] A few months later, *Life* ran another set of before-and-after photographs, this time with a more permanent improvement. As the headline explained, "Radio-Iodine Halts One Type of Cancer. Radioactive Chemical Brings about History-Making Recovery of Patient Dying from Thyroid Tumors."[82] The pair of small but impressive portrait photos was captioned simply, "Bernard Brustein in 1942, left; [and] as he looks today." The unclothed man on the left was pathetically emaciated; the one on the right, in a business suit with full features, smiled with confidence and gratitude.

CANCER RESEARCH IN THE 1950s

Cancer had long fascinated *Life*'s editors, and in the 1950s the magazine was able to report on new evidence linking tobacco with cancer. In late 1953, the headline of a two-page news story with nine photographs announced, "Smoke Gets in the News: Doctors Report Tobacco Tar Induces Mouse Cancer, Note Rise in Cigaret Use and Human Lung Cancer."[83] A bizarre laboratory machine dominated the splash page. The device, as a simulation of human smoking, puffed on sixty cigarettes at a time to collect the residues needed for the animal tests. The tumors that resulted from painting smoke residue on the skin of mice were illustrated, but the article was not limited to this direct causal link. It also bought to the fore the role of statistics in appreciating a correlation between smoking and human disease.[84]

Three years later, *Life* declared a causal link between smoking and cancer: "New Cigaret-Cancer Link: Study Shows That as the Smoking Rate Rises, Damage Rises Too."[85] The article provided images showing how cancers were born, grew, and finally invaded the lungs. But the most important feature of this report was in making an early shift from correlation to cause, eight years before the surgeon general's

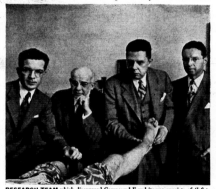

DRAMATIC IMPROVEMENT effected with new drug is shown in the movie clips above and at right. Before treatment arthritic grimaces with pain when doctor touches

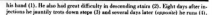

his hand (1). He also had great difficulty in descending stairs (2). Eight days after injections he jauntily trots down steps (3) and several days later (*opposite*) he runs (4).

HORMONE STOPS DISEASE

For a number of years a few researchers have suspected that the adrenal gland had something to do with rheumatoid arthritis. One clue came from the fact that women suffering from the disease showed a marked improvement during pregnancy, a period during which the gland is stimulated. On the theory that the adrenal in arthritic victims might not be performing all of its functions, Dr. Philip Hench and associates of the Mayo Clinic spent nine years testing the effects of several of the hormones which that complicated gland secretes. One of these, a substance now known as Compound E, brought immediate and dramatic results. Of the 14 patients treated with the new drug, all were relieved of pain and swelling within a few days and some who could scarcely walk were actually able to run (*opposite page*).

In all but three patients the original symptoms returned after injections were stopped, indicating that Compound E, like insulin, might have to be given regularly. Another problem is that Compound E, isolated by Dr. E. C. Kendall, can be produced at present only by a very long and costly process. It may be two years before the drug is synthesized and enough of it is available for the general public at a reasonable price. Nonetheless the discovery may come to be considered a landmark in medical history comparable to the discovery of insulin or penicillin. When Hench and Kendall appeared recently before the Association of American Physicians after the showing of the now famous movie from which these sequences on this page were printed, the usually cool membership gave them an ovation seldom seen in medical gatherings.

RESEARCH TEAM which discovered Compound E and its use consists of (*left to right*) Drs. C. H. Slocumb, E. C. Kendall, P. S. Hench and H. F. Polley, all of Mayo's.

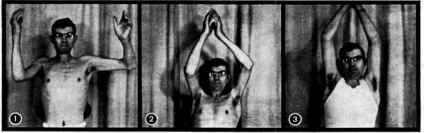

USE OF ARMS RETURNS to the 34-year-old arthritic after treatment with Compound E. Before being injected he was unable to raise his arms above his shoulders (1). Four days after being treated he could easily raise his arms above his head (2). Three months later he had gained considerable flesh and could use his arms normally (3).

FIG. 102. Interior page, "Hormone Stops Disease," *Life,* June 6, 1949, 110. Upper caption reads, "Dramatic improvement effected with new drug is shown in the movie clips. . . . Before treatment arthritic grimaces with pain when doctor touches his hand (1). He also had great difficulty in descending stairs (2). Eight days after injections he jauntily trots down steps (3)." Lower caption reads, "Use of arms returns to the 34-year-old arthritic after treatment with Compound E. Before being injected he was unable to raise his arms above his shoulders (1). Four days after being treated he could easily raise his arms above his head (2). Three months later he had gained considerable flesh and could use his arms normally (3)." Center photograph by Alfred Eisenstaedt; patient photographs uncredited. Page © 1949 Life, Inc. Reprinted with permission. All rights reserved. Author's collection.

report solidified that understanding. Thanks to the release of tobacco-industry documents because of litigation, it is now clear that the cigarette industry saw this article, with its pronounced claims of a causal connection, as extremely dangerous. Among the possible responses they considered were "a strong protest" in a release to the general press, a full-page ad in *Life* to balance the story, a counteracting story in *Look* magazine, an immediate press conference, and a private approach to Henry Luce. Choosing the last option, they secured a meeting with Luce and his editors in less than two weeks, and they left the discussion feeling optimistic.[86] Within a year, however, in April 1957, *Life* published more research news about one of the chemical compounds in tobacco leaves that becomes carcinogenic after it is burned in pipes and cigarettes. In practical terms, the work of Dr. Ernest Wynder at Sloan-Kettering suggested the possibility that removal of the waxy substance that he identified from smoking tobacco could greatly reduce the risk of cancer from smoking. In scientific terms, it offered further confirmation that the cancer risk was undeniable.[87] The article's photograph of Wynder posed the scientist looking upward at a flask containing the "cancer-causing agent," another instance of a *Life* photographer employing an increasingly common iconography for the heroic medical scientist. In 1964, *Life* capped its earlier coverage about the increasing evidence for a link between smoking and cancer with a strong and visually dramatic story on the surgeon general's report on cigarettes and cancer, "Verdict on Cigarettes: 'Guilty as Charged.' Government Report Nails Down Smoking Hazards."[88]

GAMMA GLOBULIN, RESPIRATORS, AND THEN A VACCINE FOR POLIO

By the 1950s, decades of laboratory research on the polio virus had improved scientists' ability to study it and to cultivate it in animals, but practical improvements were limited. Prevention consisted mostly of advice to avoid beaches, swimming pools, and crowds during the summer polio season. Available therapies were Sister Kenny's muscle rehabilitation and the mechanical respirator that kept many people alive in the hope that in time they might recover the ability to breathe on their own. None of these measures gave much solace to worried parents. Yet over the years, ordinary citizens continued to contribute to the March of Dimes, expressing their confidence that science could be counted on to find a solution, as it had found solutions for smallpox and rabies and diphtheria and diabetes. The laboratory had produced vaccines and serum therapy and, recently, sulfa drugs and penicillin. People hoped and wished.

By the early 1950s, a form of serum therapy for polio, extracting a natural resistance from one animal's body and injecting it into another's, seemed to show some promise, just as serum injections had reduced diphtheria deaths in the 1890s. In this case, the source was not horses but human beings, whose extracted and puri-fied gamma globulin would be given to children as a test to determine whether it could provide some resistance to infection, thereby reducing the number of cases and their severity. In September 1951, *Life* reported such an experiment in Utah, in which nearly three thousand children were injected with gamma globulin and a similar group received an inactive serum substitute. "One fearless 3-year-old offered himself up with a display of valor reminiscent of a yellow jack volunteer. 'I want a shot,' he announced. 'I don't want polio.'"[89]

Results were encouraging, and two years later, under the threat of a growing epidemic, a large-scale application of gamma globulin was made in Montgomery, Alabama. *Life* headlined its article "$625,000 Inoculation: 33,000 Children Get Gamma Globulin in a Southern Polio Epidemic."[90] This instance was the first pre-ventive use in an actual epidemic. The left-hand page of the *Life* article offered four photos of children being inoculated; the entire right-hand page had one huge photo of a health official standing behind a pyramid of empty serum bottles, which was just two days' worth. With a cost of twenty dollars a dose, the serum bottles were carefully destroyed after use "to prevent black marketeers' using the labels and bot-tles of the scarce drug" (fig. 103). Once again, a *Life* photographer structured an image by means of a geometric arrangement of repeated small elements.

In mid-October of the same year, as the polio season was winding down, *Life* ran a short article about a redesigned iron lung. These large machines were a frequent reminder of polio's devastating power, if also a symbol of courage and determina-tion on the part of heroic patients and their nurses and physicians. Patients whose muscles could not sustain adequate breathing were locked into these mechanical respirators from the neck down. Two-thirds of the splash page for "A Better Break for Polio Patients: Improvements Give a Respite from Iron Lung Life" was given over to an extreme close-up of a person's head extending from the metal canister and encased in a large, clear bubble of rigid plastic.[91] Respirators worked by increasing and decreasing air pressure on the patient's torso, rhythmically drawing air into the lungs and forcing exhalation out. As the article explained, the new bubble around the head could be used to force air down into the lungs for a short time, which would allow nurses to pull the metal apparatus away from the patient and provide therapy to the patient's body and limbs.

In the early 1950s, iron lungs were becoming more common and more visible all across the United States. Their growing presence was both reassuring and troubling. They symbolized medical progress at the same time as they reminded parents of the epidemics of paralysis and death among American children. It was at just this moment that decades of laboratory work on culturing the polio virus offered the possibility of a breakthrough that might prevent infection before it could wreak its damage on the nervous system. In the summer of 1952, *Life* proclaimed, "The End of Polio Is in Sight at Last. Two Sets of Scientists Come Up with Vaccines Which Promise Conquest of This Disease in This Decade." Twelve photos were used to show aspects of the laboratory work and a test on one child, who was photographed

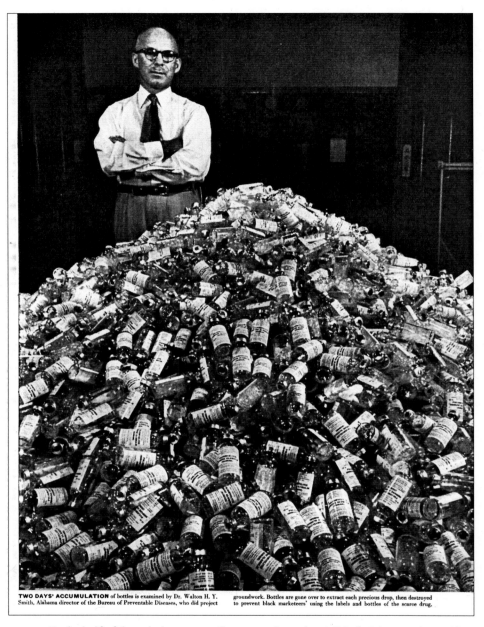

TWO DAYS' ACCUMULATION of bottles is examined by Dr. Walton H. Y. Smith, Alabama director of the Bureau of Preventable Diseases, who did project groundwork. Bottles are gone over to extract each precious drop, then destroyed to prevent black marketeers' using the labels and bottles of the scarce drug.

FIG. 103. Right half of the splash opening, "$625,000 Inoculation," *Life,* July 13, 1953, 33. Photograph by John Zimmerman. Page © 1953 Life, Inc. Reprinted with permission. All rights reserved. Author's collection.

in shadow to remain anonymous. One approach, developed at Johns Hopkins with funding from the March of Dimes, used killed virus. Six children received the vaccine and were shown to have developed antibodies. The other vaccine, being developed by Lederle Laboratories, was a "cooled-off" virus, prepared by inoculating a series of hamsters, a species not normally susceptible to polio virus. The article announced that "unless progress is far slower than now seems likely, the preventive will be available before 1960."[92]

But much sooner than expected, a workable killed-virus vaccine was developed by Jonas E. Salk of the University of Pittsburgh, another researcher supported by the March of Dimes. In March 1953, the *Journal of the American Medical Association* published Salk's report of a promising trial with ninety subjects, and the success made front-page news. His approach was to use an emulsified product that offered protection against all three major viral strains in one vaccine. The *New York Times* reported that "it may take at least another year, and more likely two to three years, before the vaccine can be made available with safety for general use."[93]

In less than a year, steps were under way to test the new Salk vaccine's value in the general population, with an unprecedentedly large experimental trial involving millions of people. *Life* flagged the story on a cover in February 1954: "How Polio Vaccine Was Found: A Great Medical Detective Story." The editors chose a well-known science writer, Robert Coughlan, for a piece they titled "Tracking the Killer" and subtitled "Production of New Polio Vaccine Brings a Great Medical Mystery-Drama, with a Cast of Thousands, Up to Its Climactic Act."[94] In this long report, most of the images were just small illustrations. It was certainly no *Life* photoessay. But the splash pages that opened the story were classics of *Life*'s photographic style. The entire left-hand page was given over to an Andreas Feininger photograph of a sea of test tubes; nothing else was in the picture. This created much the same effect as the unbounded crowd of mice on *Life*'s earliest medical cover photograph in March 1937. The image was an appealing, if rather abstract, composition of ovals and parallel lines, modulated by glassy transparency and reflections. "Test tubes symbolize endless experiments that led to discovery," explained the caption. The facing page presented two photo portraits of Jonas Salk and John Enders, taken by Alfred Eisenstaedt and Verner Reed, respectively (fig. 104). Like a re-creation of Edelfelt's Pasteur gazing into a bottle of rabies virus, Eisenstaedt's Salk contemplated the contents of a large glass flask holding polio virus.

In the spring of 1955, the world anxiously waited for the results of the prior summer's polio-vaccine trial, which included nearly two million people as experimental subjects and controls. Even before the results were known, new vaccine was being manufactured and stockpiled so it would be ready to protect children for the 1955 polio season if the trial had a successful outcome, as *Life* reported in the issue dated April 11, one day prior to the scheduled announcement of results but in distribution a full week before its cover date.[95] As promising results would create a sudden demand for the new preventive, twenty-seven million doses were being readied in advance (fig. 105).

TRACKING THE KILLER

Production of new polio vaccine brings a great medical mystery-drama, with a cast of thousands, up to its climactic act

by Robert Coughlan

THE biggest experiment in U.S. medical history will take place during the next few months when at least 500,000 children will be injected with a vaccine against poliomyelitis. Inoculations probably will get under way next month, in towns throughout the country, and will continue into June. Then local medical teams under the National Foundation for Infantile Paralysis will wait and watch as the annual curve of polio begins to climb, slowly in June, higher in July, highest in August and September, then falls steeply again with cool weather. Comparing the amount of polio among the inoculated children with that among the uninoculated ones, a committee of leading scientists will be able to judge the vaccine's effectiveness.

In theory it should produce immunity against polio in most or all of the inoculated children. The expectation is that it will produce at least some. Conceivably, it may produce none.

Suppose it should produce little or none. That would be a disappointment but would not alter the fact that an effective polio vaccine can be and will be made. This is the important news about polio, obscured in the public excitement about the forthcoming field trial of the vaccine. As Dr. Jonas Salk, under whose direction it was developed, has said, "The question . . . has not been what needs to be done to develop an immunizing agent against poliomyelitis but rather how this can be accomplished." In other words, the conquest of polio is now only a matter of technique.

A few years ago polio researchers were as far from this stage as cancer researchers are now from the basic answers in their field. Beginning in 1949, however, an amazing series of discoveries has occurred, culminating for the moment in the vaccine about to be tested. It is the purpose here to bring that forthcoming event into perspective for Life's readers by showing 1) what lies behind it and consequently what can reasonably be expected of it, and 2) what the near future may bring in polio vaccine research.

It is a dramatic story—one of the great medical detective stories of all time. It involves thousands of scientists, notably the two on the right of this page. We shall tell it here as it developed, clue by clue, not omitting the false clues. It is not, however, a simple story or one easy to follow. The search necessarily takes us into the world of microscopy and beyond, into a subsection of that world which until recently had been entirely invisible. To start with we must understand the nature of infectious diseases and the mechanism by which the body normally protects against them.

Antibodies vs. "germs"

IT was Robert Koch and Louis Pasteur who, in the 1880s, showed that infections are caused by bacteria, commonly known as "germs," which are in perpetual assault on the body. Occasionally, under conditions which make the body susceptible, they cause active infection and the individual may sicken and die. But ordinarily he does not, because the invading germs and substances which they produce stimulate the body to manufacture tiny chemical entities called "antibodies." For each kind of germ there is a corresponding antibody specially designed to deal with it. Moreover, these antibodies stay in the blood stream for a while, in some cases for the rest of the individual's life, and protect against future attack by that kind of germ. A vaccine consists of germs which have been so weakened (or killed) that they can no longer cause damage but which still can stimulate the body into pouring out antibodies. Vaccination has the same practical effect as a mild case of the disease.

Accordingly, Pasteur and those who followed him were soon able to give protection against a number of infectious diseases. But others would not yield because no causative germs could be found. In 1892 a Russian named Iwanowski showed the reason: the infectious material was so small that it passed through the finest laboratory filters; so small that even when it could be isolated it could not be seen because

CONTINUED ON NEXT PAGE

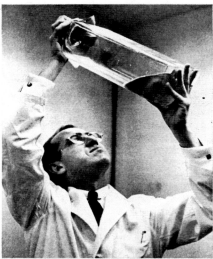

DR. JONAS E. SALK heads group at University of Pittsburgh which developed the vaccine now to be tried. Bottle holds a batch of the virus that causes polio.

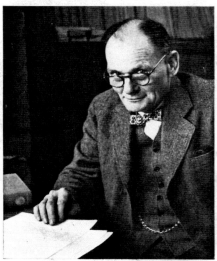

DR. JOHN ENDERS and his associates at Harvard made crucial breakthrough in 1949 with a method for growing the polio virus in test tube tissue cultures.

FIG. 104. Right half of the splash opening, "Tracking the Killer," *Life,* February 22, 1954, 121. Photographs by Alfred Eisenstaedt (upper) and Verner Reed (lower). Page © 1954 Life, Inc. Reprinted with permission. All rights reserved. Author's collection.

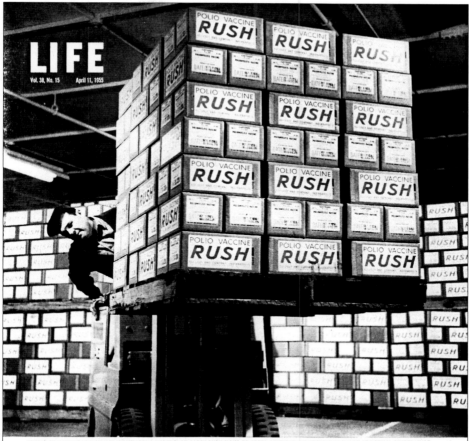

CRATES OF VACCINE IN A CHILLED INDIANAPOLIS WAREHOUSE CARRY RUSH SIGNS TO SPEED SHIPMENT AND PREVENT SPOILAGE AT NORMAL TEMPERATURE

U.S. GETS SET FOR POLIO VACCINE

Nobody knew for sure that the news would be good, but the U.S., which has so often wearily waited to hear the worst, last week excitedly hoped to hear that the day of infantile paralysis epidemics has been ended at last.

The word would come on April 12 from the University of Michigan where statisticians (next page) are completing evaluation of the polio vaccine developed by Dr. Jonas Salk of the University of Pittsburgh, which was given a test involving 1,830,000 children last year.

There were strong reasons for hope. In the laboratory the vaccine had protected monkeys and chimpanzees against massive doses of injected polio virus. And in a preliminary trial in 1954, in which 5,000 Pittsburgh schoolchildren were vaccinated, the level of protective antibodies was significantly raised. This set off a sudden flurry of optimistic speculation. Last week newspaper stories, trying to jump the gun, said the report would endorse the vaccine as 100% effective. But these stories were criticized as both premature and unfounded. The final count had not yet been made and a few children in last year's mass test are reported to have subsequently contracted polio.

Most optimistic of all were the drug makers who had gambled millions by plunging into full production. Already, crated stockpiles of the fluid stacked their cooled warerooms to the rafters (above), ready to go to drugstores all over the U.S. at a moment's notice. As long ago as October the National Foundation for Infantile Paralysis, which spent $22,400,000 in 17 years on polio research, had contracted to buy $9 million worth of the Salk vaccine.

FIG. 105. Splash page, "U.S. Gets Set for Polio Vaccine," *Life,* April 11, 1955, 35. Photograph by Albert Fenn. Page © 1955 Life, Inc. Reprinted with permission. All rights reserved. Author's collection.

249

Expectations were heightened by the fact that two million families had been involved in the vaccine trial. The daily press reinforced the anticipation. The *New York Times,* for example, primed its readers for the big day with regular articles: "Physicians Will Get Salk Report via TV" (April 7), "An Outline of the Medical Prospects on Eve of Report on Salk Vaccine" (April 10), "Vaccine Report Set for Tuesday; Dr. Francis to Give Facts to U.S. on Whether It Can Prevent Paralytic Polio" (April 10), "Verdict on the Salk Anti-Polio Vaccine Is Awaited with Widespread Interest" (April 10), "Vaccine Report Awaited by U.S." (April 11), and "Finding Due Today on Polio Vaccine; Francis to Report If Salk Method Is Effective" (April 12).

On the morning of April 12, 1955, the positive results were released to a meeting of scientists in an auditorium at the University of Michigan, where Thomas Francis Jr., in charge of the evaluation, was chairman of the Department of Epidemiology in the School of Public Health. This was no ordinary press conference. The meeting was broadcast nationwide by closed-circuit television to fifty-two thousand doctors who gathered at their local TV stations to watch the proceedings. Reporters rushed to telephones, and their afternoon and evening papers carried news of the great polio breakthrough in oversized headlines. In the *Baltimore Sun,* a huge banner headline proclaimed, "Polio Vaccine Safe and Effective."[96] Everyone got excited. Even an activist paper such as the daily *People's World* in Los Angeles reported "Polio Vaccine a Success" on its front page the very next morning.[97] The positive results created exhilaration all around the country.

After the deluge of newspaper coverage in the dailies, the weekly *Life* could add little to the climactic event. "Polio Vaccine Gets Go-Ahead: Doctors Hear Cheering Statistics" was the headline on a modest two-page news story in the next issue. The photographs were strong but hardly memorable.[98] But in the following issue, *Life* recovered some of its characteristic enthusiasm and style in "A Hero's Great Discovery Is Put to Work: Mass Polio Inoculations Get Under Way and a Nation Thanks Dr. Jonas Salk" (fig. 106).

The polio-vaccine breakthrough of 1955 was a major event in the media and in public sentiment. It was felt to be a greater achievement than pneumonia therapy or tuberculosis drugs, greater even than sulfa drugs and penicillin—though in fact it did not save nearly as many American lives as those advances did. Recognizing the disparity between the vaccine's initial achievement and its enthusiastic reception in popular culture does not deny its great value, but it helps to make clear some of the features that have shaped the reception of medical advances since the first breakthrough in 1885. Although polio sickened and killed far fewer people than pneumonia and tuberculosis did, it was a well-known ailment, it struck children, and it was sometimes fatal. Its potential to surprise any family, just as an unexpected dog bite would, made it widely feared far out of proportion to the limited number of actual cases. Just as Pasteur seemed able to wipe out the threat from hydrophobia, Salk seemed able to vanquish polio, simply by administering to children a series of little injections made in the laboratory. It was the biggest-of-the-big medical

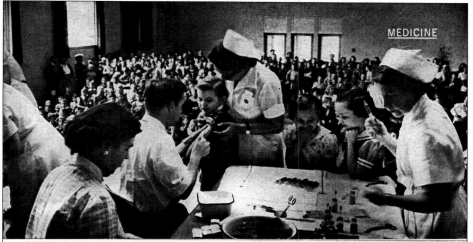

A HERO'S GREAT DISCOVERY IS PUT TO WORK

Mass polio inoculations get under way and a nation thanks Dr. Jonas Salk

As the nation's children began to queue up for Salk polio vaccine and a conference in Washington sought to devise the best ways of putting limited supplies to use, Dr. Jonas Salk, developer of the vaccine, found himself last week in the role of national hero.

Tributes ranged down from a citation from the President and a proposal that he be given a special Congressional Medal of Honor to offers of farm equipment. Newspapers in several cities were raising Salk funds and a U.S. senator introduced a bill to give him an annual stipend of $10,000. Salk, 40, who lives on a University of Pittsburgh research professor's salary and hopes to increase the effectiveness of his vaccine from 80% to 100%, said he would take no money for himself but indicated it would be used for further research. Meanwhile, demands for the vaccine created some confusion and raised the possibility that the government would help guide its distribution.

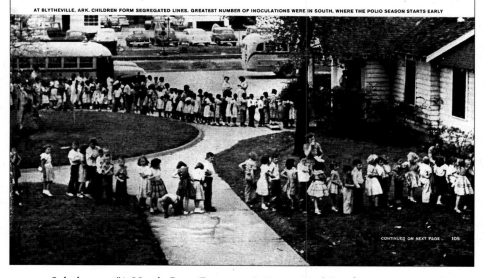

CONTINUED ON NEXT PAGE   105

FIG. 106. Splash page, "A Hero's Great Discovery Is Put to Work," *Life*, May 2, 1955, 105. Photographs by Ross Madden from *Black Star* (upper) and Charlie Bell for *Memphis Commercial Appeal* (lower). Page © 1955 Life, Inc. Reprinted with permission. All rights reserved. Author's collection.

breakthroughs, and though others followed, medical triumphs were never this big, this clear, or this universally appreciated again.

LIFE'S UNIQUE CONTRIBUTION TO SCIENCE POPULARIZATION

Life taught the American public about science and medicine with an unprecedented richness of detail packaged in an effective format. Part of that format was memorable photography. Another part of it was well-conceived and elegantly designed charts and drawings. Another ingredient was entertainment; humor, cleverness, surprise, and sheer visual beauty leavened the learning in *Life's* medical stories. All these features of *Life's* approach to medicine and its other subjects accounted for its achievements as an informal science teacher for Americans. *Life's* role as a major science popularizer has not been recognized, and its contribution may have been overlooked because it is so easy to think of *Life* magazine's pages as populated primarily by starlets and celebrities, by fashion and frivolity. The same assumption might also account for *Life's* being slighted in scholarly examinations of medicine in popular culture.[99]

In *Life's* first decade, it pioneered a new kind of science popularization and created an audience for it. In the 1930s and 1940s, radio was a very popular medium, but it was not a good medium for science education. Specialized magazines such as *Science News* and *Popular Science* reached only readers already engaged with science. Comic books popularized science and medicine, but they reached only children for the most part. Articles on science, medicine, and history of medicine were hardly absent from competing publications such as *Look* magazine and the *Saturday Evening Post* or from the widely distributed weekend newspaper supplements, but most of their articles lacked the consistent high quality of *Life's* information, layout, and illustration. Additionally, the medical coverage in the other periodicals was much less frequent than it was in *Life* and it lacked the consistent point of view that strengthened *Life's* presentation.[100]

Because the magazine had a unified approach to science and nature underlying its stories, *Life's* contribution to U.S. culture was greater than the sum of impressions gleaned by millions of individual readers glancing over myriads of miscellaneous facts. In *Life,* nature was wonderful, and equally so were people's efforts to understand it and turn its powers to human benefit. *Life's* curiosity was never satisfied, and there was always more to discover, more amazing things to see, more neat achievements to describe and appreciate. *Life* articulated no formal philosophy beyond the watchwords in its prospectus that its science should be "honest" and that "*Life* likes life." But it had an intellectual commitment to a kind of thinking that might formally be regarded as naturalism or, more broadly, as a form of "secular humanism."[101] In fact, Luce's general goals for *Life*—and especially for its coverage of nature and science—could almost have been taken from a 1937 book by Alfred C. Kinsey about biology teaching, in which he argued that teachers should help students see that "it is an interesting world in which they are living."[102] Kinsey's approach was that developed by the scientists who were active in creating the new high school subject of biology in the early decades of the twentieth century, and those teachers believed that handling organisms would help students "recognize that life was neither dirty nor mysterious. In biology class squeamish or vulgar expressions about bodies would give way to neutral scientific description, and intellectual honesty and autonomy would replace superstition."[103]

Life sustained the goals that these reforming teachers set for honest information about living systems—even in presentations of sexual topics, a major area in which high school reformers had to compromise in the face of external pressures. Schoolbooks "could not include, for example, detailed diagrams of the reproductive tracts for fear the books would fall into inappropriate hands."[104] In contrast, *Life*, on several occasions, provided those diagrams and photographs, as well as open discussions of venereal disease. Another example of *Life*'s commitment to a philosophical naturalism was the antimysterious approach the magazine took to photographs. Although *Life* pursued spectacular photographs to impress its readers, the editors explicitly demystified photography by illustrating behind-the-scenes techniques and explaining how the effects and illusions were achieved through lighting, camera position, editing, and so forth.[105]

For science coverage, the editors and writers realized early on that patient and generous cooperation from scientists would be essential for securing the kind of photographs the magazine wanted, especially in laboratories or clinical settings. These images could not be captured on the fly, no matter how candid they looked. Sometimes the photographer might spend a full week in a laboratory, getting the scientists to repeat their activities and poses again and again in the midst of cameras, photography assistants, and lighting equipment. This cooperation was founded in part on a trust that the magazine earned by the way it treated science stories. In a striking departure from normal journalistic practices, the editors at *Life* let scientists review the copy before a story was published. The editors learned that scientists were different from others in the news and that this vetting improved the stories, caused no problems, and helped to open doors.[106]

Life editors unexpectedly learned something else about scientists that proved invaluable to the magazine. Gerard Piel, the magazine's first long-term science editor (1938–1944), discovered that scientists and doctors were among the most avid readers of the science stories in *Life*. These professionals were hungry to learn about work in other fields of science; outside their own specializations, even scientists or physicians were general readers. But a scientist, physician, or engineer was a reader with a difference, with no patience for cant or obfuscation, exaggeration or sensation. Those readers encouraged *Life* to maintain accuracy and clarity in its science coverage, even while that coverage was being packaged in spectacular photographs and elegantly concise drawings and charts.[107]

LIFE'S PICTURE OF MEDICAL PROGRESS

Over *Life*'s first twenty years, it published hundreds of medical articles on diseases, discoveries, doctors, and patients—both past and present. Although the subject matter was diverse and wide ranging, a fairly consistent picture of medical progress came into focus and held steady through the 1950s. Above all, medicine in *Life* was inherently progressive in both senses of the word; that is, it continually gained understanding and power, and it embodied humane and democratic values. *Life* was optimistic about medicine; it honored the profession and celebrated its accomplishments, especially those based in science. *Life*'s picture had much innocence, little skepticism, and less cynicism. Before the late 1950s, *Life*'s coverage did not include public scandals about the profession, greedy doctors, drug-company shenanigans, or needy patients without access to care. It portrayed hardworking individuals, some in clinical medicine and others in the laboratory. *Life*'s very few negative stories reported on social and institutional failures, such as chronic and custodial care for patients in mental hospitals, and even these reformist articles were not angry or cynical.

The magazine gave far more attention to medical research than to patient care. It defended researchers' needs for experimental subjects, both animal and human, and it applauded funding for research. Millions of Americans who did not attend college learned from *Life* that research, especially in the laboratory, was the only source of new therapies and vaccines. To *Life*'s readers, research was no mere abstraction or empty slogan; it was something they examined in countless articles and photographs that allowed them "to see strange things; . . . to see man's . . . discoveries; to see things . . . hidden behind walls and within rooms, things dangerous to come to."

Through *Life*'s powerful black-and-white photography, the individual doctors and scientists responsible for medical advance were enlarged into heroic figures. In these stylish photographic portraits, they became like icons, worthy of veneration. *Life* did not bring their personalities and private lives to the fore, as it often did with celebrities and politicians. The pictured scientists, like the saints in paintings and sculpture, were at once both visually familiar, with their recognizable attributes, and mysteriously distant, in their arcane activities and unusual environments. Through many such photographs over the years, readers of *Life* learned to recognize the scientist as a special kind of person, whose selfless work was valuable to everyone and who merited respect, even awe. In *Life,* as in the comic books of the same era, the maker of a medical discovery was often regarded as a hero.

Because so many of *Life*'s articles were devoted to visual exploration of the natural world, merely turning the pages fostered an enthusiasm for nature and for the scientific understanding of it. The magazine's highly naturalistic portraits of the body, normal and pathological, including tumors and molds and germs and cells, encouraged readers to see that medicine, like science, trafficked in a nature filled with wonder and that medical knowledge was wonderful too.

Life's articles also demonstrated that scientific medicine was a central presence in American life; it was not something beyond comprehension or dangerous. Though clearly a specialized activity, esoteric in its details, it was not alien, something apart from ordinary people. The optimistic image of medical research and medical practice as entirely benevolent and unconflicted was not as naive as it might appear in retrospect. The doubts and scandals, cynicism and frustration that came to mark the media image of American medicine were still in the future. Much was demanded of medicine, but its sometimes halting steps were not seen as failures. The expectations had not risen so high as to invite complaints that it was failing by not making miracles fast enough. Through the 1950s, the public had few ethical or political quibbles about the United States' medical research or its health care practices—although this was to change substantially in the 1960s.

CHAPTER 10

THE MEANING
OF AN ERA

THE YEAR 1955 was a great moment for medical research and for the American public. Millions of cheering American families warmly welcomed the triumph of the Salk polio vaccine, and the media celebrated it grandly. Enthusiasm for medical progress had never been higher. It seemed that more breakthroughs were ready at hand and that medical progress had no limit. Over the prior seventy years, medicine had improved immeasurably, breakthroughs had become bigger and bigger, setbacks and failures had gone unnoticed, and criticism of medical research had been largely unimaginable. An editorial cartoon of 1955 embodied the easy optimism about steady medical innovation when it depicted Father Time inscribing an ever-longer list of victories over disease (see fig. 2 in chapter 1). This image captured the cultural outlook of the United States in the mid-1950s. Americans had no reason to think that the pattern of achievements might not continue or that their universal confidence in ever more medical progress was misplaced. But unforeseen change was in the offing, and the era of untarnished enthusiasm would soon draw to a close.

Over the following few years, negative elements began to complicate people's attitudes, even if popular expectations for medical research did not vanish entirely. Doubters started to question whether medicine was still honorable and worthy of the public's trust. Unprecedented failures commanded attention right alongside advances, and in contrast to the prior era, there was no consistent imagery of medical progress over the second half of the twentieth century. Although most people still wanted the most advanced treatments when they could afford them, they often regarded medicine with an ambivalence unknown in the century's first half. In the

1950s, some Americans worried that the sympathetic family doctor was being re-placed by faceless specialists. For example, a *Life* magazine cover asked if "bedside manner was a thing of the past."[1] The "wonder-drug makers" were challenged, as well, for taking "handsome profits from their captive consumers."[2] The size of drug-companies' profits was not closely tied to the public's sentiment about doctors, but other scandals were. During the 1960s, the credibility of the medical profession was repeatedly smeared by exposure of abusive procedures such as physicians' making profits from their own prescriptions. The ethical failings arose directly out of medicine's achievements: "Pills like these cure illness. But some doctors seize the chance to make money from them."[3]

Sometimes advances themselves created iatrogenic problems or had unexpected consequences. For example, powerful new drugs such as reserpine and chlorproma-zine introduced in the mid-1950s enabled many mentally ill patients to emerge from institutions and find new lives in the community. But in time, many of these peo-ple became burdens to themselves, their families, and society because anticipated community-support systems were never put into place. Then, in the early 1960s, the birth defects caused by thalidomide, a sedative newly in use by pregnant women in Europe to combat morning sickness, made clear the risks of modern drugs and raised major doubts about the responsibility of manufacturers and the government in protecting the public's safety. Widespread awareness of thousands of deformed babies also gave new urgency to worries about abortion and euthanasia as the public was facing major birth defects in large numbers. Americans were deeply affected by these events, even though most of the tragedies occurred aboard.[4]

Medical advances meant not only better treatments but also more treatments for more people, and the change of scale in health care institutions after World War II created problems without precedents. For example, with the rapidly growing num-ber of blood transfusions, new risks carried by transfused blood became apparent. The expansion of medical care, increasingly in high-technology settings such as hos-pitals, raised costs beyond the capacity of traditional payment systems. The rapid escalation of medical expenses led to periodic crises and repeated calls for solutions. Proposals that the federal government start paying for health care services of cer-tain groups of Americans provoked angry opposition from organized medicine. The aggressive opposition to reform, however, not only failed to prevent the establish-ment of Medicare and Medicaid but also weakened many people's faith in doctors. A growing cynicism compounded the effect of other questions raised about medical ethics and professionalism. The exposure of a long-running but ethically dubious study of syphilis in poor southern blacks, known as the Tuskegee study, created a public outcry and government inquiries. Scandals such as this one further chipped away at medicine's special status in American culture.

Once the old confidence and optimism were lost, even triumphs might produce media criticism. In the late 1960s, when the South African surgeon Christiaan Bar-nard removed the heart from an accident victim and successfully implanted it in the chest of a patient who survived, this operation became the most impressive medical breakthrough since the Salk vaccine.[5] Within several years, it also became medicine's most visible failure. Popular excitement about giving a new human heart to a person arose from its novelty, its technical achievement, and the questions it raised about what defined a person's individuality if one had another person's heart. This unprecedented surgical and humanitarian triumph—"Gift of a Human Heart" was the caption for *Life* magazine's cover photograph of the smiling patient—generated breathless headlines and television coverage around the world a few weeks before Christmas in 1967.[6] It was a great media bonanza, the "rabies shots" story for the television era. When this first patient died after only eighteen days, it did not significantly dampen the popular acclaim for this medical milestone. Over time, however, pessimism about medical progress crept into the heart-transplantation story, not only with the deaths of successive recipients but also because of publicity about unprofessional competitiveness between two Texas heart surgeons: Denton Cooley and Michael DeBakey.[7]

In the fall of 1971, as sentiment increasingly turned against heart-transplant operations as medically premature and ethically questionable, *Life* magazine flaunted the sorry outcome of the procedure with a shocking cover. A photomontage placed six heart-transplant patients gathered together for a celebration against a background photograph of a beating heart. The smiling patients expressed the optimism that had come under siege. Bold words printed on the photograph left no doubt as to the story's content: "A New Report on an Era of Medical Failure. The Tragic Record of Heart Transplants. Six Recipients of Transplants Shown Here . . . Were All Dead within Eight Months of Being Photographed Together."[8] Americans' sense of medical progress had changed greatly from halcyon days not long before. Fittingly, *Life* confirmed the change with powerful words right on the cover, signaling "medical failure" not as an isolated incident but as characteristic of a new "era," in contrast to the long period of medical success that had preceded it.

Many developments in the popular culture of that prior era, a time without "medical failure," have been examined in these pages. But it remains to delineate for the period as a whole the characteristic features in the picture of medical progress. And perhaps surprisingly, the imagery had remarkable stability and consistency despite the enormous changes in medical science between the days of Louis Pasteur and those of Jonas Salk.

A breakthrough's most important visual symbol was almost always a vial of some hitherto unknown material—the new cure—that saved lives visibly and quickly. Dependably effective remedies had not been something people expected of doctors before 1885. The initial breakthroughs that overthrew that old assumption were all therapies. But an enthusiasm for therapeutic powers, for curative potions that rescued people when death was lurking, overshadowed such great preventives as vaccination or antisepsis. Smallpox vaccination, for example—historically important as it was in saving lives and preventing sickness—never became a prime example in the public's notion of medical progress. Only several decades into the twentieth century did smallpox vaccination and such discoveries as adding yeast to people's diet to prevent pellagra become visible in the common imagery. In 1885, when Americans became excited about the new rabies shots, they were inaccurately seeing them as a cure even though the actual mechanism was to prevent an infection. That it was innocent children being pulled back from death's door by this new product and shortly thereafter by the use of diphtheria antitoxin made these therapies especially impressive.

The research laboratory—but not the study, the library, the hospital, or the bedside—was another main feature of the image, as the place from which these miracle cures emerged. In popular consciousness, the advances seemed to owe little to hard thinking or clinical experience and everything to manipulation of physical entities and the testing of their effects on animal and human bodies. Prints in the popular media made the laboratory familiar to the public, including its workbench, shelves of bottles and flasks, and cages of rabbits. In the 1880s, laboratories were far less common in hospitals and medical schools than they were in the media. This workplace setting became a major component of the iconography of medical progress, in sharp contrast to the earlier graphic images of physicians. Edelfelt's painting of Pasteur standing in his laboratory, so widely reproduced and imitated, was a revolutionary new image at the time, but one that quickly came to dominate the conception of the medical scientist in the minds of the public as well as in the imagination of artists and photographers. From Pasteur through Salk, in newspapers, magazines, books, and films, the image of a man standing in a laboratory contemplating a glass bottle of his remedy was the easiest way to show that the person was a hero of medical progress.

Experimental studies also required multitudes of animals, along with the laboratory's flasks, bottles, burners, and microscopes. These visual indicators remained part of the popular imagery even as new and large equipment came to be employed during the twentieth century. The microscope and the circle in which artists depicted the minute structures revealed by the microscope remained prominent. After the turn of the twentieth century, the thermometer, the stethoscope, and surgical whites came to symbolize the clinician, but they were rare in depictions of medical research, corroborating the public's assumption that progress arose in the laboratory. The use of experimental animals and human subjects to test new ideas, procedures, and products was visible to the public from the beginning. Rabbits living in cages and being dissected on the table were illustrated in the daily press and family magazines. The use of dogs for experiments was widely shown. Horses entered the picture of medical progress in the 1890s because the life-saving diphtheria antitoxin was made in their bodies and extracted from blood drawn from their veins. After about fifty years, cats and monkeys were added to the visible menagerie. In the public mind, medical progress was unimaginable without animal subjects. For research on certain diseases, human subjects were also necessary, and they, too, were highly visible in popular graphic images throughout the period.

New substances caught the public's eye far more effectively than new ideas did. Almost always, the breakthrough was something that could be held in the hands, and often something injected from a syringe. In this respect, ordinary people's understanding of medical progress and their list of great moments differed from the thinking of historians of medicine, who celebrated such intellectual achievements as the setting aside of spontaneous generation, the analysis of immune reactions, the differentiation of filterable viruses, and the understanding of metabolism and the role of hormones in the body's self-regulation. Although conceptual advances were not entirely ignored by the media and the public, they were less prominent. De Kruif and the comic-book writers did include stories about germs and vitamins and the vectors of transmission for yellow fever and Texas cattle fever. The films about Pasteur and Ehrlich did highlight the germ theory of disease, the role of certain cells within the body as active agents in resisting foreign particles and germs, and Ehrlich's theory of how a chemical molecule can be modified to be lethal only to a specific microbe. Yet these films' biggest moments were the successful injections of anthrax vaccine, rabies vaccine, antitoxin, and Salvarsan.

All through the era from Pasteur to Salk, the public's active engagement with the latest in laboratory research was another part of the picture, even though it usually took place outside the pictorial frame. Right from the first episodes in the 1880s, ordinary people saw the novelties as exciting. They read about them, they tested them in their bodies, they honored the men who discovered them, they gave money to help patients receive the new remedies, and they tried to see firsthand those who had been saved by them. As early as the 1890s, grateful parents and philanthropists contributed funds—and horses—to support laboratory work. That was the moment at which medical charity was first redirected to include research rather than just patient care for the poor. With the help of the popular media, the public kept itself informed about laboratory medicine, even when its enthusiasm exceeded that of the medical profession itself. This was no passive spectatorship; the public actively cheered the advances, invented new ways to support research, celebrated the participants, and memorialized them too.

Institutional settings for research were visibly present in the public's picture of medical progress throughout the era. In 1890, the New York Pasteur Institute was often front-page news, and it was the first research institute to benefit from donations and philanthropic gifts. A decade later, the Rockefeller Institute for Medical Research drew even more media coverage. Later, the National Foundation for Infantile Paralysis became the most familiar institution known for fostering medical innovation. But in the media and in people's hearts, such corporate entities were represented by familiar individuals, not by buildings or organizations. The American public recognized in the press the faces of interesting individual scientists such as Paul Gibier, George Rambaud, Simon Flexner, Alexis Carrel, and Hideyo Noguchi as stand-ins for their institutions, just as President Roosevelt and Jonas Salk became living symbols of the March of Dimes.

Individual men and women, far more often than institutions, were celebrated in popular culture as the engine of medical progress. At first it was Pasteur and Koch who became the celebrities of the day, quickly followed by Gibier and Flexner. Then Carrel and Noguchi of the Rockefeller Institute and later Marie Curie and Sister Kenny became media stars. They were all popular figures about whom the public sought to know their personalities and their personal lives. Fortunately for them, the press usually accorded the medical heroes somewhat more respect and privacy than other fashionable people received. Still, the fact that they were part of popular culture as individual persons with families, emotions, and ambitions—not just names that identified theories and discoveries—was the key to ordinary people's engagement with the excitement of medical research over the first half of the twentieth century. Even as the individual was being replaced by the research team and the apparatus was gaining size and complexity during the mid-twentieth century, the public's vision centered on the solitary discoverer, seeing Jonas Salk as a modern-day Pasteur, injecting children with a life-saving fluid. The pictorial convention established by Edelfelt's painting was used again and again because it conveyed all the key elements of the medical breakthrough: a thoughtful individual, surrounded by apparatus and holding aloft a miracle-working injection.

De Kruif capitalized on this desire for heroic individuals. Using a novelistic style, he brought the mechanics of medical research to life through dramatized narratives of particular scientists. Although he wrote about both the present and the past, it was his historical narratives that first made medical history a popular genre and its heroes widely familiar. His stories of discovery were devoured by the public. For about twenty-five years, medical history remained a familiar subject in all the mass media, and people's picture of medical progress was enriched by delineations of breakthroughs from before their time. This awareness of an ever-lengthening series of research triumphs aggrandized the status of the recent discoveries by placing their makers in a pantheon of medical heroes. In this era, medical history and its famous names were a living part of mass culture. Unfortunately, the general public's familiarity with earlier medical discoveries did not continue much past midcentury. College students, for example, can no longer reliably identify Louis Pasteur; and when one professor inquired about the Louis Pasteur film at a video-rental store, the clerk asked her whether he was the actor or the director.

CODA

If Helen Hayes, long honored as the "first lady of the American theater," seems an unlikely figure to illuminate the popular understanding of medical progress, her life nonetheless reveals how intimately developments within medicine were connected with media performances about medicine and medical history, helping to shape the way ordinary folks' pictured medical progress. Not only an exceedingly popular actress, Hayes was also a beloved public figure from the 1920s until her death in the

1990s. Her presence extended through a wide swath of the mass media for half a century, with innumerable appearances, not only on the stage but in the newspapers and magazines, on the screen, and on radio and television. Several episodes in her career highlight the complex entanglements of medical discovery with popular culture.

The 1931 film of *Arrowsmith* was Helen Hayes's first Hollywood success after she had established a huge reputation on the stage. She played Leora Tozer Arrowsmith, the good-hearted, but doomed, wife of the heroic Dr. Arrowsmith (played by Ronald Colman), who moved from small-town practice to the heights of research achievements.[9] In both the book and the film, Leora—as nurse, devoted wife, and victim of a laboratory accident—was the most sympathetic character. Hayes replayed this role over the following two decades in at least three radio versions of "Arrowsmith"—as dramatized by Orson Welles in 1939, on the *Helen Hayes Theater of the Air* in 1940 and 1941, and on *Electric Theater* in 1948 and 1949.[10] Furthermore, the book and the dramatizations based on it, while known to be fiction, seemed as real as history to many Americans, due to the many parallels with the popular microbe-hunter stories and such contemporary discoveries as insulin, vitamins, miracles drugs, and the causes of hookworm and pellagra. The conflating of fiction with reality was further reinforced by such marketing decisions as the use of a photograph of real people, Hayes and Colman, on the dust jacket of the novel. Other photographs of the actors in the film served as illustrations within the book (as in fig. 58 in chapter 6).

In the summer of 1949, when Americans were facing one of the worst polio epidemics they had seen, Helen Hayes and her eighteen-year-old daughter Mary were performing together in a summer-stock company.[11] Mary took ill and was sent home to New York City with what seemed like the flu. Soon she was hospitalized. By the time her mother arrived, Mary was already in an iron lung with bulbar polio, and she lived only a few more days.[12] The publicity surrounding Mary's death increased donations in support of polio research, and Helen Hayes became active in fundraising activities for the National Foundation, such as chairing its fashion show in 1950.[13] During the 1950s, Hayes narrated "The Breath of Life," about a young victim of poliomyelitis in a radio drama series called "Biographies in Sound." NBC radio also presented a program called "Helen Hayes Talks about Polio."[14] Hayes later recalled with pride that "Jonas Salk told me I was one of the biggest assets he had in getting his vaccine to the world."[15] In addition to frequently appearing on radio both as Leora Tozer and also as herself to educate the public about polio, Hayes starred in two fact-based medical history dramas in the mid-1950s. In April 1953, NBC broadcast "The Fight against Pain," in a series entitled *Medicine U.S.A.*[16]

Then, in November 1954—during the dark fall and winter when the results of the Salk vaccine trial were being silently tabulated by an army of statisticians—Hayes took on the role of a California woman doctor whose long career included several signal moments in medical history dating back to the 1880s. The broadcast was

carried nationally in the *Hallmark Hall
of Fame* on the CBS radio network.[17]
This biographical drama was presented
as a true story. In this performance, the
actress whose film career started as the
fictional nurse Leora Tozer was now
playing the real-life physician Rebecca
Lee Dorsey (fig. 107), who had died just
months before. Dorsey had bizarrely
—if perhaps unconsciously—borrowed
scenes and situations from Hollywood's
medical history films when writing her
memoirs, thereby turning her autobiography into fiction. She was almost like
Tozer/Hayes in reverse, with historical
facts transformed by fantasy, rather than
fiction appearing as real to an audience.
Her culturally enriched "memories" were
fully accepted as authentic by the media,
and the historical importance of this
1954 radio play is not in any facts it gets
right or wrong but in the way it confirms
both the popular picture of medical

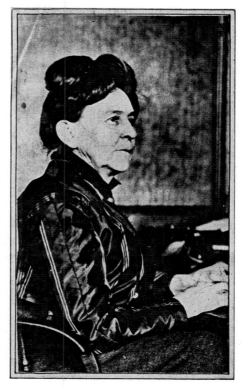

FIG. 107. Dr. Rebecca Lee Dorsey at age sixty,
in a photograph published in the *Los Angeles
Times,* January 12, 1919, in a large article entitled "Some of the Brainy Business Women
of Los Angeles." Author's collection.

progress and the familiarity with medical history that ordinary listeners in that
era brought to the story. And Dorsey offered the 1950s public a continuous link
all the way back to Louis Pasteur and
the first rabies shots.

As the play opens, Dorsey is a young American doctor suffering from tuberculosis some time around 1880. When informed that she can be saved only by Robert
Koch's new serum, she hurries to Berlin. There she has to overcome Koch's hesitation to undertake a human trial by boldly asserting that, if she must die, she would
rather die from his serum than from the disease. Then, having been cured by Koch's
tuberculin, she somehow manages to secure a place in Pasteur's laboratory during
the historic summer of 1885. Fortuitously, when Joseph Meister and his mother des-
perately seek treatment for the boy, Dorsey can use the story of her personal experience with Koch's serum to overcome Pasteur's hesitation about a human trial of
his rabies treatment. In the second act, just as Dorsey is trying to start a practice in
Los Angeles, she is rebuffed by a father with two diphtheritic sons who refuses to
let her stick them with a needle because a girl in the community had recently died
after receiving a diphtheria inoculation.[18] She tells him of how she had been cured

by a needle, as was Joseph Meister, and how she herself worked with Behring on developing the antitoxin treatment, yet he relents only after one of his sons dies. The other son is then saved with the help of Dorsey's needle, and this success makes headlines in Los Angeles papers and gives her career a needed boost. At the end of the performance, radio host Lionel Barrymore explained to listeners that Dorsey had still been practicing when she recently died at the age of ninety-five. He also reported that when a film-studio representative had met with her and mentioned possibly making a movie of her life, she said, "If you do, I hope you'll have my favorite actress play me, Helen Hayes."

Dorsey's version of her life touched so many chords with popular expectations that her distortions and fantasies were readily taken for truth just because these scientists' names and the situations in which she placed herself were already familiar in the mass culture of the era. Though her story cannot be taken as history for those early decades, its easy credibility in the 1950s helps reveal the sense of medical history current at that time. To historians, the inaccuracies and impossibilities in this story are simply grotesque. Koch's tuberculin did not precede Pasteur's rabies vaccine but followed it by five years. Dorsey never worked with Pasteur. In the dramatization, Dorsey and Pasteur speak with a chummy informality that would have appalled the great chemist. His collaborators never spoke to him in this way, and it is unlikely that even his wife did. In fact, the tonality of the repartee between Dorsey and Pasteur more closely resembles the on-screen relationship between Paul Ehrlich and his wife, Hedwig, in *Dr. Ehrlich's Magic Bullet*, with Hedwig having to manage the distracted scientist, who is so forgetful that he neglects mundane things such as eating. And distortions such as these were not limited to the dramatization. Dorsey's obituary in the *New York Times* placed her squarely into the seminal milieux of medical history: "Dr. Rebecca Lee Dorsey, whose career spanned the development of modern medical science, died today at her home. She was 95 years old and had practiced [in Los Angeles] since 1886. She had studied under Louis Pasteur, Joseph Lister, Profs. Rudolph, Virchow, Billroth, Kaposi, Konradt and others who were pioneers in bacteriology, cellular pathology and endocrinology."[19] The same day's obituary in the *Los Angeles Times* ran about twenty column inches. To the teachers just listed "for the young woman doctor in Europe between 1883 and 1886," this unsigned obituary added Rokitansky, Loeffler, Klebs, Brown-Séquard, and others. She was said to have administered the first diphtheria antitoxin used in Los Angeles before 1893, delivered the first baby in a hospital in Los Angeles, and so forth.[20] Of course, any such use of antitoxin in 1893 was impossible since none was available in the United States until about two years later. In fact, this same newspaper had reported on January 16, 1895, that the first antitoxin for patients had just arrived in Los Angeles, coming from Gibier's Pasteur Institute in New York.[21] Although it is possible that Dorsey had been involved in the antitoxin's administration and that her recollection was simply off by two years, her claim was less likely to be a memory slip about the order of events than unrestrained self-aggrandizement and self-deception, given the impossibly rich collection of teachers she claimed for herself.

Only a few weeks before Dorsey's death in 1954, the *Los Angeles Times* published a letter to the editor from her, speaking to current discussions about the preventive use of regular rabies shots for animals. But she used the bulk of the letter to describe her youthful experience with Louis Pasteur:

> In 1885 I was a medical student at the old Pasteur Institute in Paris. . . . I have the formula for the inoculations that Prof. Pasteur used at this time. . . . I also am the only living person who was present when the first inoculation for rabies was ever given to a human being—little Joe Meister, July 9, 1885. . . . At this first use of the serum on a human being Prof. Pasteur was very nervous—I supported his right elbow with my right hand and held the arm of the patient with my left hand when the injection was given.[22]

Of course, the chemist Pasteur never gave the injections himself. No evidence confirms any American woman doctor studying or working in Pasteur's laboratory at this time. Meister was not treated at the Pasteur Institute, which opened only three years later. And although Pasteur was certainly nervous about the risks of giving Meister these injections, he employed only his very closest associates in the treatments and kept everything secret for several weeks until the boy's life seemed out of danger.[23]

The *Hallmark Hall of Fame*'s dramatized "true story" of Rebecca Lee Dorsey linked Louis Pasteur's rabies vaccine and the potent "serums" injected by modern doctors' needles to other pioneering feats of twentieth-century medicine. Having Helen Hayes play the role even fulfilled the hopes of the late Dr. Dorsey, who had died before the broadcast. Performing this role of a modern healer, Hayes was able to unite the medical stories in which she had often appeared onstage with her offstage engagement in the struggle against polio. Like most Americans at the time of this broadcast, Helen Hayes, who had lost her daughter to polio, was waiting for the results of the controlled experiment in which more than a million children served as guinea pigs receiving either the Salk vaccine or a placebo.

The following spring, Salk was crowned a hero, as a man whose magic shots from the laboratory saved the lives of children, just like Louis Pasteur seventy years before (with or without the steady hand of Rebecca Lee Dorsey). Leading lady Helen Hayes, who had played Mrs. Arrowsmith, who had volunteered for the March of Dimes, and who had brought the story of Dr. Dorsey to U.S. airwaves, shared a natural rapport with the man who conquered polio with support from the March of Dimes. Salk and Hayes were almost the same age, and they had both come of age within a popular culture enthusiastic about medical history and medical research. Within a few years of Salk's triumph, he, like Pasteur, opened a research institute bearing his name, and when the entertainment industry was raising money to support the Salk Institute for Biological Studies, Helen Hayes added to the luster of the celebration

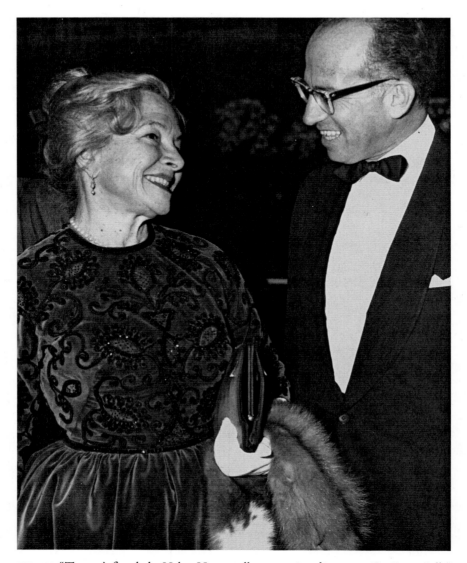

FIG. 108. "Theatre's first lady, Helen Hayes, talks to vaccine discoverer, Dr. Jonas Salk," at the gala premiere of Darryl F. Zanuck's film *The Longest Day,* a benefit for the Salk Institute. Sunday magazine of the *New York Daily News,* December 2, 1962, 11. Photograph by Daniel Jacino © 1962 New York Daily News. Used with permission. All rights reserved.

(fig. 108). It is more than coincidence that the triumphs of Pasteur and Salk each prompted an outpouring of public generosity in support of medical research or that out of the publicity emerged permanent institutions of research named for the men who made the key discoveries. The unique and unprecedented events of 1885 had set in place an enduring pattern of public excitement and gratitude.

ENCORE

If the late twentieth century abandoned the fervent faith in medical progress that had dominated American culture for seventy years, many people in medicine and in philanthropy have never lost their conviction that research in medical science is the most effective way to contribute to the world's health and well-being. One recent expression of that confidence resonates with this book's argument connecting a French rabies cure to American support for laboratory research. In the spring of 2005, the Pasteur Foundation honored former president William J. Clinton for his work on behalf of developing nations and their fight against HIV/AIDS. At a gala banquet, Bill Clinton received the Pasteur Foundation's 2005 award from the ambassador of France to the United States, Jean-David Levitte, and the director general of the Institut Pasteur, Philippe Kourilsky.[24] Their gift to Clinton made explicit the historical connection between Clinton's twenty-first-century global campaign against AIDS and the new era of medical progress that started with Louis Pasteur's treatment in Paris of four little American boys (see color plate 22). They presented him with "*Judge*'s Wax Works—The Political Eden Musée," a political cartoon published in 1886 (seen in color plate 6). In this colorful caricature, an earlier Democratic president, Grover Cleveland, had been portrayed as "Pasteur Cleveland," inoculating Democracy with civil service reform against the spoils system of rabies in an image that illustrated the general public's ready familiarity with Pasteur's rabies breakthrough.

In the early years of the twenty-first century, few people other than historians of medicine and some history-loving physicians would still recognize a picture of Louis Pasteur inoculating for rabies. The long-lived cluster of widely shared images about medical progress is no longer familiar. For seventy years, however, all the popular media educated a wide audience about the power of reason and objectivity in science and about such core ideals as naturalism and social utility. And many ordinary citizens clearly came to share those values with scientists. If the American public first became thrilled with laboratory research through giddy human-interest journalism about dogs, boys, and a chemist far across the Atlantic, the newly established enthusiasm for science continued to expand, reinforced by recurrent images of the benefits of laboratory research for medicine. The public's curiosity fostered a new publishing genre of popular medical history and supported the movement of these stories into films, radio drama, and comic books. In thousands of ways, these diverse media evoked for their audiences the value of carefully controlled experiments. These media images encouraged people to honor the laboratory worker as a hero who made contributions to society as real as those of the statesman, the soldier, or the entrepreneur. For seven decades, American popular culture kept circulating—with remarkable consistency and little dissent—the unprecedented notion of medical advance that first emerged with Pasteur's breakthrough. And Jonas Salk, like Louis Pasteur before him, became a household name when he too used a needle to inject killed virus to protect children from the most feared ailment of his time.

RADIO DRAMAS OF MEDICAL HISTORY IN CAVALCADE OF AMERICA

DuPont's *Cavalcade of America* broadcast hundreds of thirty-minute dramas from October 1935 to March 1953, first on CBS and then on NBC. (A television series of the same name aired from 1952 to 1957.) Because program titles often do not indicate the subject of the drama (e.g., "The Giant in the Meadow" or "Make Way for the Lady"), it is possible that this compilation has overlooked some relevant programs.

PROGRAMS FEATURING THE MEDICAL HEROES WHOSE STORIES WERE COMMONLY DRAMATIZED

"Heroism in Medical Science" (in two parts, about Crawford Long discovering anesthesia and William Crawford Gorgas fighting yellow fever; December 4, 1935)

"The Story of Dr. Reed" (June 25, 1940)

"Arrowsmith" (February 23, 1942)

"Yellow Jack" (with Tyrone Power; April 6, 1942)

"Clara Barton" (June 1, 1942)

"The Colossus of Panama" (William Gorgas fighting yellow fever; June 8, 1942)

"Sister Kenny" (November 30, 1942)

"Conquest of Pain" (ether anesthesia; December 11, 1944)

"Garden Key" (Samuel Mudd fighting yellow fever while in prison; November 8, 1948)

PROGRAMS FEATURING LESS FAMILIAR FIGURES FROM
THE HISTORY OF MEDICINE

"Pioneer Woman Physician: Elizabeth Blackwell" (January 27, 1937)

"The Ounce of Prevention" (Cotton Mather and Zabdiel Boylston introducing smallpox inoculation; February 17, 1937)

"The Red Death" (Joseph Goldberger working on pellagra; October 30, 1940)

"The Mystery of the Spotted Death" (the Public Health Service researching Rocky Mountain spotted fever; July 7, 1941)

"Josephine Baker" (a public-health doctor dealing with "Typhoid Mary"; August 4, 1941)

"Angels on Horseback" (the Frontier Nursing Service, with Myrna Loy; March 23, 1942)

"The Giant in the Meadow" (Theobald Smith puzzling out Texas fever; August 24, 1942)

"That They Might Live" (Marie Zakrzewska; October 19, 1942)

"Lifetide" (Norman Bethune inventing the mobile blood bank; March 22, 1943)

"Make Way for the Lady" (Mary Putnam Jacobi; June 14, 1943)

"The Weapon That Saves Lives" (sulfa drugs; August 23, 1943)

"The Story of Penicillin" (Fleming and Florey; April 24, 1944)

"Conquest of Quinine" (chemists trying to synthesize this wartime scarcity; July 31, 1944)

"Doctor in Crinoline" (Elizabeth Blackwell, with Loretta Young; December 18, 1944)

"The Doctor with Hope in His Hands" (Harvey Cushing pioneering brain surgery; March 11, 1946)

"With Cradle and Clock" (Knud Stowman immigrating in 1702 to champion obstetric medicine; September 2, 1946)

"That They Might Live" (Chevalier Jackson inventing the bronchoscope; October 7, 1946)

"The Doctor and the President" (Benjamin Waterhouse vaccinating Thomas Jefferson; April 21, 1947)

"No Greater Love" (Clara Maass, army nurse who died fighting yellow fever; March 8, 1948)

"Experiment at Monticello" (Thomas Jefferson vaccinating his family, servants, and slaves; January 10, 1949)

"Sir Galahad in Manhattan" (J. Marion Sims founding the first women's hospital in the United States; November 14, 1950)

"Militant Angel" (Annie Warburton Goodrich campaigning for professional standards in nursing; May 15, 1951).

"A Medal for Miss Walker" (Mary Walker being captured by the Confederate Army during the Civil War; January 6, 1953)

CHAPTER 1. MEDICINE IN THE PUBLIC EYE, THEN AND NOW

1. *Chicago Daily News,* April 12, 1955, 1. The most recent account of all these developments is David M. Oshinsky, *Polio: An American Story* (New York: Oxford University Press, 2005).

2. "She's First to Get Polio Vaccine Here" and "President Acts to Share Vaccine Data with the World: Red Countries Included in Eisenhower's Plan to Send Out Reports on Salk Tests," *Los Angeles Times,* April 14, 1955, 1.

3. "Dr. Jonas E. Salk: Portrait by Karsh of Ottawa," *Wisdom: The Magazine of Knowledge for All America* 1:8 (August 1956), cover (photograph by Yousuf Karsh). This issue contains a number of articles linking the present and the past in a continuous chain of medical progress, including, for example, "Great Men of Medicine," "To the Men of Medicine" by William Osler, "Jonas E. Salk, Medical Researcher," "The Story behind the Polio Vaccine," "History of Pharmacy in Pictures," "Why They Became Doctors," "Doctors, Diseases, and Drugs," and "Ars medica."

4. Robert Coughlan, "Tracking the Killer: Production of a New Polio Vaccine Brings a Great Medical Mystery-Drama, with a Cast of Thousands, Up to Its Climactic Act," *Life,* February 22, 1954.

5. Murray B. Light, *From Butler to Buffett: The Story behind the Buffalo News* (Amherst, N.Y.: Prometheus Books, 2004), 135–136.

6. The image was published without a date or any citation to the original source (only a picture credit to "Center H. Roger Viollet") in *Health and Disease* by René Dubos, Maya Pines, and the Editors of Time-Life Books (New York: Time-Life Books, 1965), 70–71. The caption had a quite misleading error, indicating that the boy shown was Joseph Meister, the first person treated under Pasteur's guidance. In fact, Meister's treatment in July 1885 was a tightly guarded secret because it was so risky and the outcome was uncertain; no onlookers, reporters, or newspaper artists were there to witness Meister's injections. Only two months later, after Meister survived the treatment and seemed out of danger of developing rabies, did Pasteur begin to share word of the experiment, and only after his public announcement in late October did newspaper coverage stir up public interest.

7. "Vakcination hos Pasteur," *Nutiden* 507 (June 6, 1886), 359. This weekly Danish newspaper reprinted the image published a few weeks earlier in a French magazine, *Le Journal Illustré* of March 28, 1886, where it was captioned, "Séance de vaccination contre la rage au laboratoire de l'Ecole Normale Supérieure en présence de L. Pasteur, du dr Grancher et d'Eugène Viala. Dessin d'après une nature de Meyer, grave par Meaulle." For a contemporary U.S. publication of people watching Pasteur observing the inoculation of a standing boy, see "Pasteur's Treatment of Rabies," *Scientific American Supplement* 21:544 (June 5, 1886), 8692.

CHAPTER 2. BEFORE THERE WERE MEDICAL BREAKTHROUGHS: DISEASES AND DOCTORS IN THE PICTORIAL PRESS, 1860–1890

1. Epigraph quoted from Charles Neider, *Mark Twain* (New York: Horizon Press, 1967), 43.

2. *Judge* 9:217 (December 12, 1885), 2.

3. *Judge* 9:220 (January 2, 1886), 10.

4. Charles E. Rosenberg, "The Therapeutic Revolution: Medicine, Meaning, and Social Change in Nineteenth-Century America," in *The Therapeutic Revolution: Essays in the Social History of American Medicine,* ed. Morris J. Vogel and Charles E. Rosenberg, 3–25 (Philadelphia: University of Pennsylvania Press, 1979).

5. Frank Luther Mott, *A History of American Magazines,* 5 vols. (Cambridge, Mass.: Harvard University Press, 1938–1968), 2:453–465; Joshua Brown, *Beyond the Lines: Pictorial Reporting, Everyday Life, and the Crisis of Gilded Age America* (Berkeley: University of California Press, 2002); and Andrea G. Pearson, "*Frank Leslie's Illustrated Newspaper* and *Harper's Weekly*: Innovation and Imitation in Nineteenth-Century American Pictorial Reporting," *Journal of Popular Culture* 23:4 (Spring 1990), 81–111.

6. Pearson, "*Frank Leslie's*," 82–86.

7. Mott, *History of American Magazines,* 2:469–487; Pearson, "*Frank Leslie's.*" Brown, *Beyond the Lines,* is centered on *Frank Leslie's,* but it provides significant material on *Harper's Weekly* as well.

8. Pearson, "*Frank Leslie's*," 92, 103.

9. Mott provides overviews of both magazines in *History of American Magazines,* 3:520–534 (for *Puck*), and 3:552–556 (for *Judge*). On both, see also Richard Samuel West, *Satire on Stone: The Political Cartoons of Joseph Keppler* (Urbana: University of Illinois Press, 1988).

10. On the *National Police Gazette,* see Mott, *History of American Magazines,* 2:325–337; and Elliott J. Gorn, "The Wicked World: The *National Police Gazette* and Gilded Age America," *Media Studies Journal* 6:1 (Winter 1992), 1–15.

11. On the *Daily Graphic,* see Frank Luther Mott, *American Journalism, A History: 1690 to 1960,* 3rd ed. (New York: Macmillan, 1962), 502, 666–667; and Brown, *Beyond the Lines,* 267.

12. For the pictorial component of public-health agitation in this era, with cartoons from several of these magazines and newspapers, see Bert Hansen, "The Image and Advocacy of Public Health in American Caricature and Cartoons from 1860 to 1900," *American Journal of Public Health* 87:11 (November 1997), 1798–1807.

13. Philip P. Choy, Lorraine Dong, and Marlon K. Hom, eds., *Coming Man: 19th Century American Perceptions of the Chinese* (Seattle: University of Washington Press, 1994),

164–165. On circulation figures in the early 1880s for the *Police Gazette* and many other magazines, see Mott, *History of American Magazines,* 2:6–9.

14. Because this book is concerned with the changing perception of medicine in general, it focuses on the mainstream profession in all its variety, but it leaves aside the images of quacks and quackery as a distinct subject of inquiry. The visual records of quack medicine have been beautifully recorded and illustrated in William H. Helfand, *Quack, Quack, Quack: The Sellers of Nostrums in Prints, Posters, Ephemera and Books* (New York: Grolier Club, 2002).

15. The broadcloth phrasing comes from *Puck* magazine in 1883 and is quoted at greater length later in this chapter.

16. *Puck* 25:632 (April 17, 1889), back cover (128).

17. *St. Louis Globe-Democrat,* February 14, 1886, 4.

18. The coverage was unprecedented, and it played an important role in the success of one newspaper. Mrs. Frank Leslie, soon after her husband's death, managed quickly to raise the circulation of the paper she took over and to pay off inherited debts through aggressive pictorial coverage of the situation of Mr. Garfield in bed and Mr. Guiteau in jail; see Brown, *Beyond the Lines,* 172.

19. Although illustrations published only abroad would not support the arguments made in this book, this one is included because it repeats an image from a U.S. paper, while also illustrating how the pictorial weeklies often copied from one another, even across the Atlantic. And although the copying was more often done by the Americans, the traffic ran both ways.

20. The related article in *Harper's Weekly* (508) also describes how the paper's artist, William A. Rogers, made a drawing of the scene without disturbing the President. A longer account is found in his memoirs: W. A. Rogers, *A World Worth While: A Record of "Auld Acquaintance"* (New York: Harper and Brothers, 1922), 20–24.

21. "A Board of Health Doctor in a New York Tenement," *Harper's Weekly* 33:1703 (August 10, 1889), cover (637), wood engraving by William A. Rogers; story on 651.

22. "J. Marion Sims, M.D.," *Harper's Weekly* 20:1017 (June 24, 1876), 517–518.

23. *New York World,* January 5, 1886, 1.

24. *Puck* 18:443 (September 2, 1885), 4.

25. Morris J. Vogel, *The Invention of the Modern Hospital, Boston, 1870–1930* (Chicago: University of Chicago Press, 1980); David Rosner, *A Once Charitable Enterprise: Hospitals and Health Care in Brooklyn and New York, 1885–1915* (Cambridge: Cambridge University Press, 1982); and Charles E. Rosenberg, *The Care of Strangers: The Rise of America's Hospital System* (New York: Basic Books, 1987).

26. Among the many such illustrations, a few typical ones may be noted. Exterior and interior views of New York Hospital's new building at Stuyvesant Square are seen in *Frank Leslie's Illustrated Newspaper* 44:1122 (March 31, 1877), 61, and in *Harper's Weekly* 21:1058 (April 7, 1877), 272. Wide-angle architectural views are seen in *Harper's Weekly* 18:896 (February 28, 1874), 193 (State Homeopathic Asylum for the Insane, Middletown, Orange County, New York, and Hudson River State Hospital for the Insane, Poughkeepsie, Dutchess County, New York); *Frank Leslie's Illustrated Newspaper* 48:1226 (March 29, 1879), 61 (The Mary Fletcher Hospital, Burlington, Vermont); *Frank Leslie's Illustrated Newspaper* 68:1752 (April 13, 1889), 152 (The New York Cancer Hospital); and *Harper's Weekly* 37:1881 (January 7, 1893), 17 (The New York Post-Graduate Medical School and Hospital and The New St. Luke's Hospital).

27. Joseph Hirsh with Beka Doherty, *Saturday, Sunday, and Everyday: The History of the United Hospital Fund of New York* (New York: The Fund, 1954).

28. John J. Fialka, *Sisters: Catholic Nuns and the Making of America* (New York: St. Martin's, 2003).

29. C. J. Taylor, "Remember Hospital Sunday!" *Puck* 20:511 (December 22, 1886), cover (271). The following year, *Puck* again devoted a cover to this cause: Joseph Keppler, "An Outside Ally," 22:563 (December 21, 1887).

30. C. J. Taylor, "Charity—False and True: Let the Long-Suffering Public Discriminate between Worthy and Unworthy Objects, and Not Let the Worthy Lack Support," *Puck* 26:667 (December 18, 1889), 294–295.

31. For a later example, see "The Beneficent Work of the Ladies Hospital and Prison Association among the Criminal and Unfortunate at Blackwell's Island," *Frank Leslie's Illustrated Newspaper* 64:1657 (June 18, 1887), 285, full-page wood engraving from "sketches by a staff artist."

32. The image was published in Albert S. Lyons and R. Joseph Petrucelli II, *Medicine: An Illustrated History* (New York: Harry N. Abrams, 1978), 545; in Ann Novotny and Carter Smith, eds., *Images of Healing: A Portfolio of American Medical and Pharmaceutical Practice in the 18th, 19th, and Early 20th Centuries* (New York: Macmillan, 1980), 71; in M. Patricia Donahue, *Nursing, the Finest Art: An Illustrated History* (St. Louis: Mosby, 1985), 272; and in Rosenberg, *Care of Strangers,* facing 182. This engraving was also used on the cover of three successive editions of a popular teaching anthology, Judith Walzer Leavitt and Ronald L. Numbers, eds., *Sickness and Health in America: Readings in the History of Medicine and Public Health* (Madison: University of Wisconsin Press, 1978, 1985, and 1997).

33. Charles E. Rosenberg, "Social Class and Medical Care in Nineteenth-Century America: The Rise and Fall of the Dispensary," *Journal of the History of Medicine and Allied Sciences* 29:1 (January 1974), 32–54. See, for example, "Doctors Robbed of Fees: Free Dispensaries, They Say, Treat Gratuitously Rich Patients; Which Ought to Be Stopped; Abuse of Medical Charity," *New York Times,* May 25, 1897, 1.

34. For two later dispensary images, see "Scenes at the New York Free Dispensary, Centre Street, Near Canal," *Frank Leslie's Illustrated Weekly* 72:1866 (June 27, 1891), 357, full-page wood engraving of drawing by J. Durkin; and "In a Public Dispensary—Treating Patients of La Grippe," *Harper's Weekly* 36:1831 (January 23, 1892), 73, front cover, wood engraving from drawing by C. S. Reinhart; the related story is on p. 90. In the second image, no doctor is seen, no examination area or table is visible, and people sit in pews waiting for a turn at the window of a counter from which medicines are dispensed.

35. Vern L. Bullough and Bonnie Bullough, *The Care of the Sick: The Emergence of Modern Nursing* (New York: Prodist, 1978), 113. An exact count of nurses in the United States in the late nineteenth century is not available, but the timing of the rise in their numbers to the closing decade may be confirmed by the changing number of nursing schools: 15 schools in 1890 and 432 in 1900 (118).

36. Examples of eminent men in politics dressed as children's nurses may be found in *Judge* (September 26, 1885; May 23, 1896; and July 3, 1897) and in *Puck* (January 18, 1882; September 2, 1896; and November 17, 1897).

37. The paucity of nurse images seems implicitly confirmed by their virtual absence from an eight-hundred-page study (including 541 figures) of the image of women from 1876 to 1918: Martha Banta, *Imaging American Women: Idea and Ideals in Cultural History* (New York: Columbia University Press, 1987), has only one figure with nurses in it, "Women in War" by Daniel MacMorris, dating from 1955 (575). Further confirmation that images of trained nurses were rare until the end of the nineteenth century is found in an important exhibit on the image of nurses and nursing, in which only three of the eighty-five items are from the U.S. popular media for this era; see William H. Helfand, *The Nightingale's Song: Nurses and Nursing in the Ars Medica Collection of the Philadelphia Museum of Art* (Philadelphia: Museum of Art, 2000). Although it is possible that there were U.S. printings of "The Lady with the Lamp" image of Florence Nightingale at Scutari in the mid-1850s, I have not yet found any.

38. The article is "New York Medical College for Women," *Frank Leslie's Illustrated Newspaper* 30:759 (April 16, 1870), 71. The illustrations for this article appear on 65 (the cover), 72 (two images), and 73 (one image). Separately, on pp. 66–67, the paper ran "Women Doctors," an essay by Augustus K. Gardner, M.D., who comments on the images of the female medical students and praises women doctors in general. He confesses that he had made unkind and unfair judgments about them twenty years earlier and admits that he had been wrong. His new praise for women doctors is strong, if expressed in ways that maintain sexist assumptions about sex differences.

39. The arrangement of this corpse and its coverings, including an exposed foot and hand, are echoed in a political cartoon by Thomas Nast published on the cover of *Harper's Weekly* several years later. There might have been some traditional image from which both artists worked. Nast's scene has a female body representing New York City laid out on the slab of a morgue; the image is titled "Foully Murdered." The corpse is being viewed through large glass windows by smiling spectators indicated as the "Tammany Hall Ring" (July 7, 1877, p. 1071).

40. This set of images has been largely overlooked by historians, garnering no mention in such important books as Regina Markell Morantz-Sanchez, *Sympathy and Science: Women Physicians in American Medicine* (New York: Oxford University Press, 1985), and Michael Sappol, *A Traffic of Dead Bodies: Anatomy and Embodied Social Identity in Nineteenth-Century America* (Princeton, N.J.: Princeton University Press, 2002). Only the front cover in this group of images seems to be present in the sixty-thousand-item database of photographs and graphic art at the National Library of Medicine called "Images from the History of Medicine." The cover image was reprinted in Ruth J. Abram, ed., *"Send Us a Lady Physician": Women Doctors in America, 1835–1920* (New York: Norton, 1985), 94. This generously illustrated collection of essays printed two other images of women medical students and mistakenly attributed them to this *Frank Leslie's* issue. I have identified one of these (a dissection scene on p. 94) as being taken from the *National Police Gazette* 36:134 (April 17, 1880), 16 (with story on 14), and the other (a commencement ceremony printed on p. 95) as being originally published in *Frank Leslie's Illustrated Newspaper* 36:915 (April 12, 1873), 73.

41. That women doctors were assimilated into negative as well as positive stereotypes of the medical profession was made clear in a satire that appeared as one of nine "Cartoons on Current Topics" on the front page of the *New York Daily Graphic*, April 6, 1878. Two well-dressed women, carrying their diplomas and their surgical instruments, are shown leaving a commencement ceremony at a medical college; the caption ridicules them as "The New Women Doctors Licensed to Cure or—Kill." This is no different in tone or imagery than mockery that was commonly directed at male physicians.

42. "The Transfusion of Blood—An Operation at the 'Hôpital de la Pitié,'" *Harper's Weekly* 18:914 (July 4, 1874), 570 (illustration) and 569 (article); and "Performing the operation of transfusion of blood at the hospital of Pity Paris France," *Scientific American* n.s. 31:10

(September 5, 1874), 147. The *Scientific American* article included two additional small images, "The Transfusion of Blood, A.D. 1667," and "Blood Globules Magnified" (both on 146).

43. Newspapers reported from time to time on individual doctors' attempts to save desperate individuals with transfusions of human or animal blood. The *New York Times,* for example, ran short articles on animal experiments on July 17, 1856, and January 21, 1859, and several longer articles in 1874, 1875, 1877, and 1880. On August 18, 1881, the *New York Times* reported on page 1 that the wounded President Garfield was recovering from his relapse and that there were no thoughts of using a blood transfusion. On February 21, 1886, the *St. Louis Globe-Democrat* published "Transfusion of Blood: The Dream of Early Medicine Made a Reality of Modern Surgery." This five-column article with three drawings of the apparatus and its connections to the blood vessels appeared in a weekly series of unsigned Sunday articles about medical progress.

44. On the history of these catalogues and of the Tiemann company more generally, see the introduction by James M. Edmonson and F. Terry Hambrecht to the 1889 centennial reprint of the *American Armamentarium Chirurgicum* (San Francisco and Boston: Norman Publishing and The Printers' Devil, 1989), 1–65. I have not determined how early the blood transfusion devices appeared in Tiemann publications or in those of other makers; in the 1889 edition, the transfusion section is on 117–119.

45. *New York Times,* April 30, 1880, 4 (untitled editorial), and June 19, 1880, 2 ("Transfusion of Blood").

46. *New York Times,* September 11, 1877, 4.

47. "The Transfusion of Blood—May the Operation Prove a Success," *Puck* 16:404 (December 3, 1884), center spread (216–217), chromolithograph by Joseph Keppler.

48. "The Transfusion of Blood—A Proposed Dangerous Experiment," *Judge* 14:350 (June 30, 1888), back cover (196).

49. *A Facsimile of Frank Leslie's Illustrated Historical Register of the Centennial Exposition, 1876* (New York: Paddington, 1974); for the lists of exhibit categories, see p. 36.

50. James D. McCabe, *The Illustrated History of the Centennial Exhibition Held in Commemoration of the One Hundredth Anniversary of American Independence: With a Full Description of the Great Buildings and All the Objects of Interest Exhibited in Them* (Philadelphia: National Publishing, 1876; reprinted 1975), 216.

51. McCabe, *Illustrated History,* 216. In *Frank Leslie's Illustrated Historical Register,* this painting is not mentioned. The only remark about Eakins is that a portrait of his was poorly hung (204).

52. "Cartoons and Comments," *Puck* 7:162 (April 14, 1880), 88.

53. "Old School Etiquette," *Puck* 13:327 (June 13, 1883), cover (225), drawing by F. Graetz.

54. For more on the era's controversy within the medical profession about consulting with "irregulars," see John Harley Warner, "Ideals of Science and Their Discontents in Late Nineteenth-Century American Medicine," *Isis* 82:3 (September 1991), 454–478.

55. "Cartoons and Comments," *Puck* 13:327 (June 13, 1883), 226.

56. "Our Merciless Millionaire. Vanderbilt:—'The Public Be—Doctored!'" *Puck* 16:399 (October 29, 1884), cover (129), drawing by Frederick Opper.

57. William H. Vanderbilt (1821–1885), railroad magnate, was the eldest son of Commodore Cornelius Vanderbilt. In the mid-1870s, he inherited nearly one hundred million dollars and increased it to about two hundred million before his death, making him the richest man in the United States. This particular gift to the College of Physicians and Surgeons was indeed five hundred thousand dollars, consisting of his purchase of twenty-nine city lots for two hundred thousand dollars and a check for three hundred thousand dollars tendered to the medical school on October 17, 1884. Vanderbilt made many other six-figure charitable gifts. See John Shrady, *The College of Physicians and Surgeons, New York, and Its Founders, Officers, Instructors, Benefactors and Alumni: A History*, 2 vols. (New York/Chicago: Lewis, 1903), 1:160–162.

58. A bowdlerized reference to the quotation opens an article in the *New York Times*: "In his famous interview with a Chicago reporter, in which Mr. Vanderbilt was represented as saying, 'The public be blanked,' or words to that effect . . ." (October 30, 1882, 4).

59. Thomas P. Hughes, *American Genesis: A Century of Invention and Technological Enthusiasm, 1870–1970* (New York: Penguin Books, 1989); Wyn Wachhorst, *Thomas Alva Edison, an American Myth* (Cambridge, Mass.: MIT Press, 1981).

60. "A Sun of the Nineteenth Century," *Puck* 11:269 (May 3, 1882), back cover (146), drawing by F. Graetz.

61. In a number of prints, the scalpels and saws were part of an autopsy scene, whether in news drawings or in political cartoons. There were only a few serious illustrations of either a postmortem examination or a class in gross anatomy such as those in figs. 13 and 14. Several prints showed the autopsy of President Garfield in the fall of 1881 after he succumbed to the bullet wound inflicted by Charles Guiteau. Sometimes cartoons of political or social commentary also provided autopsy scenes, and in these cartoons the instruments were often more visible. Images of the Garfield autopsy may be found in *New York Daily Graphic* of September 29, 1881, and October 6, 1881, and in *Frank Leslie's* of October 8, 1881. *Puck* satirized the problems of collecting on life insurance in a remarkable full-page vignette, "The Popular American Life Insurance Autopsy," June 14, 1879, back cover (160), in which Puck asks the agent, "Is this the sort of treatment you insure your late customers?" Years later, *Puck* offered a front-cover autopsy of a bloated Republican Party elephant, "A Final Autopsy —Verdict: Died from Swallowing an Utterly Indigestible Object [the McKinley Bill]," February 15, 1893, 409. (This chromolithograph was drawn by W. A. Rogers, whose work may be seen in fig. 16.) On July 25, 1891, an issue of the *National Police Gazette* offered a double-page spread of "Four Murderers Killed by Electricity," which included one scene of "Making the Autopsies."

62. Martin S. Pernick, *A Calculus of Suffering: Pain, Professionalism, and Anesthesia in Nineteenth-Century America* (New York: Columbia University Press, 1985).

63. A more schematic half-page drawing appeared a week earlier: "The Wounded President: Ascertaining the Location of the Bullet—From a Sketch by W. Shinkle [*sic*]," *Harper's Weekly* 25:1286 (August 13, 1881), 557. For a neurologist's well-illustrated and disquieting historical account of Garfield's treatment and death, see George Paulson, "A Long and Lonely Dying: President James A. Garfield," *Timeline* 22:3 (July-September 2005), 44–53. For illustrations of media coverage of the shooting, the convalescence, the trial of Guiteau, and his execution, see Russell Roberts, "Strangled for the Republic: The Assassination of President Garfield," *Timeline* 22:3 (July-September 2005), 30–43.

64. "The Execution of Criminals by Electricity. Experiments with Electric Currents at the Columbia College School of Mines. 'Trying It on a Dog,'" *Frank Leslie's Illustrated Newspaper* 66:1717 (August 11, 1888), cover (405; with story on 411); based on a sketch by a "staff artist."

65. I have not yet found an identical group of these images on one page in another publication, but the fact that three U.S. papers and one British paper all carried the same image of Pasteur among the rabbit cages during one week strongly suggests that they were all working off the same French publication, probably the weekly magazine *L'Illustration,* credited by name in the *Daily Graphic.* The illustrations appeared in the *Daily Graphic* of June 16, 1884, and in *Harper's Weekly, Frank Leslie's,* and the *Illustrated London News* in issues dated June 21, 1884. (The *Illustrated London News* also included a portrait of Pasteur.)

CHAPTER 3. HOW MEDICINE BECAME HOT NEWS, 1885

1. Many people wrongly assume that Pasteur became known to the general public in the United States from pasteurized milk. Although Pasteur did develop heat treatments to improve the keeping quality of beverages two decades prior to the rabies vaccine, he applied them to beer and wine, not milk. As a means of improving the safety of milk, the process that later came to be called pasteurization achieved prominence in the United States only well after the turn of the century; see S. Henry Ayers, *The Present Status of the Pasteurization of Milk,* rev. ed., U.S. Department of Agriculture Bulletin No. 342 (1922).

2. Because of the high frequency of references to newspaper articles throughout the book, they are often cited directly in the text. Note, too, that the year of an article is sometimes omitted in this chapter, as dates from September to December are for 1885 and those from January through July are for 1886.

3. The terms *rabies* and *hydrophobia* may both be used for a single disease shared by animals and people. In older usage, hydrophobia was usually applied to the human malady and rabies to cases in animals. The symptom that prompted the name hydrophobia is frequently, but not always, present in human cases and is not characteristic of animal cases. That *rabies* has generally replaced *hydrophobia* in most usage may well be a result of Pasteur's introduction of an animal vaccine. In this book, the two words are used interchangeably except in quotations.

4. For extended attention to the historiographical issues, see Bert Hansen, "America's First Medical Breakthrough: How Popular Excitement about a French Rabies Cure in 1885 Raised New Expectations for Medical Progress," *American Historical Review* 103:2 (April 1998), 373–418.

5. In Michael Schudson's vivid phrasing, "Pulitzer plugged his Western voice into the amplifier of the East, New York City"; see *Discovering the News: A Social History of American Newspapers* (New York: Basic Books, 1978), 92. Schudson indicates that Pulitzer expanded circulation from 15,000 at purchase in 1883 to 60,000 in 1884, then to 100,000 in 1885 and, by the fall of 1886, to 250,000, or roughly one of every five New Yorkers.

6. The pattern was similar in Russia, where "it was not Koch's celebrated work on the anthrax bacillus, but Pasteur's anti-rabies vaccine that initially attracted Russian interest," according to John F. Hutchinson, "Tsarist Russia and the Bacteriological Revolution," *Journal of the History of Medicine and Allied Sciences* 40 (1985), 422. And just as in the U.S. case, the scientific interest was fostered by the attention given to local patients who traveled to Paris for treatment, in this case a number of Russian peasants who had been bitten by a rabid wolf in Smolensk province and then treated in Pasteur's laboratory in early 1886.

7. Consumption was the greatest single killer of the era, even though it was not feared as a contagious disease until some years after Koch's 1883 discovery of the tubercle bacillus. About one-seventh of all reported deaths were due to tuberculosis, and among people who died in middle age, it claimed one in three, according to Thomas D. Brock, *Robert Koch: A Life in Medicine and Bacteriology* (Madison, Wisc.: Science Tech, 1988), 117.

8. New York City, for example, experienced no hydrophobia deaths in 1885 and only thirty-nine over the preceding fifteen years (*New York Herald,* January 7, 1886, 6). These were official figures of the Registrar, made public upon a request from ex-governor Hoffman. In 1890, Hermann M. Biggs told the New York Academy of Medicine that New York City had reports of only nine rabies deaths over the prior ten years; see Biggs, "The Present Experimental Aspect of Pasteur's Prophylaxis for Rabies," *Transactions of the New York Academy of Medicine,* 2nd ser., 7 (1890–1891), 367. (Although Biggs's figures include the postvaccine years, the vaccine did not become readily available in New York City until 1890.) For Philadelphia, the numbers were comparable, with sixty deaths over the twenty-five years ending in 1884; see John G. Lee, "The Mortality from Rabies in the Last Twenty-five Years in Philadelphia," *Medical Times* (April 3, 1886), 494–495. For Paris, Louis Pasteur's own figures showing an average of twelve deaths per year in the years preceding introduction of the new inoculation technique are cited in Gerald L. Geison, *The Private Science of Louis Pasteur* (Princeton, N.J.: Princeton University Press, 1995), 332–333.

9. J. F. Smithcors, *The American Veterinary Profession: Its Background and Development* (Ames: Iowa State University Press, 1963), 402. At that time, New York City had over 1.25 million human inhabitants and about ten thousand horse stables.

10. "Half a Million Dogs," *New York Herald,* December 27, 1885, 5.

11. A similar illustration, entitled "Shooting a Mad Dog," appeared a few years later in *Harper's Weekly* on August 2, 1879.

12. For news illustrations of a cage of dogs being lowered into the river to drown them, see *Daily Graphic* 14:1343 (July 7, 1877), 36; *Harper's Weekly* 24:1232 (August 7, 1880), 508; *Frank Leslie's Illustrated Newspaper* 54:1398 (July 8, 1882), 316; and *Daily Graphic* 39:[3995a] (January 10, 1886), 4. For the use of this scene in political cartoons and caricatures, see *Puck* 3:63 (June 26, 1878), 3; and *Puck* 9:225 (June 22, 1881), 276–277.

13. *New York Times,* June 9, 1881, 2; paragraph breaks have been inserted.

14. The cause of rabies was a "filterable virus," that is, something so small that it passed through the finest filters then available. It was too small to be seen by any optical microscope. In more recent usage, we restrict the word virus to such particles. But in Pasteur's era, *virus* (whether in French or English) could be applied to any infectious agent, including the much larger (and quite different) bacteria and yeasts. To avoid confusion, historians usually avoid using the word virus in a nineteenth-century context except in quotations. Sometimes when nonhistorians notice the word being used by Pasteur for the rabic agent, they mistakenly give him credit for discovering its character as a virus in the modern sense.

15. This account depends on Gerald L. Geison, "Louis Pasteur," *Dictionary of Scientific Biography,* vol. 10 (New York: Charles Scribner's Sons, 1974), 350–416; Gerald L. Geison, "Pasteur, Roux, and Rabies: Scientific versus Clinical Mentalities," *Journal of the History of Medicine and Allied Sciences* 45 (1990), 341–365; Geison, *Private Science*; and René Vallery-Radot, *The Life of Pasteur,* trans. R. L. Devonshire (Garden City, N.Y.: Doubleday, 1924), 390–444. See also Patrice Debré, *Louis Pasteur,* trans. Elborg Forster (Baltimore: Johns Hopkins University Press, 1998); this book unaccountably omitted the list of bibliographic references found in the French edition of 1994.

16. Brilliant research by the late Gerry Geison using Pasteur's private laboratory notes showed that the route to success was neither so short nor sure and that at several points important discrepancies exist between what had been achieved empirically and what Pasteur either reported or led others to believe about his work. The actual achievements in Pasteur's laboratory and some key failures were not known, however, except to Pasteur and a very small number of associates until Geison's archeology of the notebooks made them plain in recent years. The emphasis of my narrative is on what was publicly known, reported, or believed in the 1880s about Pasteur's rabies work, rather than on Pasteur's now accessible "private" science. For the rabies research and its application to human patients, see chapters 7–9 of Geison, *Private Science*.

17. "Hydrophobia—M. Pasteur's Experiments," *Harper's Weekly* 28:1435 (June 21, 1884), 392. This article might have been prompted by an article that appeared a few weeks before: "Professor Pasteur's Laboratory for the Study of Rabies," *Scientific American Supplement* 17:440 (June 7, 1884), 7015–7016. The same dog-cage drawing appears in both articles, but two other images in each are not repeated. This magazine was not an occasional supplement but a weekly sister publication to *Scientific American* for a specialized audience and requiring a separate subscription.

18. In *Private Science,* Geison shows that the first experimental inoculations ran from most virulent to least, rather than the reverse, and that Pasteur did not begin trying the least-to-most order until late May 1885 (see Geison's chart on p. 244). Geison also identifies two prior trials on humans that were never publicly acknowledged; official and popular accounts treat Joseph Meister's injections in July 1885 as the premier human experiment.

19. Vallery-Radot, *Life of Pasteur,* 414. Significantly, the dog experiments reported by Vallery-Radot as "constantly successful" have been shown by Geison's analysis of the laboratory notebooks to have been far less successful. Geison shows, in table 9.1 on page 241 of *Private Science,* that 62 percent (sixteen of twenty-six) of the dogs receiving treatment after being bitten survived. Not only is 62 percent somewhat less than the 100 percent implied by Vallery-Radot's phrasing (38 percent died even with treatment), but 62 percent is only slightly better than the 57 percent survival rate of the seven untreated dogs held as controls.

20. For the months preceding the Newark episode in December, I have reviewed six newspapers: the *New York Herald,* the *New York Times,* the *New York Tribune,* the *Chicago Tribune,* the *St. Louis Globe-Democrat,* and the *St. Louis Post-Dispatch.* For December 1885 through the spring and into the summer of 1886, I systematically examined those newspapers, and also the *Boston Evening Transcript*; the *Brooklyn Eagle*; New York's *Daily Graphic, Evening Post, Sun,* and *World*; and the following Newark papers: *Daily Advertiser, Daily Journal, Evening News, Morning Register,* and *Sunday Call.* Other papers, checked in a less systematic way, include the *Daily American* (Nashville, Tenn.), *Danbury (Conn.) Evening News,* the *Florida Times-Union,* the *Florida Weekly Times,* the *Honolulu Daily Bulletin,* the *Los Angeles Daily Herald,* the *Los Angeles Daily Times,* and the *Pacific Commercial Advertiser* (Honolulu).

Post-Newark visuals are discussed later in the chapter. Prior to the Newark episode, the only rabies visuals in the U.S. press during 1885 were in the *New York Daily Graphic,* which, on November 19, 1885, printed an image of Pasteur watching the injection of Jupille (apparently copied from *L'Illustration* of November 7, 1885) and then, on December 1, published two images of Pasteur in his laboratory (both of them taken from the *London Graphic* of November 21).

21. Similar stories ran in all the New York and Newark papers, and they were picked up widely across the country, running daily, for example, in the *Boston Evening Transcript,* the *Chicago Tribune,* and both major St. Louis papers, the *Globe-Democrat* and the *Post-Dispatch.* My citing or quoting from any particular newspaper at any point should not be taken to imply that that paper is the only source on the matter.

22. For more about Billings, see the opening section of chapter 4.

23. "The Boys Who Were Bitten. More Than $1,000 Subscribed to Send Them to Paris. The Views of Dr. Billings on Cauterization for Mad Dog Bites. The Boys Go Aboard the Steamship Canada This Afternoon," *New York Sun,* December 8, 1885, 1; "The Children's Farewell. Dr. Pasteur's Patients Sail on the Steamer Canada. They Bid Good-By to America with Tears in Their Eyes. Dr. Billings Accompanies Them, and Promises to Take Every Care of Them. One of the Dogs Shows Symptoms of Hydrophobia," *New York World,* December 10, 1885, 5; and an unsigned editorial, *New York Evening Post,* December 10, 1885, 2.

24. "Pasteur's Discovery," *St. Louis Globe-Democrat,* December 13, 1885, 19.

25. "The New Scheme," *Puck* 18:458 (December 16, 1885), 243.

26. For more information on the rhythms of weekly publications' delivery and a confirmation that weeklies might have appeared on a newsstand seven days ahead of the cover date, see Joshua Brown, *Beyond the Lines: Pictorial Reporting, Everyday Life, and the Crisis of Gilded Age America* (Berkeley: University of California Press, 2002), 254–255. I have also observed evidence for earlier delivery in the "date received" information sometimes stamped onto library copies of these magazines.

27. *Puck* 18:458 (December 16, 1885), cover (241).

28. The best orientation to cartoonists' views of Grover Cleveland and James G. Blaine is Stefan Lorant, *The Presidency: A Pictorial History of Presidential Elections from Washington to Truman* (New York: Macmillan, 1953), 364–391. See also Samuel J. Thomas, "The Tattooed Man Caricatures and the Presidential Campaign of 1884," *Journal of American Culture* 10:4 (Winter 1987), 1–20; Richard Samuel West, *Satire on Stone: The Political Cartoons of Joseph Keppler* (Urbana: University of Illinois Press, 1988); and Harlen Makemson, "One Misdeed Evokes Another: How Political Cartoonists Used 'Scandal Intertextuality' against Presidential Candidate James G. Blaine," *Media History Monographs* 7:2 (2004–2005), 1–20.

29. "Pasteur's Latest Discovery," *Harper's Weekly* 29:1513 (December 19, 1885), 836–837.

30. "An Inoculation for Hydrophobia," *Scientific American* 53:520 (December 19, 1885), 391 (crediting the *Herald* as the source for its story).

31. The article entitled "Dr. Pasteur, with Portrait" ran on p. 14, and the portrait captioned "Dr. Pasteur, the French chemist who is to treat the six [*sic*] dog-bitten children of Newark, N.J." appeared separately on p. 4 in a group of portraits.

32. Pasteur among the rabbit cages was published in *L'Illustration* of May 31, 1884, *Harper's Weekly* of June 21, 1884, and *La Science Illustré* of September 15, 1888. Pasteur peering through a microscope was in the *London Graphic* of November 21, 1885, the *New York Daily Graphic* of December 1, 1885, and *L'Universe Illustré* of December 12, 1885.

33. "M. Pasteur and His Patients," *Frank Leslie's Illustrated Newspaper* 61:1578 (December 19, 1885), 300.

34. "What We Are Coming To: Fifteen Cents Worth of Hydrophobia Virus for Pa," detail from full-page spread of ten cartoons, "Hydrophobia!" by H. C. Coultaus, *New York Daily Graphic* 39:3976 (December 19, 1885), cover (1). For a reproduction of the entire page, see Hansen, "America's First Medical Breakthrough," 392.

35. *St. Louis Globe-Democrat,* December 22, 1885; other papers, including the *Chicago Tribune* and the *New York Herald,* carried the same report. In the quoted section, I have silently corrected the spelling of the doctor's name from "Granchet."

36. Kaufmann's portrait even appeared on the front page of the *New York World,* along with pictures of three dogs being held in captivity because they had been bitten by the dog that bit the Newark children (December 15).

37. *Boston Morning Journal,* December 29, 1885, 2.

38. "Pasteur's Experiments," *St. Louis Globe-Democrat,* January 3, 1886, 9.

39. The story is "Pasteur Methods in America," *New York Daily Graphic* 39:3989 (January 3, 1886), 4. Along with "Inoculating the Rabbit," the other images on this page illustrated "one of the medical men," "the dog garret: dogs that have been bitten by rabid dogs," and "the tools used in operations."

40. The *New York Tribune* (January 9, 1886, 7) carried the earliest ad that I have found for the Pasteur inoculation group.

41. *Monthly Catalogue of the Eden Musée: Price Ten Cents* (New York, April 1886), 29. I have not determined how long the Pasteur group remained on exhibit in New York City, though the description is still found in the August 1886 catalogue. In Chicago's Eden Musée (whose relation to New York's is uncertain), the Pasteur group was still on exhibit at least as late as September 1889, as the monthly catalogue with that date carries the same text as in the New York catalogue quoted here.

42. For more on the cartoonist and his sources, see Hansen, "America's First Medical Breakthrough," 400–401. A color reproduction may be found at http://www.pasteurfoundation. org/pictures_gala2005.html (accessed October 28, 2007). The iconography of this image, a seated Pasteur holding a squirming young child to inoculate him, is unlike any known Pasteur image and was clearly derived from a widely known 1870s sculpture by Giulio Monteverde of Edward Jenner vaccinating his son.

43. Andrea Stulman Dennett, *Weird and Wonderful: The Dime Museum in America* (New York: New York University Press, 1997).

44. Very popular freaks could, however, command two hundred dollars a week, and perhaps far more. Brooks McNamara, in " 'A Congress of Wonders': The Rise and Fall of the Dime Museum," *ESQ: A Journal of the American Renaissance* 20:3 (1974), 224, gives two hundred dollars as a high figure. The St. Louis proprietor who exhibited the Newark children claimed in a letter to the editor that the weekly payment for the more unusual freaks could be as much as seven hundred dollars (*St. Louis Globe-Democrat,* April 18, 1886).

45. McNamara, "Congress of Wonders," 224.

46. A copy of this handbill was graciously shared with me by Annick Perrot, curator of the Musée Pasteur. Broadway and Treyser's Palace Museum was in St. Louis, Missouri (in "America's First Medical Breakthrough," I mistakenly wrote that this museum was in Philadelphia).

47. Dr. Martin A. Couney displayed premature babies in his incubators on Coney Island for decades. He staged presentations at national and international fairs including Paris in 1900, Chicago in 1933, and New York in 1939–1940. Since the latest techniques of care for premature babies were hard to find and expensive to secure, worried and needy parents offered their babies to Dr. Couney and he provided the best nursing and medical care available, paying for it all with showmanship and ticket sales. See William A. Silverman, "Incubator-Baby Side Shows," *Pediatrics* 64:2 (August 1979), 127–141; and Gary R. Brown, "The Coney Island Baby Laboratory," *American Heritage of Invention and Technology* 10 (Fall 1994),

24–33. On Alexis St. Martin and Phineas Gage, see Hansen, "America's First Medical Breakthrough," 399; and Reginald Horsman, *Frontier Doctor: William Beaumont, America's First Great Medical Scientist* (Columbia: University of Missouri Press, 1996).

48. This was big news in the United States. The papers first announced a day or two in advance that Pasteur was going to present a report on his treatments to the Paris Académie des Sciences at the Institute of France and that he was going to propose a subscription to fund a permanent institute. See, for example, the *Chicago Tribune* and *St. Louis Globe-Democrat* on February 28, and *Boston Evening Transcript* on March 1. After his presentation, papers reported the same ideas at greater length on March 2 (*Boston Evening Transcript, Chicago Tribune, St. Louis Globe-Democrat,* and *St. Louis Post-Dispatch*).

49. Pierre Provoyeur and June Hargrove, eds., *Liberty: The French-American Statue in Art and History* (New York: Harper & Row, 1986).

50. Two February 1886 articles in a weekly series of long, unsigned essays on medical topics published in the *St. Louis Globe-Democrat* seem significant markers of a growing sense of change in medicine: "Medical Progress: The Path of Discovery from Superstition to the Germ Theory" (February 7) and "Surgical Progress: The Stages Leading Up to Anaesthetics and Listerism." In response to a reader's inquiry, the paper identified the author as Dr. William B. Hazard of St. Louis (*St. Louis Globe-Democrat,* January 24, 1886).

51. The *New York Herald*'s first published listing of donors appeared on Sunday, December 6, in a three-column article on p. 7. The list appeared on the same day in the *Newark Register* and the *New York World.* A shorter list ran in the *New York Times.*

52. Pasteur's rabies work made its way into the *National Police Gazette* at least three times: "Dr. Pasteur" (story and portrait, December 19, 1885); "Inoculated by Pasteur" (an American naval surgeon treated by Pasteur in Paris was considering the establishment of a U.S. treatment facility, January 29, 1887); and "Rivaling Pasteur" (illustrated story on hot iron cautery, April 7, 1888). On the historical significance of this seemingly marginal newspaper, see Elliott J. Gorn, "The Wicked World: The *National Police Gazette* and Gilded Age America," *Media Studies Journal* 6:1 (Winter 1992), 1–15.

53. Relevant examples include British or U.S. writings about Darwin's evolution theory and the French debates about spontaneous generation. On the latter, see Anne Diara, "Un débat français vu par la Presse, 1858–1869: L. Pasteur—F. A. Pouchet et la génération spontanée," *Actes du Muséum de Rouen* 6 (1984), 176–210.

54. Striking examples appeared not only in *Puck* and *Judge* as indicated earlier but also in *Harper's Weekly* and *Life.* The most famous political cartoonist in the United States, Thomas Nast, took up the topic on several occasions, usually to mock the mania and blame it on editors. For a list of Nast's hydrophobia cartoons, see Hansen, "America's First Medical Breakthrough," 404.

55. The sheer number of jokes (and the way they were copied and recopied) confirms the ubiquity of references to this fad. On December 27, for example, the *Newark Sunday Call*'s "Humors of the Day" column with its "Dogmatic Humor" offered six quips from out-of-town papers about the rabies mania, including the following three samples: "Paris has lost 115,000 population in the last four years, but if the emigration of dog bitten Jerseymen continues, she will soon make it up (*Pittsburg Chronicle*)"; "It is not enough, it appears, to be bitten by a mad dog in New Jersey, but the New York papers add to the victims' agony by printing their pictures (*Pittsburg Telegraph*)"; "Down in Newark, N.J., the population devotes its time to the chasing of mad dogs. Amateur marksmen have an excellent chance to practice, while of course, the dogs escape uninjured (*Boston Globe*)" (7). One example appeared in at least four publications, nicely illustrating how widely the papers cannibalized one another's material and even commented on the borrowing. On January 12, 1886, the *New York Times* ran this short item in a column called "Jottings Here and There": "More people die in one year from trichiniasis than in 20 years from hydrophobia. Yet the owners of hogs pay no tax, buy no muzzles, and have no hogs shot down.—*Milwaukee Sentinel*" (4). Three days later, the joke was tightened a little and alliteration was added in the *Daily Graphic*: "It is asserted that more people die in one year from trichinosis than in twenty years from hydrophobia. If this is so, M. Pasteur might better devote his attention to the hogs instead of letting it go to the dogs" (2). Three days after that, *Puck* tightened the joke more and made it self-referential: "An exchange says that more people die in a year from trichiniasis than in twenty years from hydrophobia. Here is a chance for some enterprising journalist to turn the dog-scare into a hog-scare" (323).

56. Both ads appeared on page 3 of the December 20 issue: "Hydrophobia Cured. It is now the fashion to go to Paris to seek a cure. Better stay at home, saving your $1,000, and using a 25c. box of Henry's Carbolic Salve, the best healing ointment in the world"; "Mad Dogs. . . . Dr. Tobias' celebrated Venetian Liniment applied immediately upon being bitten eradicates all danger of Hydrophobia."

57. One scholar's quantitative examination of Darwin's appearance in the *New York Times* showed a similar pattern in which the "event orientation" of the press meant that quiescent intervals alternated with bursts of attention prompted by publication of the *Origin of Species,* Thomas Huxley's visit to the United States promoting it, Darwin's death, the centenary of Darwin's birth, and the Scopes trial. See Ed Caudill, "A Content Analysis of Press Views of Darwin's Evolutionary Theory, 1860–1925," *Journalism Quarterly* 64 (Winter 1987), 782–786, 946.

58. One article from a few years later confirmed both the depth of penetration of Pasteur's image as a symbol of the triumph of science in medicine and the familiarity he achieved as a "household name." An article illustrated with a portrait photograph, "Pasteur—The Famous French Chemist, One of the World's Practical Benefactors," ran in a magazine named *The Household* ("devoted to the interests of the American housewife"), issue of November 1895. The article closed this way: "We shall do well to keep in mind Pasteur's saying: 'It is in the power of man to cause all parasitic maladies to disappear from the world.' This is his best epitaph; for the world owes all that may come of the 'germ theory' in the future to Louis Pasteur" (11).

CHAPTER 4. POPULAR ENTHUSIASM FOR LABORATORY DISCOVERIES, 1885–1895

1. Frank Seaver Billings, *The Relation of Animal Diseases to the Public Health, and Their Prevention* (New York: Appleton, 1884). See also Bert Hansen, "America's First Medical Breakthrough: How Popular Excitement about a French Rabies Cure in 1885 Raised New Expectations for Medical Progress," *American Historical Review* 103:2 (April 1998), 408.

2. American doctors' cautious interpretations of Pasteur's rabies treatment were examined in Jon M. Harkness, "The Reception of Pasteur's Rabies Vaccine in America: An Episode in the Application of the Germ Theory of Disease" (master's thesis, University of Wisconsin, April 1987, 31 pages), and in Leonard J. Hoenig, "Triumph and Controversy: Pasteur's

Preventive Treatment of Rabies as Reported in *JAMA*," *Archives of Neurology* 43 (April 1986), 397–399.

3. Medical history scholarship on the changing place of science in U.S. medicine has usually focused on physiology as the major instance, with far less attention to pathology and its stepchild bacteriology; see Hansen, "America's First Medical Breakthrough," 409. For a review of discussions within the profession about these changes, see John S. Haller Jr., "'The Artful Science': Medicine's Self-Image in the 1890's," *Clio Medica* 19:3–4 (1984), 231–250.

4. Veterinarians were an exception; their interest picked up about a decade earlier, according to Patricia Peck Gossel, in "The Emergence of American Bacteriology, 1875–1900" (Ph.D. diss., Johns Hopkins University, 1988), 108–110. On the medical profession's hesitations about bacteriology, see Russell C. Maulitz, "'Physician versus Bacteriologist': The Ideology of Science in Clinical Medicine," in *The Therapeutic Revolution: Essays in the Social History of American Medicine,* ed. Morris J. Vogel and Charles E. Rosenberg, 91–107 (Philadelphia: University of Pennsylvania Press, 1979), 96; John Harley Warner, *The Therapeutic Perspective: Medical Practice, Knowledge, and Identity in America, 1820–1885* (Cambridge, Mass.: Harvard University Press, 1986), 277–281; and Gossel, "Emergence of American Bacteriology," 164–165. None of these studies mentions the rabies enthusiasm, but it is included by Gossel in her later study of changes within the discipline of bacteriology in the United States; see Patricia Peck Gossel, "Pasteur, Koch, and American Bacteriology," *History and Philosophy of the Life Sciences* 22:1 (March 2000), 81–100.

5. Gossel, "Emergence of American Bacteriology," 282, citing Charles V. Chapin, *Municipal Sanitation in the United States* (1901), 556–559. See also Victoria A. Harden, *Inventing the NIH: Federal Biomedical Research Policy, 1887–1937* (Baltimore: Johns Hopkins University Press, 1986); and David Anthony Blancher, "Workshops of the Bacteriological Revolution: A History of the Laboratories of the New York City Department of Health, 1892–1912" (Ph.D. diss., City University of New York, 1979).

6. In fact, Biggs had gone to Paris to learn about the rabies work at Pasteur's laboratory at roughly the same time as the Newark boys' treatment, although he did not accompany the Newark children—despite statements that he did in Blancher, "Workshops of the Bacteriological Revolution," 28, and in Elizabeth Fee and Evelynn M. Hammonds, "Science, Politics, and the Art of Persuasion: Promoting the New Scientific Medicine in New York City," in *Hives of Sickness: Public Health and Epidemics in New York City,* ed. David Rosner, 155–196 (New Brunswick, N.J.: Rutgers University Press, 1995), 158. Biggs probably arrived on a later steamer, but he did meet with Pasteur in late December, before visiting laboratories in Germany. That Biggs's colleague T. Mitchell Prudden had a serious interest in press coverage of medical breakthroughs is illustrated in a scrapbook of extensive newspaper clippings of the tuberculin episode, labeled "Koch's Tuberculin," in the Library of the New York Academy of Medicine. The scrapbook was received by the library as a gift from a Miss Prudden, who I assume was probably one of Dr. Prudden's nieces. I am grateful that in 1986 my student David Leibowitz called this item to my attention. Formerly in the stacks, this item is now in the academy's Rare Book Room.

7. See, for example, several pathetic photographs of children taken before their miraculous recoveries and reprinted in Michael Bliss, *The Discovery of Insulin* (Chicago: University of Chicago Press, 1982). The examples of children's images used in campaigns against polio are legion.

8. Although this image might well have first appeared in France during 1884 in reports on the dog experiments, prior to the human treatments, I have not been able to find earlier printings than those in the *London Graphic* of November 21, 1885 (p. 561) and the *New York Daily Graphic* of December 1, 1885 (p. 205). According to the *Daily Graphic,* writing on December 6, its print had already been copied and published by the *New York Telegram.* It was also printed months later with several other illustrations in *Frank Leslie's Monthly Magazine* 22:3 (September 1886), 345, in an article entitled "Pasteur's Life and Labours," 341–349.

9. *New York Herald,* December 31, 1885; see also Hansen, "America's First Medical Breakthrough," 413. On Bergh's life in general, see the nonscholarly account by Zulma Steele, *Angel in Top Hat* (New York: Harper, 1942), supplemented by useful information in two books about Bergh's sometime opponent P. T. Barnum: Neil Harris, *Humbug: The Art of P. T. Barnum* (Boston: Little, Brown, 1973); and A. H. Saxon, *P. T. Barnum: The Legend and the Man* (New York: Columbia University Press, 1989).

10. This process helps to explain why an antivivisection movement arose much later in the United States than in Britain and why it failed to achieve either popularity or legislative success. Decades earlier, starting in 1866, the New York physiology researcher Dr. John Call Dalton Jr. had faced off with some antivivisectionists, but the skirmishes were small and local. See W. Bruce Fye, *The Development of American Physiology: Scientific Medicine in the Nineteenth Century* (Baltimore: Johns Hopkins University Press, 1987), 35–53. The first important battle of American doctors with antivivisectionists took place only at the end of the century, followed by a second conflict in the 1910s. See Patricia Peck Gossel, "William Henry Welch and the Antivivisection Legislation in the District of Columbia, 1896–1900," *Journal of the History of Medicine* 40:4 (October 1985), 397–419; Susan E. Lederer, "The Controversy over Animal Experimentation in America, 1880–1914," in *Vivisection in Historical Perspective,* ed. Nicolaas A. Rupke, 236–258 (London: Croon Helm, 1987); Susan E. Lederer, *Subjected to Science: Human Experimentation in America before the Second World War* (Baltimore: Johns Hopkins University Press, 1995); and Bernard Unti, "'The Doctors Are So Sure That They Only Are Right': The Rockefeller Institute and the Defeat of Vivisection Reform in New York, 1908–1914," in *Creating a Tradition of Biomedical Research: Contributions to the History of the Rockefeller University,* ed. Darwin H. Stapleton, 175–189 (New York: Rockefeller University Press, 2004).

11. For a full account of Edelfelt's work and its place in French art more generally, see Richard E. Weisberg, "The Representation of Doctors at Work in Salon Art of the Early Third Republic in France" (Ph.D. diss., New York University, 1995), chap. 5 (573–729); for Edelfelt's study of painting, see 610.

12. In addition to the examples illustrated herein, one relatively unfamiliar image in this mode may also be noted. In *Simon Flexner* (pastel on paper, ca. 1920) by Adele Herter, Dr. Flexner holds a flask up at the level of his face, with his attention directed not toward the viewer but at the liquid in the flask. For a color reproduction, see William H. Gerdts, *The Art of Healing: Medicine and Science in American Art* (Birmingham, Ala.: Birmingham Museum of Art, 1981), 85.

13. "M. Pasteur in His Laboratory," *Harper's Bazar* 23:30 (July 26, 1890), 584–585; this large image is printed in portrait orientation running sideways across the two pages, with a modest amount of text below it. The image and the article have the same title, but the article covers rabies research and treatment more broadly, reviewing Joseph Meister's treatments and Pasteur's international recognition. It includes an enthusiastic endorsement of Dr. Paul Gibier ("in the prime of life, with the calm face and serious eyes of a student, and with a modesty as rare as Pasteur's contempt for wealth") and of the New York Pasteur Institute, where sixty-one patients had already been treated.

14. "Pasteur in His Laboratory," *Once a Week: An Illustrated Weekly* 5:25 (October 7, 1890), cover (1). The magazine did not name either the painter or the engraver of this image. This issue included on p. 3 a story by Alfred I. H. Crespi about his visit to Pasteur's laboratory.

15. *Frank Leslie's Illustrated Weekly* 76:1948 (January 12, 1893), 29.

16. Ida M. Tarbell, "Pasteur at Home: With an Account of the Work Done at the Pasteur Institute in Paris," *McClure's Magazine* 1:4 (September 1893), 335.

17. *Harper's Weekly* 93:2025 (October 12, 1895), 970. The *Review of Reviews* 12:5 (November 1895) ran the image on p. 540, facing the article "Louis Pasteur, Scientist. His Life-Work, and Its Value to the World, as Interpreted by Professor Percy Frankland [541–547] and The Late John Tyndall [547–552]"; here, the image was cropped to make the figure larger in the frame. It was titled "M. Pasteur at Work," and no artist was credited as painter or engraver.

18. Charles F. Horne, *Great Men and Famous Women: A Series of Pen and Pencil Sketches of the Lives of More than 200 of the Most Prominent Personages in History* (New York: Selmar Hess, 1894). This collection was published in sixty-eight fascicles; copies today may be unbound, bound in eight volumes, or bound in four volumes under these rubrics: soldiers and sailors, statesmen and sages, workmen and heroes, and artists and authors. Pasteur was included in installment number 50, along with Queen Victoria, Thomas Edison, and Florence Nightingale, all of them found in the "workmen and heroes" group. An engraved version of the Edelfelt portrait (in a left-to-right reversal) appeared in Ainsworth Rand Spofford, Frank Weitenkampf, and J. P. Lamberton, *The Library of Historic Characters and Famous Events of All Nations and All Ages*, 12 vols. (Boston: J. B. Millet, 1902), facing p. 173 in vol. 10. I have not yet confirmed that Edelfelt's painting was also included in the 1894–1895 edition of this book, though it was present in the ten-volume 1897 edition published in Philadelphia. It also appeared in books on art, such as Richard Muther, *The History of Modern Painting*, 4 vols. (New York: Dutton, 1907).

19. For the art historical context, see Linda Nochlin, *Realism: Style and Civilization* (Harmondsworth, U.K.: Penguin, 1971), chap. 4, "The Heroism of Modern Life," and especially the section entitled "Realist Heroes," 181–192, which concludes with a discussion of paintings of physicians and surgeons.

20. This point has been meticulously established by Weisberg, "Representation of Doctors at Work," 57–163. See also Ludmilla Jordanova, *Defining Features: Scientific and Medical Portraits, 1666–2000* (London: Reaktion Books, 2000), in which Jordanova notes of a watercolor made in the 1850s, "this unusual and delicate image showing Faraday in his laboratory is noteworthy because there had been few depictions of men of science at work" (39). The rarity of such images before the 1880s is confirmed in Gerdts, *Art of Healing*, and in Willem Dirk Hackmann, *Apples to Atoms: Portraits of Scientists from Newton to Rutherford* (London: National Portrait Gallery, 1986). The same pattern held true in photographic portraits of physicians, according to Daniel M. Fox and Christopher Lawrence, *Photographing Medicine: Images and Power in Britain and America since 1840* (New York: Greenwood, 1988), 23: "The backgrounds which photographers used for making portraits at this time [i.e., 1840 to 1890] very often represented libraries and never places of medical work. Doctors were rarely photographed with medical instruments although this was not an invariable rule."

21. Brown-Séquard was born a British subject of an American father and French mother; he later became a French citizen. On this episode, see Newell Dunbar, *The "Elixir of Life":*

Dr. Brown-Sequard's Own Account of His Famous Alleged Remedy for Debility and Old Age, Dr. Variot's Experiments . . . To Which is Prefixed a Sketch of Dr. Brown-Sequard's life, with Portrait (Boston, 1889); J.M.D. Olmsted, *Charles-Édouard Brown-Séquard: A Nineteenth Century Neurologist and Endocrinologist* (Baltimore: Johns Hopkins University Press, 1946), 205–239; Merriley Borell, "Brown-Séquard's Organotherapy and Its Appearance in America at the End of the Nineteenth Century," *Bulletin of the History of Medicine* 50:3 (Fall 1976), 309–320; and Michael J. Aminoff, *Brown-Séquard: A Visionary of Science* (New York: Raven, 1993), 163–173.

22. "Note on the Effects Produced on Man by Subcutaneous Injections of a Liquid Obtained from the Testicles of Animals by Dr. Brown-Sequard, F.R.S., Etc.," *Scientific American Supplement* 28:710 (August 10, 1889), 11347–11348. See also an editorial, "Dr. Brown-Sequard's Recent Experiments," *Scientific American* 61:6 (August 10, 1889), 80.

23. For example, just in the *New York Times*: "Doctors Who Disagree: The Brown-Séquard Elixir Divides the Medical Profession" (August 23, 1889); "Another Victim of the Elixir" (September 3, 1889); and "No More Elixir for Him" (September 13, 1889). The third of these articles reports that a man's physician used lamb spinal cord to prepare the injection rather than testicles, perhaps confusing Pasteur's method with Brown-Séquard's. A lengthy story in the *Brooklyn Eagle* observed that "experiments have been tried throughout the country on an extensive scale" and enumerated negative results and near tragedies of people who had "fallen victim to quacks and charlatans as a direct consequence of the craze" (August 18, 1889).

24. *Frank Leslie's Illustrated Newspaper* 69:1771 (August 24, 1889), 39.

25. William A. Hammond, "The Elixir of Life," *North American Review* 149:394 (September 1889), 257–264. For more on Hammond's scientific and commercial work in organotherapy, see Bonnie Ellen Blustein, *Preserve Your Love for Science: Life of William A. Hammond, American Neurologist* (Cambridge: Cambridge University Press, 1991).

26. "A Muncie Snake Story," *National Police Gazette* 54:628 (September 21, 1889), 7, with illustration on 5.

27. Words and music by J. Winchell Forbes. I wish to thank William H. Helfand for sharing with me a copy of this song.

28. *Judge* 16:411 (August 31, 1889), 336–337, "Hopeless Cases," center-spread chromolithograph by Grant Hamilton.

29. The figures in the center are Charles A. Dana (with a tag to identify him as owner-editor of the *New York Sun*) and Joseph Pulitzer (proprietor of the *New York World*, apparently recognizable without a label), who have brought the Democratic Party (see tag on the tiger's tail) in for Doctor Randall's protectionism treatment. At the right, the enervated body of "Free Trade" is being carried in by two men coming from the U.S. Capitol, visible behind them through the doorway: Roger Quarles Mills, congressman (later senator) from Texas, and Henry Watterson, editor of the *Louisville Courier-Journal*.

30. For many examples of clysters, see William H. Helfand and Sergio Rocchietta, *Medicina e farmacia nelle caricature politiche Italiane, 1848–1914* (Milan and Rome: Edizioni scientifiche internazionali, 1982); William H. Helfand, *The Picture of Health: Images of Medicine and Pharmacy from the William H. Helfand Collection* (Philadelphia: Philadelphia Museum of Art, 1991); Eugen Holländer, *Die Karikatur und Satire in der Medizin* (Stuttgart: Enke, 1921); and Helmut Vogt, *Medizinische Karikaturen von 1800 bis zur Gegenwart, mit 315 Abbildungen* (Munich: J. F. Lehmann, 1962).

31. G. Archie Stockwell, "The Brown-Sequard Discovery," *Scientific American Supplement* 28: 720 (October 19, 1889), 11509–11510.

32. Olmsted, *Charles-Édouard Brown-Séquard,* 209.

33. David Leibowitz, "Scientific Failure in an Age of Optimism: Public Reaction to Robert Koch's Tuberculin Cure," *New York State Journal of Medicine* 93:1 (January 1993), 41–48; for the image of Koch as St. George, see p. 43. On tuberculosis research more generally, see Thomas D. Brock, *Robert Koch: A Life in Medicine and Bacteriology* (Madison, Wisc.: Science Tech, 1988); Mark Caldwell, *The Last Crusade: The War on Consumption, 1862–1954* (New York: Atheneum, 1988); Georgina D. Feldberg, *Disease and Class: Tuberculosis and the Shaping of Modern North American Society* (New Brunswick, N.J.: Rutgers University Press, 1995); Christoph Gradmann, "Robert Koch and the Pressures of Scientific Research: Tuberculosis and Tuberculin," *Medical History* 45:1 (January 2001), 1–32; and Gradmann, "Money and Microbes: Robert Koch, Tuberculin and the Foundation of the Institute for Infectious Diseases in Berlin in 1891," *History and Philosophy of the Life Sciences* 22:1 (March 2000), 59–79.

34. In my collection is a three-hundred-page scrapbook of newspaper clippings entirely on medical subjects, primarily from Hartford, Connecticut, newspapers dating from 1885 to 1892 (with a few more from 1900). A full nineteen pages have articles about the tuberculin episode, from mid-December 1890 to late March 1891. Unfortunately, the book lacks a name for its compiler or any other indications of provenance or purpose. A much smaller anonymous scrapbook of newspaper clippings of the tuberculin episode, labeled "Koch's Tuberculin," is held in the Rare Book Room of the New York Academy of Medicine. The library records it as a gift from a Miss Prudden, probably a niece of Dr. T. Mitchell Prudden.

35. "Away with Koch's Lymph," *Medical News* 58:23 (June 6, 1891), 625.

36. A small version of this portrait appeared in the *Danbury Evening News,* November 22, 1890, 1.

37. "The Prevention and Cure of Consumption—Dr. Koch's Great Discovery," *Frank Leslie's Illustrated Newspaper* 71:1839 (December 13, 1890), 349. The associated article, "A Visit to Dr. Koch," appears on p. 353. The same portrait had been used six years earlier in *Harper's Weekly* 28:1445 (August 30, 1884), 563. In 1890, it was republished on the cover of the *Illustrated American* of December 6, 1890, and by *Harper's Weekly* 34:1771 (November 29, 1890), 932, to illustrate the article "Dr. Koch and His Great Work" by Amos W. Wright (on p. 934), with a related editorial, "Dr. Koch's Discovery" (on p. 923). A week later, the portrait and the lab scene appeared together in "Cure of Consumption—An Interview with Professor Koch by Dr. Charles Hacks in *L'Illustration,*" in *Scientific American* 63:23 (December 6, 1890), 358–359. Since the *Scientific American* article was a translation from the report in a French weekly, *L'Illustration,* the French report was perhaps the source of the U.S. versions of the scene in *Scientific American, Frank Leslie's Illustrated Newspaper,* and the *New York Herald* of January 16, 1891. Small sketches of a pipette, a bottle of lymph, "The Needle," and "The Injection" (into the back of a seated patient) ran in the *New York Herald,* December 28, 1890. In May, *The Cosmopolitan: A Monthly Illustrated Magazine* 11:1 (May 1891), 90–95, printed two images in the story "Doctor Koch and His Lymph" by Julius Weiss, M.D.: the same commonly reproduced portrait and a photograph entitled "Inoculating a Patient," with two men handling the injection high up on a patient's back near the spine and five other men observing the procedure; all are wearing dark suits.

38. *Puck* 26:676 (February 19, 1890), cover (431), "The Smallest Specimen Yet," chromolithograph by Frederick Opper, in which a tiny President Benjamin Harrison is positioned on a microscope slide; for a reproduction, see Bert Hansen, "New Images of a New Medicine: Visual Evidence for Widespread Popularity of Therapeutic Discoveries in America after 1885," *Bulletin of the History of Medicine* 73:4 (December 1999), 636.

39. *Frank Leslie's Illustrated Newspaper* 71:1842 (January 3, 1891), 408, "Dr. Koch's Treatment of Consumption.—Examination by Dr. George F. Shrady, at St. Francis Hospital, of the Patient Sent to Berlin by 'Frank Leslie's Illustrated Newspaper.'—From a Sketch by C. Bunnell"; for a reproduction, see Hansen, "New Images of a New Medicine," 661.

40. In an earlier issue, *Frank Leslie's Illustrated Newspaper* had reprinted a European engraving of "Sir Morell Mackenzie Injecting Dr. Koch's Lymph at the Throat Hospital, London." That image appeared in a cluster of illustrations under the rubric "Pictorial Spirit of Leading Foreign Events," *Frank Leslie's Illustrated Newspaper* 71:1841 (December 27, 1890), 400.

41. *Puck* 28:718 (December 10, 1890), 276–277, "A Bad Case of Consumption—Reciprocity Lymph," center-spread chromolithograph by Joseph Keppler.

42. The traditional, or prebreakthrough, images of medicine persisted for a while alongside the new ones, as, for example, in another *Puck* center spread by Joseph Keppler, about six months earlier: "Dangerous Doctors for a Desperate Case," a view of the U.S. Senate. In this scene, senators, some wearing surgical aprons, are trying to cure the McKinley Tariff Bill using saws, scissors, and "senatorial chloroform." One takes a pulse with a pocket watch. There is no thermometer or stethoscope in sight. See *Puck* 27:692 (June 11, 1890), 248–249.

43. *Judge* 19:478 (December 13, 1890), back cover (198), "The Rival Doctor Kochs. The Debilitated Party—'Begob, I have me own private opinion that yez are both quacks!'" Full-page chromolithograph by Grant Hamilton. Dr. Koch-Cleveland's bottle is marked "Humbug Reform Lymph—A Hypocritical Preparation," and Dr. Koch-Hill's reads "Hill's Spoils System Lymph with Peanut Essence."

44. Grover Cleveland was out of office at the time, having been defeated in his bid for reelection as president in 1888; he was elected to that office again in 1892. David B. Hill was governor of New York State and was Cleveland's rival for the Democratic nomination in 1892.

45. "Modern Medicine," poem signed "E. Frank Lintaber," in *Puck* 28:719 (December 17, 1890), 288. I have silently corrected the spelling of "bacillae" in the sixth line. Twelve omitted lines cover typhoid fever, rattlesnake bite, leprosy, and dyspepsia. "Lintaber" was apparently an occasional pen name of E. Franklin Taber, according to the *National Union Catalogue of Pre-1956 Imprints,* in which E. Frank Lintaber is added in parentheses to the Taber entry.

46. *Judge* 19:483 (January 17, 1891), 267, in a column of jokes.

47. *Judge* 22:534 (January 9, 1892), 34. In the cartoon, these labels appear on four large bottles standing on the floor, each in front of a man holding a huge hypodermic syringe. For more about the "gold cure," see Hansen, "New Images of a New Medicine," 664; and William H. Helfand, *Quack, Quack, Quack: The Sellers of Nostrums in Prints, Posters, Ephemera and Books* (New York: Grolier Club, 2002), 184–197.

48. Most of the primary sources from the era use the spelling *anti-toxine,* a now obsolete form. *Antitoxin,* the usual form today, is used here except in direct quotations.

49. Paul Weindling tells the international scientific story and cites further literature in "From Medical Research to Clinical Practice: Serum Therapy for Diphtheria in the 1890s," in *Medical Innovations in Historical Perspective,* ed. John V. Pickstone, 72–83 (New York: St.

Martin's, 1992). On the importance of the press and the public in Hermann Biggs's diphtheria campaign, the pioneering examination is Jean Howson, "'Sure Cure for Diphtheria': Medicine and the New York Newspapers in 1894" (graduate course paper, History Department, New York University, 1986). Citations to other studies may be found in Hansen, "New Images of a New Medicine," 665–666; and in Evelynn M. Hammonds, *Childhood's Deadly Scourge: The Campaign to Control Diphtheria in New York City, 1880–1930* (Baltimore: Johns Hopkins University Press, 1999).

50. "The New Remedy for Diphtheria," *Harper's Weekly* 38:1969 (September 15, 1894), 867.

51. The traditional page of loose type composed of individual letters and separate pictorial blocks was held together in part by the rigid rules dividing the columns. Any large image that broke these rules weakened the plate and increased the risk of its falling apart on high-speed rotary presses. When stereotyping was introduced (making a mold and then a cast of the plate) so that the same page could be run simultaneously on several presses, it had the secondary benefit of allowing images to break the column rules without the old danger, and images wider than one column became commonplace.

52. Two further examples indicate the special interest that people found in the horses' role. A long article in the *New York Times,* March 26, 1895, 3, opens with this series of headlines: "'No. 7' a Valuable Horse. Has Furnished the Health Board with 15 Quarts of Antitoxine. Bought for $10; Worth $5,000. Gaining Flesh While Losing Blood and Does Not Appear to Be at All Dissatisfied in His New Role." Even decades later, horses were still the primary image used to represent the antitoxin discovery in Robert A. Thom's (widely reproduced) painting *The Era of Biologicals,* which shows three anonymous technicians in white jackets, pants, and hats drawing blood from two horses. See George A. Bender, *Great Moments in Pharmacy: The Stories and Paintings in the Series "A History of Pharmacy in Pictures" . . . by Robert A. Thom,* 2nd ed. (Detroit: Northwood Institute Press, with special permission of Parke, Davis & Company, 1967), 173. For scholarly analysis, see Jacalyn Duffin and Alison Li, "Great Moments: Parke, Davis and Company and the Creation of Medical Art," *Isis* 86:1 (March 1995), 1–29.

53. That wide public appreciation of the way these horses were saving children's lives might have undermined antivivisection sentiment is not easily demonstrated, but the idea merits consideration.

54. "The New Diphtheria Cure," *Leslie's Illustrated Weekly* 80:2053 (January 17, 1895), 43 for text and 46 for images, had an accurate text but ran an alarmingly erroneous caption for the picture of treating the baby: "The Method of Injecting the Poison in Order to Obtain Serum." A few weeks later, *Leslie's* ran another diphtheria picture (this time without a story) and again used an incorrect or misleading caption. See "The New Treatment for Diphtheria at the Hospital for Sick Children, Paris—*L'Illustration,*" one of several images on the Foreign Press page, *Leslie's Illustrated Weekly* 80:2057 (February 14, 1895), 109, which clearly shows not the new hypodermic injection but the established intubation operation in which a seated doctor works in the mouth of a baby held on a woman's lap with an attendant standing behind the woman to hold the baby's head steady.

55. It is important to remember that photographs only seem to capture unmediated reality and that they must be understood as shaped by the conventions of producing and interpreting them, a point made by many historians and critics. See Fox and Lawrence, *Photographing Medicine,* 5–13.

56. Horace D. Arnold, "The Relation of Laboratory Research to the General Practitioner of

Medicine," *Boston Medical and Surgical Journal* 149:18 (October 29, 1903), 473–478 (quotation on 474).

57. The best single account of these nineteenth- and early-twentieth-century developments is Paul Starr, *The Social Transformation of American Medicine* (New York: Basic Books, 1982). See also James H. Cassedy, *Medicine in America: A Short History* (Baltimore: Johns Hopkins University Press, 1991); Lederer, *Subjected to Science*; Edward Shorter, *The Health Century* (New York: Doubleday, 1987); Richard Harrison Shryock, *The Development of Modern Medicine: An Interpretation of the Social and Scientific Factors Involved* (New York: Hafner, 1969, reprinting the 1947 edition); Nancy Tomes, *The Gospel of Germs: Men, Women, and the Microbe in American Life* (Cambridge, Mass.: Harvard University Press, 1998); and Ronald G. Walters, ed., *Scientific Authority and Twentieth-Century America* (Baltimore: Johns Hopkins University Press, 1997).

CHAPTER 5. CREATING AN INSTITUTIONAL BASE FOR MEDICAL RESEARCH, 1890–1920

1. Paul Gibier, *Recherches expérimentales sur la rage et sur son traitement* (Paris: Asselin et Houzeau, 1884), 87. For substantial, if perhaps not entirely reliable, biographical information, see "Paul Gibier, A.M., M.D.," an unsigned éloge in the final issue of the *Bulletin of the Pasteur Institute* 8:3 (September 1900), 9–14, followed by a bibliography of his "principal works" (with French-language titles given only in English) on 14–16. Interesting autobiographical comments occur from time to time in Paul Gibier, *Psychism, Analysis of Things Existing: Essays* (New York: Bulletin, 1899).

2. The report of Gibier's investigation is mentioned in the éloge published in the final issue of the *Bulletin of the Pasteur Institute*, 11. In the associated bibliography, it is listed (on p. 15) as "Report to the French Government on the German Laboratories of Bacteriology, Official Mission, 1885," among the works in French. I have not yet been able to locate a copy of this report or even learn its French title.

3. "Yellow Fever Microbes: Dr. Gibier of Paris, En Route for Florida, Talks about Them," *New York Times,* October 16, 1888, 3.

4. "A Pasteur Institute," *New York Times,* February 19, 1890 (about the opening reception).

5. For laboratory procedures and working conditions between 1885 and 1900, see Patricia Peck Gossel, "A Need for Standard Methods: The Case of American Bacteriology," in *The Right Tools for the Job: At Work in Twentieth-Century Life Sciences,* ed. Adele E. Clarke and Joan H. Fujimura, 287–311 (Princeton, N.J.: Princeton University Press, 1992).

6. Paul Gibier, "Experimental Research on Professor R. Koch's Fluid with Exhibition of Cultures and Effects upon Animals, Read before the Medical Society of the County of New York, February 23, 1891," *New York Medical Journal* 53 (March 14, 1891), 303–304.

7. "The Pasteur Treatment," *North American Review* 151 (August 1890), 160–166; and "Koch's Cure of Consumption," *North American Review* 151 (December 1890), 726–730. These magazine articles also reached an even wider public when summarized in the daily press. See, for example, "Pasteur and the Rabies: How the Enterprising Doctor Obtained His Idea," *Brooklyn Eagle,* August 10, 1890, 12, with acknowledgment to Dr. Paul Gibier and the *North American Review.* A few months later, a front-page article in the *Brooklyn Eagle* (December 3, 1890) reported on the enlarged December issue of the *North American Review* and listed

subjects of many of its articles, including this one: "Dr. Paul Gibier, of the New York Pasteur institute, something of what he knows about Dr. Koch from having studied under him and of his so called consumption cure."

8. "Pasteur Building Dedicated," *New York Times,* October 11, 1893, 9. Patients were already in residence as early as June; see "Saved by a Projecting Awning," *New York Times,* June 19, 1893, 1.

9. "An Hour with Paul Gibier," *New York Times,* December 23, 1893, 2.

10. Gibier's products were also listed elsewhere, as in the widely circulated *Merck's 1896 Index: An Encyclopedia for the Physician and the Pharmacist* (New York: Merck, 1895), 42.

11. This was the same James Carroll who became famous several years later as the first experimental case of yellow fever and as leader of the research group in Cuba during Walter Reed's absence. Several relevant letters from 1894 and 1895 are found in the collection of the Otis Historical Archives, National Museum of Health and Medicine, Armed Forces Institute of Pathology, Washington, D.C. In Curatorial Records: Numbered Correspondence, 1894–1917, OHA 19, see items numbered 337 and 341 (rabies treatment for James Carroll); 374 and 396 (Reed's request to Gibier for antitoxic serum and Gibier's reply); 492 (Reed's request for a culture of the bacillus diphtheriae "which will produce a powerful toxine" and Gibier's reply); 862 (Reed to Sternberg about securing sample of tetanus antitoxin made at New York Pasteur Institute); and 932 (Reed to Gibier for instructions on use of tetanus antitoxin and reply). For assistance with the Reed-Gibier correspondence, I thank Michael Rhode.

12. Additional U.S. Pasteur institutes were established in Chicago in 1890, Baltimore in 1897, and then Atlanta, Pittsburgh, and St. Louis, all in 1900. About twenty-five more institutes were opened after 1900.

13. L. Emmett Holt, "The Antitoxine Treatment of Diphtheria," *Forum,* March 1895, 112.

14. That Gibier's priority over the Health Department has generally not been noticed is probably because his work was ignored in C.-E. A. Winslow, *The Life of Hermann M. Biggs, M.D., D.Sc., LL.D., Physician and Statesman of the Public Health* (Philadelphia: Lea and Febiger, 1929), which is the mostly likely source of later repetitions of this error in John Duffy, *A History of Public Health in New York City, 1866–1966* (New York: Russell Sage Foundation, 1974), and in many more recent works. The misattribution of credit for priority is somewhat surprising because the participants must have been aware of Gibier's having success while their efforts were failing, since there was so much coverage. Among the documents showing precisely how early Gibier's antitoxin was ready is a published letter written on December 12, 1894, by a physician in Quebec City, describing how he had treated himself with Gibier's product earlier that month and that he had recovered completely by the ninth; see Charles Verge, "A propos d'antitoxine," *Union médicale du Canada* 24 (1895), 16–17.

15. "Gratitude Shown in a Practical Way," *New York Daily Tribune,* January 3, 1895, 7.

16. The quoted text is from a newspaper report, not from the legislation; see "New-York City Measures," *New York Daily Tribune,* March 28, 1895, 3. New York was not the only state to take action to support rabies treatments for indigents. I have found indications that similar laws authorizing state funds for treatments at a nearby Pasteur institute were enacted in Connecticut, Illinois, Maryland, Michigan, and Pennsylvania. It seems possible that other states had them as well.

17. Key to understanding this public funding of the rabies vaccine was its use as a therapy, not as a preventive. Prevention is consistently a harder sell. For a study of conflicts over prevention in exactly this time and place, see James Colgrove, "Between Persuasion and

Compulsion: Smallpox Control in Brooklyn and New York, 1894–1902," *Bulletin of the History of Medicine* 78:2 (Summer 2004), 349–378.

18. "Tetanus Cured by Antitoxin," *New York Tribune,* October 31, 1895, 11. On the same day, the *New York Times* ran a similar but longer article entitled "Lockjaw Cured by Antitoxine," 5.

19. This was tetanus antitoxin in dry form, which was said to retain its properties indefinitely. See back cover of *New York Therapeutic Review* 3:3 (July-September 1895).

20. It appears that the Board of Health's tetanus antitoxin was ready by mid-July 1896 but that its first use in a patient was in early September. See "Serum for Lockjaw," *New York Times,* July 19, 1896, 4; and "Antitoxine for Tetanus Administered for the First Time in the Public Hospitals," *New York Times,* September 6, 1896, 10. The latter article noted that "Dr. Paul Gibier of the Pasteur Institute has used the serum frequently in his practice, but he has obtained it from abroad."

21. Howard M. Breen, "The Defenders of the Human Body and Their Foes. What Is Being Done at the New York Pasteur Institute to Enlarge Our Knowledge of Health and Disease," *Metropolitan Magazine* 3:1 (January 1896), 25–29.

22. "The Pasteur Institute Zoo," *New York Times,* January 16, 1898, Sunday magazine, 2–3, with six photographs of animals.

23. J. Montgomery McGovern, "Martyrs of Science," *Royal Magazine* 1:6 (April 1899), 539–542; I. M. Montgomery, "The Pasteur Institute's Wonderful 'Zoo,'" *Broadway Magazine* 13:8 (November 1904), 11–16. I assume that both these articles are by Janet B. Montgomery McGovern.

24. The pharmaceutical company Parke-Davis began running a series of advertisements in the late 1920s, each telling the story of a medical breakthrough such as the Newark boys' trip to Paris for rabies shots; others covered typhoid shots and antitetanus injections. The series, entitled "Building the Fortresses of Health," is discussed in chapter 7.

25. Rambaud, like his uncle, became one of the nation's experts on rabies, both for lay people and for the medical profession. He was the author of the twenty-two-page rabies chapter in a major eight-volume surgical reference work, Joseph D. Bryant and Albert H. Buck, eds., *The American Practice of Surgery: A Complete System of the Science and Art of Surgery* (New York: W. Wood, 1906–1911).

26. "Pasteur Institute Ends: Major Rambaud, Now in Army, Says Hospitals Can Handle Rabies," *New York Times,* September 21, 1918, 7. Rambaud settled in France after the war and largely disappeared from U.S. medical history, except for his participation in the publication of Serge Voronoff, *The Conquest of Life,* trans. G. Gibier Rambaud, M.D. (New York: Brentano's, 1928).

27. See "Pasteur Institute's Work," *New York Times,* March 1, 1908, 6; and "Pasteur Institute Ends," *New York Times,* September 21, 1918, 7.

28. George W. Corner, *A History of the Rockefeller Institute, 1901–1953: Origins and Growth* (New York: Rockefeller Institute Press, 1964); Tom Rivers, *Reflections on a Life in Medicine and Science: An Oral History Memoir Prepared by Saul Benison* (Cambridge, Mass.: MIT Press, 1967); Elizabeth Hanson, *The Rockefeller University Achievements: A Century of Science for the Benefit of Humankind* (New York: Rockefeller University Press, 2000); and Darwin H. Stapleton, ed., *Creating a Tradition of Biomedical Research: Contributions to the History of the Rockefeller University* (New York: Rockefeller University Press, 2004).

29. Harry F. Dowling, *Fighting Infection: Conquests of the Twentieth Century* (Cambridge,

Mass.: Harvard University Press, 1977), 50–54; and Corner, *History of the Rockefeller Institute,* 59–62.

30. *New York Times,* May 31, 1908, 1.

31. "Blindness Vanishes before the March of Modern Science," *New York Herald,* December 5, 1909, sec. 3, p. 2.

32. Illustrations included a drawn portrait of Louis Pasteur in the center of four photos of the New York Pasteur Institute (clockwise from upper left: Dr. George G. Rambaud in the laboratory, exterior of Twenty-third Street building, laboratory bench, and portrait of Dr. George G. Rambaud). The following week's *Scientific American* 104:23 (June 10, 1911, 565–566) ran a long story by John B. Huber, "'Mad Dogs' and Hydrophobia: Rabies before and after Pasteur," which included five photographs of Rambaud's New York Pasteur Institute and the Edelfelt painting of Pasteur.

33. Corner, *History of the Rockefeller Institute,* 80–83. An interesting example of perhaps overly enthusiastic reporting appeared in the *New York Times* of March 12, 1911: "Cause of Infantile Paralysis a Germ" (7). The subheadlines read: "Animal Experiments Reveal What Even a Microscope Cannot Detect, Says Dr. Flexner. Prevention Now Possible." An editorial in the same day's paper applauded Flexner's work and declared the essential value of experiments using animals (12). The news report explained itself this way: "Dr. Flexner, who is, as a rule, silent as to the discoveries made at the institute of which he is director, consented to make this statement yesterday to *The New York Times* in explanation of one of the arguments he brought forward at a hearing at Albany last week in defense of the use of animals in medical research."

34. Edgar Allen Forbes, "Diseases Already or Almost Conquered," *Leslie's* 116:3005 (April 10, 1913), 388.

35. "Noguchi Isolates the Germ of Rabies," *New York Times,* September 7, 1913, 1. This story ran a full eighteen inches starting at the top of the page.

36. "The Rabies Germ Discovered," *Independent* (New York) 75:3381 (September 18, 1913), 694 (in which Rambaud's name was mistakenly printed as "Gambaur"); and "The Discovery of the Germ of Rabies," *Outlook* 105 (October 4, 1913), 251–252.

37. "A Discovery about Rabies," *Harper's Weekly* 58:2966 (October 25, 1913), 14. A full-page portrait photograph of Noguchi at his microscope (credited to Leon Gimpel, Paris) ran with a caption that said he had "recently cleared up one of the most baffling problems of medical science by isolating the germ of rabies" in *World's Work* 27 (January 1914), 246.

38. On Noguchi's life and work, including rabies and yellow fever, see the lively, undocumented, and idiosyncratic account by Gustav Eckstein, *Noguchi* (New York: Harper & Brothers, 1931); a very balanced and useful narrative by Isabel Rosanoff Plesset, which covers his work much more fully than its title suggests, *Noguchi and His Patrons* (Rutherford, N.J.: Fairleigh Dickinson University Press, 1980); and Paul Franklin Clark, "Hideyo Noguchi, 1876–1928," *Bulletin of the History of Medicine* 33:1 (January-February 1959), 1–20. The failed rabies "discovery" is given one sentence in Corner, *History of the Rockefeller Institute,* 188.

CHAPTER 6. THE MASS MEDIA MAKE MEDICAL HISTORY POPULAR

1. The character of the pneumonia work was recorded in a memoir by Lewis Thomas, *The Youngest Science: Notes of a Medicine-Watcher* (New York: Viking, 1983), 40–44. See also

Harry F. Dowling, *Fighting Infection: Conquests of the Twentieth Century* (Cambridge, Mass.: Harvard University Press, 1977), on serum therapy for pneumonia (44–50) and for meningococcal infections (50–54); and Scott H. Podolsky, *Pneumonia before Antibiotics: Therapeutic Evolution and Evaluation in Twentieth-Century America* (Baltimore: Johns Hopkins University Press, 2006). An important popular account of pneumonia serum in *Life* magazine, December 20, 1937, is discussed in chapter 9.

2. Incidentally, one of the most important scientific outcomes of the pneumonia-typing research was not medical but biological. In the 1910s, Rockefeller scientists discovered that certain chemicals in the cell could transform one type of pneumonia into another. Over several decades, they studied this transforming substance and eventually saw that it was DNA. It was this work by Oswald Avery, Colin MacLeod, and Maclyn McCarty that in 1944 directed attention to DNA as a carrier of genetic information. About a decade later, Watson and Crick's double-helix model showed how DNA could encode and replicate inheritable information, thereby establishing this known but not yet famous chemical compound as having a unique and fundamental role in the reproduction of living things. See René J. Dubos, *The Professor, the Institute, and DNA* (New York: Rockefeller University Press, 1976); and Maclyn McCarty, *The Transforming Principle: Discovering That Genes Are Made of DNA* (New York: Norton, 1985).

3. Daniel J. Kevles, *The Physicists: The History of a Scientific Community in Modern America* (Cambridge, Mass.: Harvard University Press, 1977), 170–174; Peter J. Kuznick, *Beyond the Laboratory: Scientists as Political Activists in 1930s America* (Chicago: University of Chicago Press, 1987), 1–70; Marcel C. LaFollette, *Making Science Our Own: Public Images of Science, 1910–1955* (Chicago: University of Chicago Press, 1990), 8–10; David J. Rhees, "A New Voice for Science: Science Service under Edwin E. Slosson, 1921–29" (master's thesis, University of North Carolina at Chapel Hill, 1979), available online at http://scienceservice.si.edu/thesis/index.htm (accessed June 4, 2008); and Ronald C. Tobey, *The American Ideology of National Science, 1919–1930* (Pittsburgh: University of Pittsburgh Press, 1971), 62–95.

4. Henry Smith Williams, *The Story of Modern Science in Ten Volumes* (New York: Funk & Wagnalls, 1923).

5. The image of Dr. Rambaud giving an injection was a cropped version of a photograph that had already appeared in Williams, *Story of Modern Science* in 1923, in *World's Work* in 1913 (fig. 50 in chapter 5), and in at least two magazine articles: John B. Huber, "'Mad Dogs' and Hydrophobia: Rabies before and after Pasteur," *Scientific American* 104:23 (June 10, 1911), 565–566, and Edgar Allen Forbes, "Diseases Already or Almost Conquered," *Leslie's* 116:3005 (April 10, 1913), 388.

6. Information on Paul de Kruif's career depends mostly on an autobiography, *The Sweeping Wind: A Memoir* (New York: Harcourt, Brace & World, 1962); a short account by a colleague, Ben Hibbs, *Two Men on a Job* (Philadelphia: Curtis, 1938); and Robin Marantz Henig, "The Life and Legacy of Paul de Kruif," *APF Reporter* 20:3 (Fall 2002), the Newsletter of the Alicia Patterson Foundation, available online at http://www.aliciapatterson.org/APF2003/Henig/Henig.html (accessed June 3, 2008). For interesting comments on the high quality of de Kruif's scientific research, see Tom Rivers, *Reflections on a Life in Medicine and Science: An Oral History Memoir Prepared by Saul Benison* (Cambridge, Mass.: MIT Press, 1967), 180–182. For de Kruif's relationship with Sinclair Lewis, see also James M. Hutchisson, "Sinclair Lewis, Paul de Kruif, and the Composition of *Arrowsmith*," *Studies in the Novel* 24:1 (Spring 1992), 48–66; James M. Hutchisson, *The Rise of Sinclair Lewis,*

1920–1930 (University Park: Pennsylvania State University Press, 1996); Charles E. Rosenberg, "Martin Arrowsmith: The Scientist as Hero," *American Quarterly* 15:3 (Autumn 1963), 447–458; Mark Shorer, *Sinclair Lewis: An American Life* (New York: McGraw-Hill, 1961); and William C. Summers, "On the Origins of the Science in *Arrowsmith*: Paul de Kruif, Félix d'Hérelle and Phage," *Journal of the History of Medicine and Allied Sciences* 46:3 (July 1991), 315–332.

7. Paul de Kruif, "An Obscure Doctor's Success against Diabetes," *Hearst's International* 44:5 (November 1923), 96–97, 131–134, and 136. In this monthly magazine edited by Norman Hapgood, de Kruif first presented a series of articles about modern quacks, which the editor claimed was as important as the famous exposé of food and drug problems by Samuel Hopkins Adams fifteen years earlier. After seven of these articles, between September 1922 and March 1923, de Kruif began writing in this magazine in October 1923 about legitimate breakthroughs such as insulin, sunlight and rickets, and radium.

8. These articles appeared in five consecutive issues of *Country Gentleman* (*CG*), a monthly magazine; all were signed Dr. Paul de Kruif, without an indication that his degree was a Ph.D., not an M.D.: (1) "Pasteur the Microbe Hunter, and How He Discovered Pasteurization and Vaccines," *CG* 90:35 (September 1925), 18–19, 47–48, 51; (2) "Pasteur and the Mad Dogs," *CG* 90:36 (October 1925), 12–13, 145–146; (3) "Koch the Death Fighter: How a Country Doctor Conquered the Curse of Anthrax," *CG* 90:37 (November 1925), 14, 119–120; (4) "The Conquest of Tuberculosis," *CG* 90:38 (December 1925), 11, 116–117; and (5) "Theobald Smith and the Texas-Fever Tick, Some Cattlemen's Wise Hunch Led Him to a Scientific Triumph," *CG* 91:1 (January 1926), 18–19, 59. These articles were illustrated by R. L. Lambdin, but these illustrations did not appear in the book *Microbe Hunters,* in which seven of the eight figures were engraved or photographic portraits and one was a drawing of two men in a field vaccinating a sheep for anthrax.

9. Paul de Kruif, *Microbe Hunters* (New York: Harcourt, Brace, 1926), 105–107. Except for a paragraph deleted after "Prussian villages," all ellipses are in the original.

10. *Life* 5:9 (August 29, 1938), 58–60.

11. Harvey Cushing, *The Life of Sir William Osler* (Oxford, U.K.: Clarendon, 1925).

12. I do not know how widely the book was syndicated or exactly how early. It received a review in the *New York Times* of February 28, 1926; by the fall, it could be found in newspapers. For example, a fourth installment of the book ran in the *Minneapolis Sunday Tribune* of September 26, 1926; it occupied a full page, including a photo portrait of Elie Metchnikoff and two drawings of research scenes. It was credited to Current News Features, Inc.

13. The *Albany Times-Union* citation is incomplete because the information comes from an eBay listing, and I have not been able to examine a copy of this newspaper from April 1934.

14. The copy I have seen described was delivered with the *Baltimore American* for Sunday, April 2, 1939, but the *American Weekly,* published in New York from 1917 to 1963, was distributed as a pictorial supplement in many different newspapers.

15. Lucy Salamanca, "G-Men of Science," a series of twelve weekly articles running on Sundays in the *Washington Evening Star* from February 21, 1937, through May 9, 1937.

16. The film, along with related stories in the mass media, made the FBI more famous and popular as the nation's crime fighter than the Justice Department, of which it is an agency. The public's enthusiasm for G-Men helped the FBI director J. Edgar Hoover (from 1924 to 1972) displace the attorney general as the country's top policeman; see Richard Gid Powers,

G-Men: Hoover's FBI in American Popular Culture (Carbondale: Southern Illinois University Press, 1983).

17. *National Geographic Magazine,* October 1937. There is no pagination in the advertising section.

18. "Physicians Honor Beaumont's Work," *New York Times,* October 6, 1933, 14.

19. "Pioneer Heroine Honored," *New York Times,* May 31, 1935, 5.

20. Sidney Howard, in collaboration with Paul de Kruif, *Yellow Jack: A History,* with illustrations by Jo Mielziner (New York: Harcourt, Brace, 1934). On the popularity of this play and the film version, see Susan E. Lederer, *Subjected to Science: Human Experimentation in America before the Second World War* (Baltimore: Johns Hopkins University Press, 1995), 133–135. The play was revived in 1944, 1947, and 1964; see Estelle Manette Raben, "*Men in White* and *Yellow Jack* as Mirrors of the Medical Profession," *Literature and Medicine* 12:1 (Spring 1993), 39.

21. Paul de Kruif, "Backstage with *Yellow Jack,*" *Stage* 15:9 (June 1938), 28–29.

22. The script was by Gilbert Laurence.

23. Barbara Melosh, "The New Deal's Federal Theatre Project," *Medical Heritage* 2:1 (January-February 1986), 47. See also Barbara Melosh, *Engendering Culture: Manhood and Womanhood in New Deal Public Art and Theater* (Washington, D.C.: Smithsonian Institution Press, 1991), 110–134; and John E. Vacha, "The Federal Theatre's Living Newspapers: New York's Docudramas of the Thirties," *New York History* 67:1 (January 1986), 67–88.

24. On movie audiences, Melosh reports weekly attendance figures as 42.9 million in 1935 and 47.8 million in 1939; see *Engendering Culture,* 8. In 1939, the total U.S. population was 139 million.

25. See Michael Shortland, *Medicine and Film: A Checklist, Survey and Research Resource,* Research Publications of the Wellcome Unit No. 9 (Oxford, U.K.: Wellcome Unit for the History of Medicine, 1989); Peter E. Dans, *Doctors in the Movies: Boil the Water and Just Say Aah* (Bloomington, Ill.: Medi-Ed, 2000); and Christopher Frayling, *Mad, Bad, and Dangerous? The Scientist and the Cinema* (London: Reaktion Books, 2005). See also Susan E. Lederer, review of *Arrowsmith,* in "Special Section on History of Science in Film," *Isis* 84:4 (December 1993), 771–772; Susan E. Lederer and Naomi Rogers, "Media," in *Medicine in the Twentieth Century,* ed. J. Pickstone and R. Cooter, 487–502 (London: Harwood, 2000); Bruce Babington, "'To Catch a Star on Your Fingertips': Diagnosing the Medical Biopic from *The Story of Louis Pasteur* to *Freud,*" in *Signs of Life: Cinema and Medicine,* ed. Graeme Harper and Andrew Moor, 120–131 (London: Wallflower, 2005); and José Elías García Sánchez and Enrique García Sánchez, "The Founders of Microbiology on Movie Posters," *Journal of Medicine and Movies* 1:2 (April 2005), 47–56, also available online at http://www.usal.es/~revistamedicinacine/Indice_2005/Revista/numero%202/ing/padres_microb_ing.htm (accessed July 17, 2008). A new collection has three essays relevant to this chapter; see Nancy Tomes, "Celebrity Diseases" (36–67); Naomi Rogers, "American Medicine and the Politics of Filmmaking: *Sister Kenny* (RKO, 1946)" (199–238); and Susan E. Lederer, "Hollywood and Human Experimentation: Representing Medical Research in Popular Film" (282–306), all in *Medicine's Moving Pictures: Medicine, Health, and Bodies in American Film and Television,* ed. Leslie J. Reagan, Nancy Tomes, and Paula A. Treichler (Rochester, N.Y.: University of Rochester Press, 2007).

26. See Thomas Elsaesser, "Film History as Social History: The Dieterle/Warner Brothers Bio-pic," *Wide Angle* 8:2 (Spring 1986), 15–31; Carolyn Anderson, "Biographical Film," chap. 18 in *Handbook of American Film Genres,* ed. Wes D. Gehring, 331–351 (New York: Greenwood, 1988); and George Frederick Custen, *Bio/Pics: How Hollywood Constructed Public History* (New Brunswick, N.J.: Rutgers University Press, 1992). For film biographies in science and medicine, see Alberto Elena, "Exemplary Lives: Biographies of Scientists on the Screen," *Public Understanding of Science* 2:3 (July 1993), 205–223. Elena's article lists 122 films, from 1908 to 1992, including films made for television. The United States was the leading producer of science biographies, with thirty-six titles overall, and especially for the years that Elena calls the "golden period" of 1939–1952.

27. This film has failed to maintain a lasting reputation, in contrast with other medical biopics such as *Arrowsmith, The Story of Louis Pasteur,* and *Dr. Ehrlich's Magic Bullet.* When released, however, it got good press. For example, Mark Van Doren, writing in the *Nation* (March 4, 1936, 292–293), praised both *Shark Island* and *Louis Pasteur* while indicating that he preferred the Mudd story for having suspense and a single big triumph. He regarded a series of separate triumphs such as those in the Pasteur film as less dramatic, though he liked both films.

28. See Alberto Elena, "El ángel inoculador: *Pasteur* y los orígenes de las biografías cinematográficas de científicos," *Arbor: Ciencia, Pensamiento y Cultura* 145:569 (May 1993), 17–37; and Shortland, *Medicine and Film,* 3–4, 25.

29. Anderson, "Biographical Film," 332. On the studio's reluctance to make a film about "the story of a milkman," in Jack Warner's words, and on the reduced fees, see Susan E. Lederer and John Parascandola, "Screening Syphilis: *Dr. Ehrlich's Magic Bullet* Meets the Public Health Service," *Journal of the History of Medicine and Allied Sciences* 53:4 (October 1998), 348.

30. A letter to the screen editor of the *New York Times* (published on Sunday, June 1, 1936, page X2) came from Leonard G. Ting at Nankai University in Tientsin, China. His letter reported that the Chinese title was *Wan Ku Liu Fang,* meaning "enduring renown through ten thousand ages." The film had a regular run at Tientsin and Peiping. There were also special very low-priced screenings for students from colleges and middle schools in these cities (at 15 to 20 percent of regular prices). "The picture evidently has a high appeal to the young Chinese and its story is easily understandable by them. China is getting 'science-minded' and welcomes pictures like 'The Story of Louis Pasteur.'"

31. See entry on *The Story of Louis Pasteur* in *The Motion Picture Guide,* ed. Jay Robert Nash and Stanley Ralph Ross, 10 vols. (Chicago: Cinebooks, 1985), 7:3145–3146. A copy of the film's pressbook in the author's collection consists of twenty-eight glossy, tabloid-sized pages offering numerous illustrations, ready-to-run articles and reviews, and suggestions for games and puzzles and also outlining in detail such ideas as promoting contests in schools (e.g., essays about medical discovery) and interviewing local physicians.

32. *Time* 27:7 (February 17, 1936), 46.

33. For observations about the use of internal, or diegetic, spectators with whom the audience in the theater can identify, see Elsaesser, "Film History," 26. Internal audiences were very important in the films about Pasteur, Nightingale, Ehrlich, Curie, and Kenny. According to Custen, it was Daryl Zanuck who pushed especially hard for writers to provide viewers with a "rooting interest" in the life of the famous person. Zanuck also advised of the need to "have clear motivation for the decisions that brought him or her greatness" (*Bio/ Pics,* 18).

34. Lorraine Noble, ed., *Four-Star Scripts: Actual Shooting Scripts and How They Are Written*

(Garden City, N.Y.: Doubleday, Doran, 1937), 392. This speech, like similar ones in the other medical biopics, had effects beyond its immediate audience in the darkened theater. Film scripts were often reused in radio dramatizations, and a 1946 radio performance of this particular speech was reissued on a long-playing record in the 1960s, "Academy Award Winners on the Air."

35. "Pasteur: The Scientist's Life as He Lived It, Not as Hollywood Imagined It," *Newsweek* 7:7 (February 15, 1936), 27. The review's title was meant as praise, not complaint, for it opens, "Last week the screen discarded prosaic formulas in favor of an untouched film source—straight biography. *The Story of Louis Pasteur* proves that thrilling cinema material lies in historic facts undistorted by romantic embellishments producers have piled on." Historians, however, see the film with different eyes, often bristling at romantic embellishments and other distortions of fact.

36. *New York Daily Mirror,* February 13, 1937, pagination unknown. This review and many others are found in a clippings file for *Green Light* at the Performing Arts Division of the New York Public Library at Lincoln Center.

37. *Dark Victory,* edited and with an introduction by Bernard F. Dick, Wisconsin/Warner Bros. Screenplay Series (Madison: University of Wisconsin Press, 1981), 76. A slightly different rendition of this dialogue was published in Glenn Flores, "Mad Scientists, Compassionate Healers, and Greedy Egotists: The Portrayal of Physicians in the Movies," *Journal of the National Medical Association* 94:7 (July 2002), 646. Note that Dr. Arrowsmith had announced a few years earlier in the movie about him, "I'm not going to be just an ordinary doctor, I want to be a research scientist. . . . I'm not interested in just giving pills to people. I'd rather find a cure for cancer" (as quoted in Flores, "Mad Scientists, Compassionate Healers," 646).

38. Lederer and Parascandola, "Screening Syphilis," 348; and Elsaesser, "Film History," 23.

39. See T. Hugh Crawford, "Screening Science: Pedagogy and Practice in William Dieterle's Film Biographies of Scientists," *Common Knowledge* 6:2 (Fall 1997), 52–68. For a brief but perceptive unpublished essay on the special contribution of Dieterle's biopics written by his friend Bertolt Brecht in about 1944, see "Wilhelm Dieterles Gallerie grosser bürgerlicher Figuren," in Bertolt Brecht, *Werke: Grosse kommentierte Berliner und Frankfurter Ausgabe,* 30 vols. (Berlin: Aufbau-Verlag; Frankfurt am Main: Suhrkamp Verlag, 1993), 23:42–44, with annotations on 23:447–448. Brecht deemed the Dieterle biopics superior to weaker examples—namely, the films about Thomas Edison (both of them), Madame Curie, Mark Twain, and Woodrow Wilson—because the historical setting was not subordinated into period details but was shown to the public as a protagonist, as the "social clockwork" of the epoch in question. An excerpt from Brecht's essay is quoted in English in Elsaesser, "Film History," 24.

40. According to Lederer and Parascandola, Warner Brothers considered and discarded ideas of doing biopics of Sigmund Freud, Joseph Lister, Joseph Goldberger, and Ignaz Semmelweis ("Screening Syphilis," 348). In 1935, Warner Brothers received a letter from a Seymour Katz proposing a film about Hideyo Noguchi. Plans for a feature film about Lister emerged at Warner's competitor, MGM, in 1939, but the film was never made; see "Story of Scientist May Be Filmed," *Los Angeles Times,* February 12, 1939, 15.

41. See also Anne Hudson Jones, "*The White Angel* (1936): Hollywood's Images of Florence Nightingale," in *Images of Nurses: Perspectives from History, Art and Literature,* ed. Anne Hudson Jones, 221–242 (Philadelphia: University of Pennsylvania Press, 1988).

42. It seems likely that the unmarried Dr. Louise Pearce (1885–1959) might have been in the scriptwriters' mind when they created the character of Dr. Sterne, the highly competent and independent woman doctor in the film. Pearce had tested the efficacy of a new drug for sleeping sickness in the Belgian Congo (Zaire) in 1920. She met with great success in the field, garnered some attention in the newspapers, and received honors from the Belgian government.

43. Typical examples of mass-media stories about Noguchi include C. Snyder, "Noguchi—The Man behind the Contagion Fighters," *Everybody's Magazine* 33 (November 1915), 554–561; and Frederick Palmer, "All the Health in the World," *Collier's* 70:18 (October 28, 1922), 15–16. Noguchi's death was reported not in an obituary but as a front-page news article in the *New York Times*: "Dr. Noguchi Is Dead, Martyr of Science. Bacteriologist of Rockefeller Institute Dies of Yellow Fever on Gold Coast. Solved Medical Riddle. Japanese, Ranked With Pasteur and Metchnikoff, Found Carrier of Own Disease" (May 22, 1928). A recent study with a worldwide scope examines how Noguchi's reputation was made and sustained: Aya Takahashi, "Hideyo Noguchi, the Pursuit of Immunity and the Persistence of Fame: A Reappraisal," in *Creating a Tradition of Biomedical Research: Contributions to the History of the Rockefeller University,* ed. Darwin H. Stapleton, 227–239 (New York: Rockefeller University Press, 2004).

44. Brief comments on *The Green Light* are found in Shortland, *Medicine and Film,* 26; Lederer and Rogers, "Media," 492; Victoria A. Harden, *Rocky Mountain Spotted Fever: History of a Twentieth-Century Disease* (Baltimore: Johns Hopkins University Press, 1990), 205; and Clive Hirschorn, *The Warner Bros. Story* (New York: Crown, 1979), 172. It has been stated incorrectly that the film's title refers to receiving permission to go ahead with vaccine trials, but in fact it is a religious metaphor used throughout the film.

45. For more on these men and on the Spencer-Parker vaccine, see Harden, *Rocky Mountain Spotted Fever.* An earlier scene in the film specifically salutes the martyrdom of several men in the laboratory who had died from the disease, naming Thomas B. McClintic, William Edwin Gettinger, George Henry Cowan, and Albert LeRoy Kerlee.

46. See Lederer and Parascandola, "Screening Syphilis." Whether de Kruif liked it or not, the film undoubtedly spurred sales of his book. The film was released in February, and in March the Pocket Books edition appeared with the actor Edward G. Robinson on the cover. This image appeared through the fourth printing in April 1940. Beginning with the fifth printing in November 1940, the film star's portrait was replaced with an unattended microscope on a plain yellow background.

47. Lederer and Parascandola, "Screening Syphilis," 358. These authors also document similar educational materials for *The Story of Louis Pasteur* and for *Arrowsmith* prepared by the Commission on Human Relations of the Progressive Education Association in the late 1930s (358). On educational materials, see also Rima D. Apple and Michael W. Apple, "Screening Science," *Isis* 84:4 (December 1993), 750–754.

48. Robert Eberwein, *Sex Ed: Film, Video, and the Framework of Desire* (New Brunswick, N.J.: Rutgers University Press, 1999), 98–99; and Lederer and Parascandola, "Screening Syphilis," 366–367.

49. *Fight for Life* was banned by the Chicago Police Department for the way it showed that city's slum neighborhoods; see Ronald R. Kline, "Ideology and the New Deal 'Fact Film' *Power and the Land,*" *Public Understanding of Science* 6:1 (January 1997), 19–30.

50. Alberto Elena, "Skirts in the Lab: *Madame Curie* and the Image of the Woman Scientist in the Feature Film," *Public Understanding of Science* 6:3 (July 1997), 269–278. Elena notes that Warner Brothers considered making a Curie film soon after the success of its Pasteur film. Marie Curie was then well known in the United States, where newspapers and magazines had published many articles about her since the early 1900s. Her visit to the United States in 1921 stimulated a huge wave of news and feature coverage. Eve Curie's book about her mother appeared in French in 1937, was serialized in English in the *Saturday Evening Post* in 1937, and then was printed by Doubleday in 1938. In time, the book sold a million copies. On Curie's U.S. visit, see any of the biographies, as well as Kevles, *The Physicists,* 204–207.

51. *New York Times,* December 17, 1943, 23.

52. This film was one of the less successful ones by Sturges, partly because of an odd mixing of comedic and tragic elements and partly because the studio substantially shortened the director's version. Shortland indicates that the studio cut nearly three reels (*Medicine and Film,* 31). For a modern appreciation of the film, based on a study of scripts, drafts, and cuts, see Frank Heynick, "William T. G. Morton and *The Great Moment,*" *Journal of the History of Dentistry* 51:1 (March 2003), 27–35.

53. A set of four twenty-one-by-twenty-eight-inch canvas-backed study charts in the author's collection were clearly made for classroom use. They take the film as a springboard for examining numerous images from the history of anesthesia before and after Morton.

54. Kenny's autobiography was published three years before the film was released: *And They Shall Walk: The Life Story of Sister Elizabeth Kenny, Written in Collaboration with Martha Ostenso* (New York: Dodd, Mead, 1943). Over the years, Kenny garnered press attention from time to time, including a major story in *Life* magazine (September 28, 1942, 73–77). For more on this film, see Shortland, *Medicine and Film,* 33; Naomi Rogers, "Sister Kenny," *Isis* 84:4 (December 1993), 772–774; Dans, *Doctors in the Movies,* 182–186; and Rogers, "Medicine and the Politics of Filmmaking." As Custen has noted, the film version of Kenny's story even managed to make medical progress seem "uniquely American" (*Bio/Pics,* 107). Shortland sees in the Sister Kenny film the beginnings of a critical view of medicine and a decline in popular appreciation of doctors, because of the negative portrayal of the medical establishment in the film (11); I do not read it that way, rather interpreting the resistance that Kenny faces from doctors as similar to the resistance that Pasteur and Ehrlich had faced in their films.

55. On audiences' tolerance for historical inaccuracies, see Custen, *Bio/Pics,* 37–38. On historical authenticity as marketing strategy, see ibid., 38; and Lederer and Parascandola, "Screening Syphilis," 354–355. For an extended examination, see Fred Andersen, "The Warner Bros. Research Department: Putting History to Work in the Classic Studio Era," *Public Historian* 17:1 (Winter 1995), 51–69.

56. Crawford observes that some films (such as the two Edison biopics) "do not explain the principles underlying their subject's technological innovations" but that Dieterle "devotes considerable time to depicting scientists at work" ("Screening Science," 53). On the Edison films, see Michael Boehnke and Stefan Machura, "Young Tom Edison—Edison, the Man: Biopic of the Dynamic Entrepreneur," *Public Understanding of Science* 12:3 (July 2003), 319–333.

57. For more-sustained analyses of the functions of biography within the popularization of science and medicine in the first half of the twentieth century, especially in the magazine literature, see LaFollette, *Making Science Our Own,* chaps. 4–6; and John C. Burnham, *How*

Superstition Won and Science Lost: Popularizing Science and Health in the United States (New Brunswick, N.J.: Rutgers University Press, 1987), chap. 5. On science more generally, see Michael Shortland and Richard Yeo, eds., *Telling Lives in Science: Essays on Scientific Biography* (New York: Cambridge University Press, 1996).

58. On the mix of success and failure in Noguchi's research, see Takahashi, "Hideyo Noguchi," 227–239, esp. 230–232. Flexner's poliomyelitis research is discussed in detail in John R. Paul, *A History of Poliomyelitis* (New Haven, Conn.: Yale University Press, 1971), chap. 12.

59. Sinclair Lewis, *Arrowsmith* (New York: Grosset and Dunlap, n.d.). The copyright page in this edition lists printings only through 1925, but this book could not have been produced before 1931 at the earliest, the date of the film starring Ronald Colman and Helen Hayes.

CHAPTER 7. "AND NOW, A WORD FROM OUR SPONSOR": MAKING MEDICAL HISTORY COMMERCIAL

1. The printed copies of the talks are each four pages, printed on a folded eleven-by-seventeen-inch sheet. That they are punched for a standard three-hole binder indicates the expectation of a regular audience of listeners who collect and save the talks. The extent of the broadcasts and the exact dates are unknown to me. Copies of seven of the talks were mailed to a listener in Montana in an envelope postmarked November 27, 1931. No. 49 shows a copyright date of 1931, but No. 50 is copyrighted 1932. How much longer the talks continued is uncertain. My collection holds fourteen talks along with the mailing envelope and a cover letter from Eastman Kodak. Haggard and his publisher later managed to serialize small pieces of *Devils, Drugs, and Doctors* into "Vignettes of History," which reached a wide readership in *Readers Digest,* such as No. 60, "Approved Treatment, but the King Died" (August 1946), 62.

2. The "Smallpox" booklet, for the broadcast of September 19, 1945, is a twenty-two-page pamphlet, just under five by eight inches. The script includes cues and even indications of the music used for atmosphere and transitions. The booklet includes a quiz to "check your reading," a list of "selected references," and a listing of stations that carried the program, grouped by time zone. It notes that the show had "won the Peabody Award as radio's outstanding educational program." The size of the listening audience is unknown to me, but the award, the number of stations, and the subscriptions for transcripts together suggest that it might have been substantial.

3. A series of radio programs by Milton Silver was adapted from Victor Robinson's *Story of Medicine* in 1938, according to a script for the first episode held by the New York Public Library.

4. It was broadcast on June 30, 1938. A copy of the script is held in the Performing Arts Collection of the New York Public Library, where it is indicated as "Men Against Death, Series 1, No. 1."

5. The broadcast date for "Louis Pasteur" was April 5, 1938. The script held in the Performing Arts Division of the New York Public Library indicates this play as "Pioneers of Science, No. 1." It is not clear whether this might be the same play as the one about Pasteur in another Federal Theatre Project radio series, *Turning Points in Famous Lives,* listed in the NYPL catalogue note on a collection of seventy-three boxes of Federal Theatre Project scripts.

6. Information about *This Is the Story* comes from a sixteen-inch record platter used for radio broadcasts. Other five-minute plays on this recording are "Galileo and the Pendulum,"

"Richard Wagner," and "Harpo Marx." Selections from the radio show were published in a book, *This Is the Story* (N.p.: Morton, 1949), but none of these four stories is in this book.

7. My information about specific radio programs derives mostly from websites maintained by fans of "old-time radio" and by people selling recordings. Because these pages are often incomplete and sometimes inconsistent, I have tried to cross-check the data when possible. I am not citing specific URLs because they are too ephemeral. Nonetheless, readers should be able to pursue information about any of these programs by doing an Internet search on a title combined with keywords such as "old-time radio." Free downloads of several of the medical history stories in *Cavalcade of America* are available online at http://www.freeotrshows. com/otr/c/Cavalcade_Of_America.html (accessed June 3, 2008). For a brief plot summary of the Dr. Zakrzewska story, broadcast under the title "That They Might Live," see Arleen Marcia Tuchman, *Science Has No Sex: The Life of Marie Zakrzewska, M.D.* (Chapel Hill: University of North Carolina Press, 2006), 257–258.

8. Besides the life of the Parke-Davis paintings as posters mailed free to physicians and as images in magazine ads, they were also collected in book form. Other companies used pictures of historical doctors in their ads, but none had the consistency, fame, and power of the paintings that were commissioned by George A. Bender of Parke-Davis from Herbert A. Thom. In considering these paintings and their poster-sized reproductions, one must keep in mind their primary audience: physicians, not the public. Although they did appear now and then in magazine ads directed at the public, their first audience was practicing physicians and pharmacists, who were encouraged to collect them and have them framed to hang in patients' waiting areas. Even if patients were expected to look at them on the wall, and perhaps compliment the doctor on them, the prints' purpose was to gain the physician's loyalty to the brand name. For a full account of the paintings, their origin, and their effects, see Jacalyn Duffin and Alison Li, "Great Moments: Parke, Davis and Company and the Creation of Medical Art," *Isis* 86:1 (March 1995), 1–29.

9. For one commercially produced device, the Pasteur-Chamberland Filter, the eponymous association was authorized and deliberate. Large and small versions of these water filters were widely advertised to the public and to establishments such as restaurants and hotels that wished to boast of the germ-free water they served patrons.

10. *Time,* April 18, 1927, 22. Lister had not merited a solo chapter in *Microbe Hunters* (1926) and received only a few passing references therein.

11. On institutional advertising, see James Playsted Wood, *The Story of Advertising* (New York: Ronald, 1958), 478–481.

12. As late as 1989, the Thom paintings were being run as ads by Warner Lambert Company, successor of Parke-Davis; see *Constitution: A Quarterly Journal of the Foundation for the U.S. Constitution* 1:2 (Winter 1989), n.p. Entitled "Standardization of Pharmaceuticals," the painting showed Messrs. Parke and Davis watching their chief chemist, Dr. Albert Brown Lyons, at his work bench with a glistening array of separatory funnels.

13. E. R. Squibb & Sons, "The Conquest of Pain," full-page magazine advertisement, June 1928 (publication history unknown).

14. E. R. Squibb & Sons, "For Us, He Fought an Endless Battle with Disease," *Woman's Home Companion,* April 1929, 52 (full page). The same ad ran in other magazines that year, including *American Magazine* and *Literary Digest.*

15. The ad was published, for example, in *Collier's,* January 13, 1935, 30–31. This artwork was also included in the *Fourteenth Annual of Advertising Art [Reproducing] the Exhibits of*

Advertising Art Displayed by the Art Directors Club of New York at Their Annual Exhibition in the Spring of 1935 (New York: Book Service Company, 1935), 65, in which it is credited to F. R. Gruger.

16. A bound portfolio of ads was produced by the company in 1929: *Building the Fortresses of Health: A Report of a Series of Advertisements by Parke, Davis and Company* (Detroit: Parke, Davis & Company, 1929). I have not found a record of this book in any library catalogue, and I am grateful to Roger K. Smith, D.D.S., of St. Joseph, Missouri, for sharing with me a complete photocopy. Some information on the placing of these ads is found in a small folder of letters at the New York Academy of Medicine Library, Special Collections MS 632.

17. Parke, Davis & Company, "3,000 Miles to Save Four Young Lives," full-page magazine advertisement published in *Collier's* (September 8, 1928), *Saturday Evening Post* (September 15, 1928), *Literary Digest* (September 22, 1928), *Hygeia* (October 1928), and *National Geographic* (October 1928).

18. Other firms tapped some of the same history in marketing rabies vaccine and other products. For example, a sales brochure of Eli Lilly and Company directed at physicians describes the company's line of "Biologicals in Preventive Medicine." Probably dating from the early 1920s, since it does not include the company's preparation of insulin, the brochure carries four portraits on its cover: von Leeuwenhoek, Jenner, Pasteur, and von Behring.

19. "Pasteur Lauded by One He Saved," *Chicago Daily News,* October 27, 1928, 3.

20. "Pasteur's First American Patient Views Unveiling of Scientist's Memorial," *Chicago Daily Journal,* October 27, 1928, 3; "Monument to Pasteur Unveiled in Grant Park," *Chicago Sunday Tribune,* October 28, 1928, 5.

21. "Tribute to Scientist's Memory: W. T. Lane Was One of the First Four Americans to Be Inoculated against Rabies," *New York Times,* November 4, 1928, sec. 9, p. 16.

22. Parke, Davis & Company, "This Picture Reunited Two Comrades Saved by Pasteur in 1885," *Saturday Evening Post,* May 23, 1931, 104. The ad was also carried in the May 1931 issue of *Child Life* (237) and probably in other magazines as well.

23. A letter dated January 28, 1936, from the Publicity Department of the New York City office of Warner Brothers Pictures to William T. Lane in Irvington, New Jersey, refers to an article about Lane and Pasteur that appeared on page 3 of the *New York World-Telegram* of January 27, 1936, and thanks Lane for helping them with the publicity. The letter notes that they were expecting Joseph Meister to arrive in New York on February 6 and that they would like Lane to join their representative "on the revenue cutter that meets Meister's ship . . . to welcome him to these shores" (typed letter signed by Gerald Breckenridge, preserved in an album of William Lane memorabilia owned by Lane's grandson, Richard F. Krentz of Tracy, California).

24. Marquis James, *The Metropolitan Life: A Study in Business Growth* (New York: Viking, 1947), 185. Although the MetLife Health Heroes series is not discussed in Bruce V. Lewenstein, "Life Insurance, Public Health Campaigns, and Public Communication of Science, 1908–1951," *Public Understanding of Science* 1:4 (October 1992), 347–365, this article provides a very useful comparison of the educational efforts of three insurance companies: MetLife, Prudential, and John Hancock.

25. James, *Metropolitan Life,* 396. The opposition to using the word syphilis in public was so strong that a radio station in 1934 told Dr. Thomas Parran, the New York State health commissioner, that he could not use it on the air when discussing venereal disease. Parran canceled the talk. See Susan E. Lederer and John Parascandola, "Screening Syphilis: *Dr. Ehrlich's Magic Bullet* Meets the Public Health Service," *Journal of the History of Medicine and Allied Sciences* 53:4 (October 1998), 360.

26. James, *Metropolitan Life*, 393.

27. Ibid., 186, 393–394. See also Louis I. Dublin, *A Family of Thirty Million: The Story of the Metropolitan Life Insurance Company* (New York: Metropolitan Life Insurance Company, 1943), 432.

28. My information about the production of Health Heroes is drawn primarily from chapter 4 of Elizabeth A. Toon's Ph.D. dissertation. I am especially grateful for her kindness in sending me a copy and exchanging ideas about MetLife's history. Much additional information and a more complete set of numbers will be available in the forthcoming book based in part on her dissertation, "Managing the Conduct of the Individual Life: Public Health Education and American Public Health, 1910 to 1950" (Ph.D. diss., University of Pennsylvania, 1998). Chapter 4 analyzes the textual content of Health Heroes on pp. 255–266. Toon points out that these books were written by Claire E. Turner and Grace T. Hallock (p. 229).

29. Elizabeth A. Toon quotes this phrasing in her dissertation (ibid., 256) from a transcript of a meeting of the Educational Advisory Group of the School Health Bureau of the Welfare Division on December 29, 1924, in the Sally Lucas Jean Papers, Southern Historical Collection, University of North Carolina, Chapel Hill.

30. Short teacher's guides did not try to amplify a booklet's content but offered suggested student projects and called attention to ancillary materials, such as Albert Einstein's tribute to Marie Curie. One teacher, a Mrs. Dougherty, stapled a teacher's guide to the inside front cover of her copy of the booklet (author's collection). Similarly, a one-page letter addressed "To school administrators" from the assistant secretary of the Welfare Division, on April 23, 1929, and perhaps enclosed with copies of the Jenner pamphlet, opens with this reminder: "May 17 is the anniversary of the birth of one of the greatest benefactors to mankind—Edward Jenner. What would be more fitting than to devote a period during the week in which this date occurs to the consideration of the tremendous value of Jenner's contribution to the whole study of disease prevention" (photocopy in author's collection). MetLife also published a sixteen-page booklet entitled "Some Ways of Using the Health Heroes Series: An Outline for Teachers" in 1927, according to the catalogue of the Countway Library at Harvard University.

31. Distribution modes of MetLife's Health Heroes series included printed booklets of various editions, filmstrips in storage cans, teacher's guides, and long-playing records that provided a soundtrack that was coordinated to the frames in the filmstrip.

32. A 1932 film, *Man against Microbe* by Iago Galdston and MetLife, is listed in the catalogue of the National Library of Medicine. Regarding access to sound projectors other than in commercial theaters, Lederer and Parascandola report that between 1937 and 1938 in West Virginia, the number of school projectors increased from 6 to 175 ("Screening Syphilis," 364). Although a public-health-service official regarded the increase as "phenomenal," it is clear that such machines were not yet readily available to schoolteachers on an ongoing basis but only for special events.

33. These numbers were kindly provided by Elizabeth Toon. MetLife later added other names to the Health Heroes roster, but in group pamphlets. Only the original seven subjects had their own individual booklets. In the 1950s, American Health Heroes abandoned the Europeans and raised the number of subjects to sixteen, perhaps in response to the era's expanded interest in biographies of figures such as these within juvenile publishing in general. Despite the new series title, two Canadians were included among the sixteen subjects: Sir William Osler, William Henry Welch, Elizabeth Blackwell, Theobald Smith, Howard Taylor Ricketts, Hans Zinsser, Walter Bradford Cannon, Sir Frederick Grant Banting, Florence Rena Sabin, William Thompson Sedgwick, Charles Value Chapin, William Crawford Gorgas, Ellen Henriette Richards, Lillian D. Wald, S. Josephine Baker, and Mabel Caroline Bragg. One booklet from the 1930s that went through several editions was *Health through the Ages,* a nonbiographical tour from the Stone Age and the ancient Hebrews and Greeks up through yellow fever and "the modern health program." In the 1960s, a booklet called "The Challenge of Health Research" offered a more wide-ranging account of twentieth-century medical discoveries; and although it did not adopt a biographical format, it did include a famous photograph of Banting and Best with a diabetic dog saved by insulin.

In 1938, a textbook publisher brought out a book for "silent reading," with the seven heroes celebrated by MetLife and the addition of Clara Barton: Charlotte Williams and Hazel A. Madison, *Heroes of Health: Thrilling Tales of Great Benefactors* (Chicago: Hall and McCreary, 1938). MetLife was not credited, but the similarity is remarkable. The 128-page soft-cover book was produced as a reader for schools, with notes on its use in silent reading for intermediate grades and remedial reading for upper grades. The heroes' stories were broken into shorter chapters, and there were tests and an explanation of how to check on reading speed and keep a record of a student's progress.

34. Anheuser-Busch, "We're Fighting Your Enemies!" *Collier's,* September 12, 1936, 55.

35. Sealtest, Inc., "He Made Life Safer for Children," *Good Housekeeping,* June 1937, 14–15.

36. National Diary Products Corporation, "Why Does Our Wine Turn Sour, M. Pasteur?" *Life* 15:24 (December 13, 1943), 17.

37. Patricia Janis Broder, *Dean Cornwell: Dean of Illustrators* (Portland, Ore.: Collectors Press, 2000; reprint of the 1978 edition with a new preface).

38. "Pioneers of American Medicine Illustrated by Dean Cornwell," *Coronet* 18:1 (May 1945), 111–117. The one painting in the series not reproduced in the magazine was that of Oliver Wendell Holmes. Another reminder of the pervasiveness of medical history in the popular media of the era is the fact that the premier issue of *Coronet* magazine in November 1936 carried an article by Paul de Kruif about a boy who died needlessly for lack of rabies shots. This magazine article, appearing the same year as Hollywood's *The Story of Louis Pasteur,* even became the subject of a news story itself: "Rabies: Paul de Kruif Exposes a Tragedy Bound with Red Tape," *Newsweek* 8:23 (December 5, 1936), 43.

39. These ads were probably widely circulated; I have found each of them in three different newspapers: the *Los Angeles Times,* the *Chicago Tribune,* and the *New York Times.* I have not seen these ads in magazines, though they might well have been printed in them as well. The dates that the ads appeared varied among the newspapers, though the order was consistent for the most part. The earliest appearance was in the *Chicago Tribune* on October 4, 1942; the latest was in the *Los Angeles Times* on August 13, 1944. The topics in the order they were published are as follows: Jenner and vaccination (1796), Withering and foxglove (1785), Behring and diphtheria antitoxin (1895), Banting and insulin (1921), "a band of army doctors" and yellow fever (1900), Koch and the tuberculosis germ (1882), Wright and typhoid vaccine (1898), Pasteur and rabies (1885), Lister and germs (1865), Auenbrugger and percussion (1761), Morton and ether anesthesia (1846), Laennec and the stethoscope (1816),

Roentgen and the X-ray (1895). For the final five ads (blood plasma, sulfa, tetanus toxoid, burn treatment, and penicillin), the association with the discovery of aspirin was dropped, and the ads were given a different rubric: "New Triumphs of Modern Medicine."

40. Ciba Pharmaceutical Products, Inc., "Heroes of the United States Medical Services: Fighter with Foods [Joseph Goldberger]," *Time,* Air Express Edition (for international mailing), May 15, 1944, 29. This ad was not present in this date's regular edition of *Time* magazine. At least ten other military doctors appeared in these two series of "Heroes" published by Ciba; three other examples that I have noted in the regular edition of *Time* magazine are "Adrift in the Arctic, Elisha Kent Kane, Med. Officer, U.S. Navy, 1820–1857" (April 27, 1942, 58); "He standardized selection of recruits, Charles S. Tripler, Brev. Brig. General, Army Med. Corps, 1806–1866" (May 25, 1942, 87); and "Surgeon of the Seas, Jonathan M. Foltz, Surg. General U.S. Navy, 1810–1877" (June 22, 1942, 48). Ads in this series also appeared frequently in medical journals.

41. Crane Valves, "Birthplace of the New Wonder Drug," *Saturday Evening Post* 217:19 (November 4, 1944), 88.

42. Shell Oil Company, Inc., "A Prayer Is Answered," *Life* 18:20 (May 14, 1945), 47. By coincidence, this issue of *Life* also contains an article, "Art in Advertising: Fine U.S. Paintings Dramatize Health Campaign" (75–77), which, despite its title, is not about public health or prevention but about the art used by commercial enterprises such as Upjohn.

43. Martha N. Gardner and Allan M. Brandt, " 'The Doctors' Choice Is America's Choice': The Physician in US Cigarette Advertisements, 1930–1953," *American Journal of Public Health* 96:2 (February 2006), 222–232. See also Alan Blum, "When 'More Doctors Smoked Camels': Cigarette Advertising in the Journal," *New York State Journal of Medicine* 83:13 (December 1983), 1347–1352. Historians' efforts to document the placement of various ads in specific journals are hampered by the common practice in medical libraries of removing advertisements from the issues before binding them.

44. R. J. Reynolds's advertising of Camels appeared in a great number of medical journals in the late 1940s, as documented by Blum ("When 'More Doctor Smoked Camels' ") and by Gardner and Brandt ("The Doctors' Choice"). In three consecutive issues of the *New York State Journal of Medicine* 47:1–3 (January 1, January 15, and February 1, 1947), a Camel ad was printed on p. 3 (or the equivalent) in each issue, a prominent location since each issue's table of contents started on p. 4.

45. The Virchow ad is reproduced in Blum, "When 'More Doctors Smoked Camels,' " 1351.

46. Some of these paintings and their descriptive texts were also reprinted in an oversized portfolio of color plates, *Know Your Doctor* (Winston-Salem, N.C.: R. J. Reynolds, 1947), which provides information about the company's goals for such ads. The portfolio carries no introduction, but a separate "Dear Doctor" letter from the company's president explains its rationale as follows: "You may recall a series of advertisements. . . . This series, sponsored by CAMEL Cigarettes, presented in graphic and dramatic form the story of the doctor. . . . Each successive advertisement brought mounting requests for reprints and copies of the illustrations for framing. . . . In the accompanying brochure KNOW YOUR DOCTOR, we have assembled the illustrations that were most frequently requested. . . . We hope that after reading this brochure you will find it merits a place on your waiting room table so that your patients may enjoy it."

47. Scott Paper Company, "Pasteur Found the Way. Now All Mankind Benefits," *Fortune* 28:1 (July 1943), 157.

48. Raycrest Fabrics, "In Cords, It's the Know How That Counts," *New York Times,* November 28, 1948, Sunday magazine, 6 (full page). I am grateful to Janet K. Mock of Bellingham, Washington, for generously providing me with this advertisement.

49. The same ad appeared in the *Saturday Evening Post,* May 23, 1953.

CHAPTER 8. POPULAR MEDICAL HISTORY IN CHILDREN'S COMIC BOOKS OF THE 1940s

1. John C. Burnham, "American Medicine's Golden Age: What Happened to It?" *Science* 215:4539 (March 19, 1982), 1474–1479. Paramount in developing and popularizing the image was Paul Starr, *The Social Transformation of American Medicine* (New York: Basic Books, 1982). For a challenge to this view's hegemony, see Rosemary A. Stevens, "Public Roles for the Medical Profession in the United States: Beyond Theories of Decline and Fall," *Milbank Quarterly* 79:3 (September 2001), 327–353. Mark Schlesinger, in "A Loss of Faith: The Sources of Reduced Political Legitimacy for the American Medical Profession," *Milbank Quarterly* 80:2 (June 2002), 185–235, provides references to a substantial secondary literature on the question. See also a five-hundred-page collection of retrospective essays about Starr's book in a special issue of the *Journal of Health Politics, Policy, and Law* 29:4–5 (August-October 2004).

2. For the United States, there seem to have been no studies of the representation of medicine or health in comic books prior to my research, published in part in Bert Hansen, "Medical History for the Masses: How American Comic Books Celebrated Heroes of Medicine in the 1940s," *Bulletin of the History of Medicine* 78:1 (Spring 2004), 148–191; and in Bert Hansen, "True-Adventure Comic Books and American Popular Culture in the 1940s: An Annotated Research Bibliography of the Medical Heroes," *International Journal of Comic Art* 6:1 (Spring 2004), 117–147. This chapter has adapted some material from the first article; readers are referred to the second article for a comprehensive listing of individual medical history stories, including many not mentioned here. For France, one may consult Philippe Videlier and Piérine Piras, *La Santé dans les bandes dessinées* (Paris: Frison-Roche, 1992). Comic books are examined in George Basalla, "Pop Science: The Depiction of Science in Popular Culture," in *Science and Its Public: The Changing Relationship,* ed. Gerald Holton and William A. Blanpied, 261–278, Boston Studies in the Philosophy of Science 33 (Boston: Reidel, 1976), and are given notice in Roger Cooter and Stephen Pumfrey, "Separate Sphere and Public Place: Reflections on the History of Science Popularization and Science in Popular Culture," *History of Science* 32 (1994), 237.

3. Cover by unknown artist, *Real Life Comics* 12 (July 1943). The unsigned story is "Famine Fighter: Dr. Joseph Goldberger," on pp. 15–22. Among the comic books discussed, very few acknowledged the writers or the artists by name. Creators are cited herein if known; but to avoid an excessive use of "anonymous," the citation of stories generally begins with the title. For comic magazines of this era, volume numbers were used rarely and not consistently, but the issue number is essential and appears in these notes immediately after the magazine title, followed by cover date of the issue and pagination of the story. To avoid confusion arising because many of the stories and the magazines have similar titles, a full reference is given even for second and succeeding citations of comic-book stories. Note that for comic books, the date on a cover or copyright page was conventional and must not be taken as a historically accurate date of publication; issues usually appeared on the newsstand one to several months earlier than the cover date. The comic books examined here have not been reprinted, and very few can be found in libraries. About half of them are held in the collection of Michigan State University Libraries; almost all of them are in the author's collection.

4. "Comicland," photographer unknown, apparently first printed in *Newsdealer* magazine in 1948 and often reprinted. For help with this image, I am grateful to Maggie Thompson, editor of the weekly *Comics Buyer's Guide* (Iola, Wisc.: Krause). Neither the Library of Congress nor the New York Public Library can locate their reported holdings of any *Newsdealer* magazine issues for 1948. The image was reprinted in *Comics Buyer's Guide* 600 (May 17, 1985) and 1131 (July 21, 1995) and in Ron Goulart, *Comic Book Culture: An Illustrated History* (Portland, Ore.: Collectors Press, 2000), 204. It was also published as an undated seventeen-by-twenty-two-inch poster by Robert Beerbohm of Fremont, Nebraska.

5. Dick Lupoff and Don Thompson, introduction to *All in Color for a Dime,* ed. Dick Lupoff and Don Thompson (New Rochelle, N.Y.: Arlington House, 1970), 11.

6. According to Will Eisner, "a visual replaces text; an illustration simply repeats or amplifies, decorates, or sets a climate for mood." See Eisner, *Comics and Sequential Art* (Tamarac, Fla.: Poorhouse, 1985), 128.

7. Eisner, *Comics and Sequential Art*; and Scott McCloud, *Understanding Comics: The Invisible Art* (New York: Harper Perennial, 1994). See also Reinhold Reitberger and Wolfgang Fuchs, *Comics: Anatomy of a Mass Medium,* trans. Nadia Fowler (Boston: Little, Brown, 1972); Robert C. Harvey, "The Aesthetics of the Comic Strip," *Journal of Popular Culture* 12:4 (Spring 1979), 640–652; Joseph Witek, *Comic Books as History: The Narrative Art of Jack Jackson, Art Spiegelman, and Harvey Pekar* (Jackson: University Press of Mississippi, 1989); and David Carrier, *The Aesthetics of Comics* (University Park: Pennsylvania State University Press, 2000). Earlier, Marshall McLuhan had suggested interesting ways that media vary in the participation they demand; see *Understanding Media: The Extensions of Man* (New York: McGraw-Hill, 1964). My interpretation of reader/listener participation for radio and comics differs markedly from McLuhan's.

8. Rudy Palais, "Walter Reed," *Science Comics* 2 (March 1946), 26.

9. "The precious drug," two panels of "Penicillin," *True Comics* 41 (December 1944), 22.

10. Reitberger and Fuchs explain it this way: "In comics, just as in fairy tales, the unreal quality of scenery and action stimulates imagination. In contrast to film and television which make an entirely passive reception possible, comics demand the co-operation of the reader in piecing together the pictures. The text alone does not furnish the story. The books for children which are always held up in preference to comics . . . are in no way superior. The after-effect on a child's imagination is probably stronger with comics" (*Comics,* 141).

11. Ian Gordon, *Comic Strips and Consumer Culture, 1890–1945* (Washington, D.C.: Smithsonian Institution Press, 1998); Amy Kiste Nyberg, *Seal of Approval: The History of the Comics Code* (Jackson: University Press of Mississippi, 1998); and Bradford W. Wright, *Comic Book Nation: The Transformation of Youth Culture in America* (Baltimore: Johns Hopkins University Press, 2001). Earlier scholarship includes Ron Goulart, ed., *The Encyclopedia of American Comics* (New York: Facts on File, 1990); John L. Fell, *Film and the Narrative Tradition* (Norman: University of Oklahoma Press, 1974); M. Thomas Inge, *Comics as Culture* (Jackson: University Press of Mississippi, 1990); Russel Nye, *The Unembarrassed Muse: The Popular Arts in America* (New York: Dial, 1970); and William W. Savage Jr., *Comic Books and America, 1945–1954* (Norman: University of Oklahoma Press, 1990).

12. The rapid growth of Superman's popularity is astounding; see Wright, *Comic Book Nation,* 14.

13. Concerns about how comic-book reading helped or hurt children's ability to do other reading surfaced early. In the 1940s, there was much public debate and quite a number of research studies, usually by educational psychologists, reading teachers, and librarians. No consensus emerged from the scientific studies, and it is important to note that a number of prominent scientists supported comics as helpful or at least not damaging to the development of reading abilities. See Nyberg, *Seal of Approval,* 5–18.

14. Nye, *Unembarrassed Muse,* 239; Nyberg, *Seal of Approval,* 3–4.

15. Wright, *Comic Book Nation,* 13–14.

16. Nyberg, *Seal of Approval,* 3–4. Nye, *Unembarrassed Muse,* 239, reports a rise to over twelve million per month for 1942.

17. Nyberg, *Seal of Approval,* 1.

18. Roger Sabin, *Comics, Comix and Graphic Novels: History of Comic Art* (London: Phaidon, 1996), 89.

19. For a comprehensive list of medical history stories in these comic books, see Hansen "True-Adventure Comic Books," which also provides name and subject indexes to specific stories.

20. On this subgenre generally, see Ron Goulart, *Ron Goulart's Great History of Comic Books* (Chicago: Contemporary Books, 1986), chap. 14; and Witek, *Comic Books as History,* chap. 1. For examples of unsubstantiated negative judgments about it, see Denis Gifford, *International Book of Comics* (New York: Crescent Books, 1984), 172–173; Reitberger and Fuchs, *Comics,* 139; and Wright, *Comic Book Nation,* 27–28, 61.

21. That three hundred thousand copies sold out in ten days was reported in "Cartoon Magazine for Children Big Success," *Publisher's Weekly,* March 8, 1941, 1127, which also noted that a run of forty thousand for Canada under the title *True Picture Magazine* was selling well and that the publisher was printing ten thousand more of *True Comics* and twenty-five thousand more of its Canadian counterpart. A history of the *True Comics* books may be found at "William E. Blake Collection of True Life 1940s Era Comics," Virginia Commonwealth University Libraries website, http://www.library.vcu.edu/jbc/speccoll/blake1. html (accessed June 3, 2008), The quotation from publisher Hecht comes from an interview in the late 1970s by William E. Blake Jr. and was presented in an unpublished lecture from 1980 now posted on the Internet; see William E. Blake Jr., "A View of History: *True Comics,* 1941–1945," Virginia Commonwealth University Libraries website, http://www.library.vcu. edu/jbc/speccoll/blake2.html (accessed June 3, 2008).

22. For information on its syndication in newspapers, see Ron Goulart, "True Comics," in *The Encyclopedia of American Comics,* ed. Ron Goulart (New York: Facts on File, 1990), 369.

23. The circulation of 750,000 was reported in "Superman Scores," *Business Week,* April 18, 1942, 54–56. The same article also noted that "advertisers have not yet realized the possibilities of these magazines for goods aimed at the juvenile demand" (56).

24. These numbers are taken from the records of the Audit Bureau of Circulation. As the bureau allowed only hand copying of data from its microfilms, the numbers were written out by Russ Maheras in a message sent to Comix-Scholars Discussion List, archived at Negative Space, http://www.hoboes.com/pub/Comics/About%20Comics/Business/Top%20Comics %20and%20Publishers/Comic%20Book%20Circulation%20Data (accessed June 3, 2008).

25. Nye, *Unembarrassed Muse,* 239; see also Gordon, *Comic Strips and Consumer Culture,* 139–151 on World War II, esp. 139–141 for data on the reading habits and comics purchases of service personnel.

26. An illuminating account of the secular humanism of *True Comics* was given in Blake, "A View of History." On Hecht, see also Nyberg, *Seal of Approval,* 31. For a photograph of publisher Hecht reviewing an advance copy with first lady Eleanor Roosevelt, see the inside front cover of *True Comics* 4 (September 1941), reproduced in Hansen, "True-Adventure Comic Books," 120.

27. Rudy Palais, "Lazear took his mosquitoes to the hospital," full page in "Walter Reed, the Man Who Conquered Yellow Fever," *Science Comics* 2 (March 1946), 29.

28. In the comic-book world, the years 1938 to 1945 are considered the "Golden Age" of comic books, the period when "superhero" comics first appeared and the industry achieved explosive growth. The second period of novelty and success, which ran from September 1956 though 1969, is designated the "Silver Age." "Modern Age" comics are those from 1980 to the present. To fill the gaps around the main eras, other terms are used: Pre–Golden Age, Post–Golden Age, Pre–Silver Age, Post–Silver Age; see Robert M. Overstreet, *The Overstreet Comic Book Price Guide,* 26th ed. for 1996–1997 (New York: Avon Books, 1996), A92–A95.

29. Goulart, *Goulart's Great History,* 263.

30. Fredric Wertham, *Seduction of the Innocent* (New York: Rinehart, 1954).

31. Nyberg, *Seal of Approval.*

32. This section is based on the roughly one hundred medical history stories that I have found in comic books of the 1940s. Since few comics are held in libraries (except at Michigan State University) and individual stories are rarely catalogued separately, it is impossible to review the corpus systematically to find them all. After years of searching and with inquiries reaching a point of diminishing returns, I am confident that I have found the majority of the relevant examples and that the main features of the phenomenon can be discerned with confidence, even if a few examples might have been overlooked. But as some comics will have been missed, any numerical statements in this section (e.g., "Sister Kenny has three stories" or "Pasteur and Reed are most popular") should not be interpreted as absolute determinations. A comprehensive listing of all the stories known to me in 2004 was published in Hansen, "True-Adventure Comic Books."

33. Harold de Lay (artist), "Yellow Jack: How the Cause of Yellow Fever Was Discovered," *True Comics* 1 (April 1941), 37–43. Wartime patriotism and militarism affected comic books' choice of subjects, but chauvinism should not be automatically assumed. For example, two issues later, *True Comics* 3 (August 1941) had a cover story entitled "Death Fighter" about Robert Koch. Even as late as 1943, a major story devoted much attention, all of it favorable, to Germans Loeffler, Behring, and Koch; see Gus Herman (artist), "The Conquest of Diphtheria," *Real Life Comics* 11 (May 1943), 30–36.

34. "The Conquest of Yellow Fever," *Real Life Comics* 19 (September 1944), 7–14 (quotation on 14).

35. Rudy Palais (artist), "Walter Reed: The Man Who Conquered Yellow Fever," *Science Comics* 2 (March 1946), 26–31; and Morris Nelson Sachs (writer) and Don Cameron (artist), "The Conquest of Yellow Fever," *Picture Stories from Science* 2 (Summer 1947), 29–32.

36. Gary Gray (artist), "Louis Pasteur," *Trail Blazers* 4 (October 1942), 11–19; and [Sam Glankoff], "Louis Pasteur and the Unseen Enemy," *Real Heroes* 7 (November 1942), 20–25.

37. Ron Goulart of Ridgefield, Connecticut, kindly identified the otherwise unknown Gary Gray as a pen name used by Jack Farr (personal correspondence, July 16, 2004).

38. These drawings were clearly indebted to the 1936 film, as some resemblances are striking, even with a strange displacement. Although the comic-book version of the young Pasteur kissing his future wife does not look like either the film Pasteur or the historical Pasteur, the drawing has a strong similarity to the publicity still on one of the lobby cards of the film, on which we see the young Dr. Jean Martel kissing Pasteur's daughter Annette, his future wife. In both images, the placement of their heads for the kiss is identical, as are the man's shirt, tie, jacket, and hairstyle. Both women have blond hair with ringlets. The film itself was in black and white, but this lobby-card photograph, like the comic book, was printed in color. Four panels of the Pasteur story from *Trail Blazers* are reproduced in black and white in Hansen, "True-Adventure Comic Books," 122.

39. "Louis Pasteur and the Unseen Enemy," *Real Heroes* 7 (November 1942), 20–25.

40. Ron Goulart kindly identified this artist as Sam Glankoff (personal communication, July 16, 2004). For more information on Glankoff's career as an artist, see *Sam Glankoff (1894–1982): A Retrospective Exhibition* (New Brunswick, N.J.: Jane Voorhees Zimmerli Art Museum of Rutgers University, 1984). A Glankoff cartoon frame from *Real Heroes* 7 is reproduced in Hansen, "True-Adventure Comic Books," 122.

41. The *True Comics* newspaper strip began in 1942 and was distributed by the Bell Syndicate, running in daily and Sunday papers. It lasted only a few years. See Goulart, ed., *Encyclopedia of American Comics,* 369. The original drawing for a four-frame Pasteur sequence on the rabies breakthrough, called "Germ Tamer" and in my collection, carries a notation of "March 16," but with no year indicated and no indication of whether that might be a date of creation or publication. I have not been able to confirm a publication date for this installment of the Pasteur story in March or April 1942, 1943, or 1944 in the newspapers I have checked.

42. *The Price of Liberty: A History of the American Jewish Committee* (New York: American Jewish Committee, 1948). Biographical information on Nathaniel Schachner, 1895–1955, was drawn from a website, Internet Speculative Fiction DataBase, "an effort to catalog works of Science Fiction, Fantasy, and Horror," edited by Al von Ruff, at http://www.isfdb.org/cgi-bin/ea.cgi?Nat_Schachner (accessed June 3, 2008).

43. Nat Schachner, "Healer of Men—A True Story of a Great Scientist," *Real Life Comics* 44 (May 1948), 28–30.

44. Schachner, "Healer of Men," *Real Life Comics* 44 (May 1948), 28–30 (quotation on 30). Schachner might have had some of his facts wrong. Haffkine studied with Metchnikoff in Odessa from 1879 to 1883, according to the obituary of Haffkine published by William Bullock in the *Journal of Pathology and Bacteriology* 34:2 (1931), 125–129.

45. Schachner, "Healer of Men," *Real Life Comics* 44 (May 1948), 28–30 (quotation on 30).

46. Nat Schachner, "The Magic Mold," *Real Life Comics* 31 (May 1946), 26–28; Nat Schachner, "Master of Medicine—A True Story of Scientific Achievement," *Real Life Comics* 41 (September 1947), 30–32; and Nat Schachner, "A Foe of Prejudice," *It Really Happened* 6 (December 1946), 22–24.

47. August M. Froehlich (artist), "Ambroise Paré: Famed Surgeon," *Real Life Comics* 33 (July 1946), 44–48.

48. "Dr. Edward Jenner: Plague Fighter," *Real Life Comics* 15 (January 1944), 34–39; and "Plague Vanquished," *Real Heroes* 15 (July-August 1946), 30–32.

49. "Catherine the Great," *Real Life Comics* 18 (July 1944), 28–33 (quotation on 32). For scholarly accounts, see Philip H. Clendenning, "Dr. Thomas Dimsdale and Smallpox Inoculation in Russia," *Journal of the History of Medicine and Allied Sciences* 28:2 (April 1973), 109–125; and John T. Alexander, "Catherine the Great and Public Health," *Journal of the History of Medicine and Allied Sciences* 36:2 (April 1981), 185–204.

50. "Plague Vanquished," *Real Heroes* 15 (July 1946), 30–32 (error on 31).

51. "Death Fighter: Dr. Robert Koch," *True Comics* 3 (August 1941), 12–19.

52. Gus Herman (artist), "The Conquest of Diphtheria," *Real Life Comics* 11 (May 1943), 30–36.

53. Herman, "Conquest of Diphtheria," *Real Life Comics* 11 (May 1943), 30–36 (both quotations on 36). The Dr. Park mentioned is William Hallock Park of the New York City Health Department, and the unspecified improvement is either the introduction of the toxin-antitoxin combination or a chemically modified toxin called toxoid. Note that the comic book reports the actual number of cases, which is much easier for ordinary readers to picture than a rate such as mortality per one hundred thousand population, which is commonly used in the expert literature. I have not confirmed these New York State numbers, but they are in line with a report that deaths from diphtheria in Manhattan and the Bronx declined from 190 in 1929 to 32 in 1934; see Louis I. Dublin and Alfred J. Lotka, *Twenty-five Years of Health Progress* (New York: Metropolitan Life Insurance Company, 1937), 60.

54. "The Conquest of Malaria: Ross + Grassi = Victory!" *Real Life Comics* 14 (November 1943), 32–37.

55. "The Discoverer of Hidden Hunger," *True Comics* 15 (August 1942), 37–41 (quotation on 38).

56. Ibid., 41.

57. "The Modest Miracle," *True Comics* 16 (September 1942), 49–53. The closing frame indicates that the comic is "a true story based on the motion picture, 'The Modest Miracle' produced by Standard Brands Inc. in the interests of the National Nutrition Program."

58. "Stephen Smith," *Real Life Comics* 30 (April 1946), 37–40 (quotation on 37).

59. Ibid., 40.

60. Ibid.

61. "Fever Fighter: Dr. Theobald Smith," *Real Life Comics* 13 (September 1943), 48–53; and "Theobald Smith and Texas Fever," *Science Comics* 5 (September 1946), 17–23.

62. "Fever Fighter," *Real Life Comics* 13 (September 1943), 48–53 (quotation on 48).

63. "Even with these facts," full page in "Theobald Smith and Texas Fever," *Science Comics* 5 (September 1946), 23.

64. Ibid., 17, 23.

65. "Conqueror of the White Plague," *True Comics* 19 (December 1942), 54–59 (both quotations on 57).

66. Ibid., 59.

67. "Famine Fighter: Dr. Joseph Goldberger," *Real Life Comics* 12 (July 1943), 15–22.

68. The Mayo brothers earned a rare two-part story, "The Mayo Family: Medicine's Miracle Men," *True Comics* 25 (July 1943), 8–12, and *True Comics* 26 (August 1943), 18–22. They appeared again in "The Mayo Brothers: Doctors Courageous," *Real Life Comics* 42 (November 1947), 13–16. The splash frame of the third of these stories strongly echoes the opening photograph of a *Life* magazine article that had appeared several years earlier: "The Mayo Clinic," *Life* 7:10 (September 4, 1939), 37–41.

69. "The Doctor Who Came Back: Dr. Samuel Mudd," *True Comics* 21 (February 1943), 36–41. Hollywood's feature film about Dr. Mudd was *The Prisoner of Shark Island* (1936), directed by John Ford. Radio versions of his story were broadcast on August 13, 1946, and November 8, 1948.

70. "Dr. David Livingstone," *It Really Happened* 4 ([August?] 1944, no month indicated), 7–15.

71. Cavell's story appeared in "Wonder Women of History," in *Wonder Woman* 3 (February-March 1943), 31–34 (quotation on 31). A Hollywood film, *Nurse Edith Cavell,* was released in 1939; a radio play of the same title was broadcast on August 20, 1946.

72. Titles include *Deeds of Daring, The Harvest of the Sea, Down to the Sea, Tales of the Labrador, Labrador Doctor,* and *Adrift on an Ice-Pan.*

73. "Adrift on an Ice Pan," *True Comics* 10 (March 1942), 26–31.

74. "Wilfred Grenfell, the Labrador Doctor," *Real Life Comics* 9 (January 1943), 41–46.

75. "Adrift on an Ice Pan," *True Comics* 10 (March 1942), 26–31 (quotation on 31).

76. In the author's collection is a scrapbook of newspaper clippings from the 1920s, apparently compiled by a child in Wisconsin, with a number of illustrated newspaper articles about Balto's triumph.

77. James Colgrove, "The Power of Persuasion: Diphtheria Immunization, Advertising, and the Rise of Health Education," *Public Health Reports* 119:5 (September-October 2004), 507, citing L. F. Bache, *Health Education in an American City* (Garden City, N.Y.: Doubleday, 1934).

78. John Vacha, "He Saved Nome—Cleveland Saves Balto," *Timeline* 22:1 (January-March 2005), 54–69. This richly illustrated article, published in a magazine of the Ohio Historical Society, reports on the rescue mission itself, contemporary coverage of it, Balto's later adventures, and the various commemorations and celebrations of Balto's leadership.

79. "Balto the Heroic Husky," *Heroic Comics* 38 (September 1946), 28–31; and "Balto of Nome," *Real Heroes* 16 (October 1946), 6–8.

80. "Canada's Pioneer Nurse: Jeanne Mance," *True Comics* 24 (May 1943), 15–18 (quotation on 16).

81. For more on this subject, see Fell, *Film and the Narrative Tradition.*

82. "The Lady with the Lamp," *Wonder Woman* 1 (Summer 1942), 29–32.

83. "The Mother of New York's East Side," *Wonder Woman* 4 (April-May 1943), 31–34. Two late examples of doctors as "wonder women of history" are noteworthy: Marie Elizabeth Zakrzewska (three pages in *Wonder Woman* 57 [February 1953]) and Florence Rena Sabin (one page in *Wonder Woman* 65 [April 1954]).

84. "Clara Barton, Angel of the Battlefield," *Wonder Woman* 2 (Fall 1942), 31–34; and "Angel of the Battlefield," *True Comics* 34 (April 1944), 16–22. She is not mentioned in "Story of the Red Cross," *Real Heroes* 4 (May 1942), 52–57. Barton was also the subject of a Hollywood short in 1939, entitled *Angel of Mercy,* and at least one radio play, which the *Cavalcade of America* broadcast on June 1, 1942.

85. "First Lady of the Army Medical Corps," *True Comics* 31 (January 1944), 30–33 (quotation on 30).

86. "Elizabeth Blackwell," *Wonder Woman* 19 (October 1946), 13–16.

87. "Penicillin," *True Comics* 41 (December 1944), 18–22; and "White Magic: The Miracle of Penicillin," *Science Comics* 1 (January 1946), 9–15.

88. In 1984, David P. Adams published an important study of media coverage of penicillin.

He used about ten magazines (not including comic books or *Life* magazine), but he did not include newspaper stories; see "The Penicillin Mystique and the Popular Press (1935–1950)," *Pharmacy in History* 26:3 (1984), 134–142. Some of the newspaper coverage was used in Adams's later book, which includes much of interest on the public's image of doctors, scientists, and medical research: *The Greatest Good to the Greatest Number: Penicillin Rationing on the American Home Front, 1940–1945* (New York: Lang, 1991).

89. "Dr. Alexander Fleming: His Penicillin Will Save More Lives than War Can Spend" (caption on cover), *Time* 43:20 (May 15, 1944), 61–62, 64, 66, 68; the article's title is "20th Century Seer."

90. Penicillin was featured in three other stories—*Marvels of Science* 2 (April 1946), *Marvels of Science* 3 (May 1946), and *Real Life Comics* 31 (May 1946)—all prompted undoubtedly by the award of the 1945 Nobel Prize to Fleming, Florey, and Chain. Ernest Chain had not been mentioned in *True Comics* or in *Science Comics* (the earliest two of the five stories), but he appeared with Fleming and Florey in the other three. And he was the main focus of the two text-only stories, namely, "Hero of Science," *Marvels of Science* 2 (April 1946), 26–27, which opens with the ominous sentence "The Gestapo had a list of wanted men," and Nat Schachner, "The Magic Mold," *Real Life Comics* 31 (May 1946), 26–28.

91. "The Fight against Infantile Paralysis," *True Comics* 32 (February 1944), 26–29.

92. Ibid., 26.

93. "Please, officer," four panels ibid., 27.

94. Ibid., 29.

95. "Australian Bush Nurse," *Real Heroes* 5 (July 1942), 22–27; "Sister Elizabeth Kenny," *Wonder Woman* 8 (Spring 1944), 32–35; and "Sister Kenny," *It Really Happened* 8 (April 1947), 14–20.

96. Whereas most of the comic-book stories followed appearances in other media and were often derived from books, films, and radio broadcasts, the pattern is a little different in this case. The initial comic-book story was dated July 1942. A radio drama followed in November 1942. The next year saw the publication of Kenny's autobiographical book, *And They Shall Walk: The Life Story of Sister Elizabeth Kenny, Written in Collaboration with Martha Ostenso* (New York: Dodd, Mead, 1943). A second comic-book story appeared in early 1944. Hollywood's film, starring Rosalind Russell, screened in 1946. Kenny's third comic-book appearance was in April 1947. Kenny was also featured in a major pictorial in *Life* magazine, and the large opening photograph from that 1942 story (reproduced in fig. 95 in chapter 9) was clearly the model for the 1947 image of Kenny in color plate 19. See "Sister Kenny, Australian Nurse," *Life* 13:13 (September 28, 1942), 73–75, 77. *Life* was scooped on Kenny's significance by an earlier story about her that ran in one of its competitors, the *Saturday Evening Post*; see "Healer from the Outback," *Saturday Evening Post* 214:29 (January 17, 1942), 18–19, 68, 70.

97. "Mom Chung and Her 509 'Fair-Haired Foster Sons,'" *Real Heroes* 9 (February-March 1943), 9–14.

98. Judy Tzu-Chun Wu, *Doctor Mom Chung of the Fair-Haired Bastards: The Life of a Wartime Celebrity* (Berkeley: University of California Press, 2005), in which figures 22 and 23 print two pages from the *Real Heroes* story. The splash page is reproduced in Hansen, "True-Adventure Comic Books," 125.

99. "Dynamic Fighter: Mabel K. Staupers," *Negro Heroes* 2 (Summer 1948), 25–28. Only two issues of *Negro Heroes* were published: Spring 1947 and Summer 1948. Although the series had been established to reprint stories from *True Comics,* the Staupers story has not been found in any other comic book, and this might be its only appearance. *Negro Heroes* was published in Chicago by the National Urban League; the second issue was produced "in cooperation with Delta Sigma Theta Sorority."

100. John G. Cawelti, *Adventure, Mystery, and Romance: Formula Stories as Art and Popular Culture* (Chicago: University of Chicago Press, 1976). As Judith Yaross Lee has observed, "Studies of popular culture have taught us to seek the clearest expression of a culture's values and assumptions in its formula literature: the highly predictable stories, factual and fictional, appearing in periodicals and books aimed at a mass audience. The stereotyped characters and plots of formula stories reveal the broadly shared attitudes that get lost amid the carefully delineated, unique characters and incidents of high literature." Judith Yaross Lee, "Scientists and Inventors as Literary Heroes: Introduction," in *Beyond the Two Cultures: Essays on Science, Technology, and Literature,* ed. Joseph W. Slade and Judith Yaross Lee, 256 (Ames: Iowa State University Press, 1990). See also Paul Theerman, "National Images of Science: British and American Views of Scientific Heroes in the Early Nineteenth Century," ibid., 259–274.

101. "You Edit This Magazine!" *True Comics* 12 (May 1942), inside back cover. One example from outside the United States offers exemplary confirmation of a comic book's influence on a child's ambition. As the Colombian biochemist Dr. Manuel Patarroyo recalled, "I was 8 years old when my father gave me a comic [book] to read. . . . And that booklet had Louis Pasteur's story and I was fascinated. Then, like any other child who wants to be a priest or wants to be a policeman or a bomber or a pilot, I wanted to be a scientist and didn't want to do anything different from what Pasteur did. Since then I have devoted my life to that." See David Spurgeon, *Southern Lights: Celebrating the Scientific Achievements of the Developing World* (Ottawa: International Development Research Centre, 1995), chap. 7, available online at http://archive.idrc.ca/library/document/101742/ (accessed June 3, 2008). Spurgeon explained that Dr. Patarroyo, a biochemist from Colombia, "developed the world's first safe and effective malaria vaccine." Since Patarroyo was born in 1947, it seems likely that the comic book he might have been reading, at least at age ten, was the Mexican comic book *Vidas Ilustres,* which ran a Pasteur story in 1957.

102. "Doctor Facts," *True Comics* 52 (September 1946), 1–5 (all quotations on 5).

103. "Presidential Aide: Bernard M. Baruch," *Real Life Comics* 39 (May 1947), 3–7 (quotation on 7).

104. Hecht's liberal humanism is described in Blake, "A View of History." That secular naturalism and a commitment to science were also core elements of the values embodied in *Life* magazine is explored in the following chapter.

105. As Reitberger and Fuchs observe, "the Second World War had a brutalizing effect on the output of all the mass media, including comics. Things that would have been judged sadistic in 1940 were deemed accurate reporting in 1945" (*Comics,* 19).

106. "Dog Dead or Alive?" *Marvels of Science* 1 (March 1946), 46–48. The opening caption explains, "A series of daring experiments by a group of Soviet scientists under Dr. Serge Bryukhonenko, pointed the way to blood-banking, transfusion and plasma separation, which has saved innumerable lives during the war."

107. In the United States, the film was introduced by J.B.S. Haldane and narrated by Walter B. Cannon. This twenty-minute black-and-white film has been made digitally available by the Prelinger Collection for free viewing or downloading online, at http://www.archive.org/details/Experime1940 (accessed June 3, 2008).

108. "Dog Dead or Alive?" *Marvels of Science* 1 (March 1946), 46–48 (quotations on 47).

109. The same year as this story in *Marvels of Science,* two different biomedical research organizations each created a prize to honor dogs that had been used in experimental work: The Whipple Prize (named for a Nobelist) and the Research Dog Hero Award (for a dog used in experimental heart surgery or cancer research). There were press conferences, and newspapers ran photographs of the happy dogs and the smiling scientists. On these awards, see Susan E. Lederer, "Political Animals: The Shaping of Biomedical Research Literature in Twentieth-Century America," *Isis* 83:1 (March 1992), 73.

110. "Experiments in Revival: Dogs Killed Then Brought Back to Life in Russia," *Life* 15:17 (October 25, 1943), 119–120, 122, 125. Years later, *Life* ran other graphic stories showing Russian experiments; see "Artificial Heart: Mechanical Device Substitutes for Living Organ," *Life* 28:19 (May 8, 1950), 90–92, and "Russia's Two-Headed Dog," *Life* 47:3 (July 20, 1959), 79–80, 82.

111. Susan E. Lederer and John Parascandola, "Screening Syphilis: *Dr. Ehrlich's Magic Bullet* Meets the Public Health Service," *Journal of the History of Medicine and Allied Sciences* 53:4 (October 1998), 350–352; and Susan E. Lederer, "Repellent Subjects: Hollywood Censorship and Surgical Images in the 1930s," *Literature and Medicine* 17:1 (Spring 1998), 91–113.

112. Paul de Kruif, *Microbe Hunters* (New York: Harcourt Brace, 1948). Part of the title page reads, "Text Edition edited by Harry G. Grover, Dickinson High School, Jersey City, New Jersey."

113. Basalla, "Pop Science"; Roslynn D. Haynes, *From Faust to Strangelove: Representation of the Scientist in Western Literature* (Baltimore: Johns Hopkins University Press, 1994). Although Basalla's sources do include some comic books, his picture is imbalanced by an overweighting of the fantasy narratives and the science fiction, and it is incomplete because he overlooks the true-adventure comics of the 1940s, with their many admirable medical scientists. He concluded that comic books' depiction of scientists was overwhelmingly negative. See also John C. Burnham, *How Superstition Won and Science Lost: Popularizing Science and Health in the United States* (New Brunswick, N.J.: Rutgers University Press, 1987); and Marcel C. LaFollette, *Making Science Our Own: Public Images of Science, 1910–1955* (Chicago: University of Chicago Press, 1990), which consider comics, however, only in relation to Basalla's observations.

114. Basalla, "Pop Science," 276.

115. To radio has been attributed the cultivation of "a tribal unity" across the United States, of which President Franklin D. Roosevelt's "fireside chats" are a prominent example. McLuhan, *Understanding Media,* is the source of the phrase "tribal unity." On the metaphor of a "common hearth" around which Americans gathered, even as they were dispersed in their homes, see Erik Barnouw, *A History of Broadcasting in the United States,* 3 vols. (New York: Oxford University Press, 1966–1970), 2:5–7. Others have extended the metaphor as a "national hearth" to describe people's connection with network-television news; see Frank Rich, "And That's the Way It Was," *New York Times,* May 19, 2002, Sunday magazine, 66, 82. On the power of shared visual images, signs, and symbols, see Warren I. Susman, *Culture as History: The Transformation of American Society in the Twentieth Century* (New York: Pantheon Books, 1984), esp. xvii; and all the essays in Erika Lee Doss, ed., *Looking at "Life" Magazine* (Washington, D.C.: Smithsonian Institution Press, 2001).

CHAPTER 9. LIFE *LOOKS AT MEDICINE: MAGAZINE PHOTOGRAPHY AND THE AMERICAN PUBLIC*

1. The chapter epigraph was quoted by David Remnick in *The Best American Magazine Writing 2003* (New York: Public Affairs, 2003), xv. The numerical data for the magazine's publication are given in Philip B. Kunhardt Jr., ed., *Life: The First 50 Years, 1936–1986* (Boston: Little, Brown, 1986), 4. See also James L. Baughman, *Henry R. Luce and the Rise of the American News Media* (Boston: Twayne, 1987); Erika Lee Doss, ed., *Looking at "Life" Magazine* (Washington, D.C.: Smithsonian Institution Press, 2001); Loudon Wainwright, *The Great American Magazine: An Inside History of "Life"* (New York: Ballantine Books, 1988); and the chapter on *Life* in Norberto Angeletti and Alberto Oliva, *Magazines That Make History: Their Origins, Development, and Influence* (Gainesville: University Press of Florida, 2004), 116–183.

2. The magazine was first reborn in the 1980s as a monthly, and it died for the second time in May 2000. It was reborn a second time in October 2004 as a thin and superficial weekly, of which twelve million copies were distributed as a weekend newspaper supplement. It died for a third time in April 2007.

3. My thinking about *Life* has benefited from Catherine A. Lutz and Jane L. Collins, *Reading National Geographic* (Chicago: University of Chicago Press, 1993).

4. Marilyn Monroe appeared on nine covers between April 7, 1952, and September 8, 1972. The accelerator, captioned "Fresh Hope on Cancer," was the cover image for May 5, 1958.

5. Edwin E. Slosson, "The Influence of Photography on Modern Life," fourth in a series of articles entitled "Science Remaking the World," *World's Work* 45:4 (February 1923), 401. The paragraph continues, "Whether this is a good or bad tendency . . . is outside of my province to consider." I was led to Slosson's article by Elspeth H. Brown, *The Corporate Eye: Photography and the Rationalization of American Commercial Culture, 1884–1929* (Baltimore: Johns Hopkins University Press, 2005), 1.

6. Quoted in Kunhardt, *Life: The First Fifty Years,* 5.

7. This text appeared in what Wainwright calls Luce's "first redefinition of Life." Wainwright provides this text in *Great American Magazine,* 100–101.

8. Both quotations are found in Wainwright, *Great American Magazine,* 104.

9. Richard Lacayo and George Russell, *Eyewitness: 150 Years of Photojournalism* (New York: Time, Inc., 1995), 67–73. On the historical development of photojournalism, see also Michael L. Carlebach, *American Photojournalism Comes of Age* (Washington, D.C.: Smithsonian Institution Press, 1997); and Marianne Fulton, *Eyes of Time: Photojournalism in America* (Boston: Little, Brown, 1988).

10. See Gerard Piel, "Reminiscences," interview transcript, 1982, Columbia University Oral History Collection, 56.

11. "Inside Job on a Big Maw: German Health Museum," *Life,* April 25, 1955, 99.

12. "University of Chicago Professor Reports on Multiple Human Births," *Life,* July 1, 1940, 43.

13. "Horse Transfusion," *Life,* July 25, 1938, 42.

14. "World's Champion Blood Donor," *Life,* February 28, 1938, 34.

15. "TB Milestone," *Life,* March 3, 1952, 21.

16. Philip Gefter, "Cornell Capa, Photojournalist and Museum Founder, Dies at 90," *New York Times,* May 24, 2008, A17.

17. These McLuhan quotations are taken from Doss, introduction to *Looking at "Life" Magazine*.

18. Little was also director of the American Society for the Control of Cancer. For more on Little and the history of the Jackson mouse, see Karen A. Rader, *Making Mice: Standardizing Animals for American Biomedical Research, 1900–1955* (Princeton, N.J.: Princeton University Press, 2004). The wider scientific context of biological materials has been explored in Adele E. Clarke, "Research Materials and Reproductive Science in the United States, 1910–1940," in *Physiology in the American Context, 1850–1940*, ed. Gerald L. Geison, 323–350 (Bethesda, Md.: American Physiological Society, 1987); and in Bonnie Tocher Clause, "The Wistar Rat as a Right Choice: Establishing Mammalian Standards and the Ideal of a Standardized Mammal," *Journal of the History of Biology* 26:2 (Summer 1993), 329–349. More on the development of the Wistar rat may be found in Jeffrey P. Brosco, "Anatomy and Ambition: The Evolution of a Research Institute," *Transactions and Studies of the College of Physicians of Philadelphia*, ser. 5, 13:1 (March 1991), 1–28.

19. Stephen P. Strickland, *Politics, Science, and Dread Disease: A Short History of United States Medical Research Policy* (Cambridge, Mass.: Harvard University Press, 1972), 1–14; James T. Patterson, *The Dread Disease: Cancer and Modern American Culture* (Cambridge, Mass.: Harvard University Press, 1987), 114–136. The *Life* article, along with other coverage in national magazines, is discussed by Strickland on p. 13, by Patterson on pp. 123–125, and by Rader, *Making Mice*, 148–150.

20. *Life* ran a boxed note "A Word about Cancer" in the following week's issue of March 8, 1937 (p. 55), and thirteen "Letters to the Editors" in the issue of March 22, 1937 (p. 76).

21. "American Medical Association and the U.S. Public Health Service Join in Syphilis War with Movie," *Life*, June 14, 1937, 29.

22. "The Frontier Nurse," *Life*, June 14, 1937, 32–35.

23. Several examples have remained familiar even after many decades. Margaret Bourke-White's photographs of people in Fort Peck, Montana, appeared in *Life*'s inaugural issue; her elegant geometric composition of the Fort Peck Dam was the cover photograph introducing *Life* magazine to the world on November 23, 1936. Dorothea Lange's enduringly famous "Migrant Mother" was taken in 1936 and first published in Dorothea Lange and Paul Schuster Taylor, *American Exodus: A Record of Human Erosion* (New York: Raynal and Hitchcock, 1939).

24. "Eye and Ear," *Life*, June 14, 1937, 62; "In an 'Iron Lung': Fred Snite, Paralytic, Starts on $50,000 China-to-Chicago Trip," *Life*, June 14, 1937, 76.

25. *Life*'s initial follow-up was on July 5, 1937. Other articles include these in *Life* (June 19, 1939 [attends Mass], and August 21, 1939 [wedding]); in *Newsweek* (June 12, 1937; November 1, 1937; August 21, 1939 [wedding]; June 24, 1940; and November 22, 1954 [obituary]), and in *Time* (June 14, 1937 [article reprinted in *Reader's Digest*, August 1937]; June 12, 1939 [at Lourdes]; August 21, 1939 [wedding]; November 18, 1946; and November 22, 1954 [obituary]). See also Leonard C. Hawkins, *The Man in the Iron Lung: Frederick B. Snite, Jr.* (Garden City, N.Y.: Doubleday, 1956).

26. "A Camera Looks inside the Egg," *Life*, October 4, 1937, 44–47. At this time, *Life* did have color in some ads, but those were colored drawings without fine detail, not photographs.

27. Lennart Nilsson, "Drama of Life before Birth," cover story, *Life*, April 30, 1965, 54–70.

28. "300,000 CCC Boys Get Pneumonia Vaccine," *Life*, October 4, 1937, 63–64, 66.

29. "Tuberculosis: A Menace and a Mystery," *Life*, November 29, 1937, 30–37.

30. "Woman Researcher Identifies Measles Virus," *Life*, November 29, 1937, 84–85.

31. "Jean Broadhurst, Educator, Is Dead," *New York Times*, September 6, 1954, 15.

32. For the history of serum therapy in pneumonia, see Scott H. Podolsky, *Pneumonia before Antibiotics: Therapeutic Evolution and Evaluation in Twentieth-Century America* (Baltimore: Johns Hopkins University Press, 2006).

33. *Life*, December 20, 1937, 9–13. Only rarely did *Life* credit a photographer in the headline rather than in the front of the magazine near the contents page.

34. See Scott H. Podolsky, "The Changing Fate of Pneumonia as a Public Health Concern in 20th-Century America and Beyond," *American Journal of Public Health* 95:12 (December 2005), 2144–2154.

35. Both letters appeared on p. 4 in the issue of January 10, 1938.

36. "Letters to the Editors," *Life*, January 17, 1938, 6.

37. "The Doctor Looks at *Life*," *Life*, January 17, 1938, 57, italics in the original.

38. For other cartoons poking fun at *Life*'s medical stories, see the tenth-anniversary issue of *Life*, November 25, 1946, 4, 8, 11, 12.

39. "You and Your Doctor," *Life*, October 12, 1959.

40. See "Red Cross Girl," *Life*, July 1, 1940; an army nurse, *Life*, May 26, 1941; volunteer nurses' aides, *Life*, January 5, 1942; "society girl" training for service as a volunteer nurses' aide, *Life*, June 8, 1942; and Jangoes, or junior nurses' aides, *Life*, April 26, 1943.

41. "Sister Kenny: Australian Nurse Demonstrates Her Treatment for Infantile Paralysis," *Life*, September 28, 1942, 73–75, 77; "Nurse Midwife: Maude Callen Eases Pain of Birth, Life, and Death," *Life*, December 3, 1951, 134–145 (with photographs by W. Eugene Smith).

42. Smith's photoessays, except for one on the missionary Albert Schweitzer, focused on people who would not have become famous without Smith's attention and eloquent photography, which conveyed their humanity to a wide public. By spending weeks with his subjects, Smith gained their trust and found ways to minimize the distraction of being photographed. Much like a painter, he conveyed not just their images but their moods and personalities, even their values. In chronological order, Smith's health-related essays in *Life* were "Country Doctor: His Endless Work Has Its Own Rewards," *Life*, September 20, 1948, 115–126; "Life without Germs: Microbe-Free Animals Grow to Maturity and Bear Young within a Strange, New Sterile Laboratory at Notre Dame," *Life*, September 26, 1949, 107–113; "Nurse Midwife: Maude Callen Eases Pain of Birth, Life, and Death," *Life*, December 3, 1951, 134–145; "A New Life for Brodie Twin: 21-Month Old Boy, Once Joined to His Brother at the Skull, Turns into a Happy Child with Surgery and Lots of 'TLC,'" *Life*, June 15, 1953, 134–140; "A Man of Mercy: Africa's Misery Turns Saintly Albert Schweitzer into a Driving Taskmaster," *Life*, November 15, 1954, 161–172; "Death-Flow from a Pipe: Mercury Pollution Ravages a Japanese Village," *Life*, June 2, 1972, 74–81. For historical and critical literature on Smith's work, see the chapter on Smith's nurse midwife photoessay in Carol Squiers, *The Body at Risk: Photography of Disorder, Illness, and Healing* (New York: International Center of Photography; and Berkeley: University of California Press, 2005), 72–93. On Smith's difficult relationship with *Life* magazine editors concerning health care subjects, see Glenn Gardner Willumson, *W. Eugene Smith and the Photographic Essay* (New York: Cambridge University Press, 1992). See also Doss, introduction to *Looking at "Life" Magazine*.

43. "Senate Hears Witnesses on Anti-Syphilis Bill," *Life*, February 28, 1938, 14.

44. "'The Birth of a Baby' Aims to Reduce Maternal and Infant Mortality Rates," *Life*, April 11, 1938, 32–36.

45. A copy of the warning letter was also printed on the splash pages of the actual story (ibid., 32–33).

46. For images of the confiscation of *Life* magazine by policemen, see Richard B. Stolley, *"Life": Century of Change: America in Pictures, 1900–2000* (Boston: Little, Brown, 2000), 288–289; and *Life*, tenth-anniversary issue, November 25, 1946, 101. For more about the making of the film and reactions to it, see Robert Eberwein, *Sex Ed: Film, Video, and the Framework of Desire* (New Brunswick, N.J.: Rutgers University Press, 1999), 59–62. Eberwein suggests that more people "saw" the film in the magazine's stills than in the theaters, and he judges the article a "major achievement," noting that "for the first time a mass audience could see . . . not just drawings but a cinematic record of the effects of desire as it results in birth" (62). On the film, see also Eric Schaefer, *"Bold! Daring! Shocking! True": A History of Exploitation Films, 1919–1959* (Durham, N.C.: Duke University Press, 1999), 51, 106, 121, 161–162, 187–191.

47. Bea Irvin (drawings) and E. B. White (text), "The Birth of an Adult," *New Yorker,* April 23, 1938, 20–21. In *Life*'s tenth-anniversary issue, the magazine republished the full *New Yorker* cartoon in fourteen frames (November 25, 1946, 11–12).

48. "Kidding *Life,* Cartoonists Have Ribbed It for a Decade," *Life,* tenth-anniversary issue, November 25, 1946, 11.

49. "Animal Experimentation: Is It Essential to Medical Progress?" *Life,* October 24, 1938, 46–53.

50. For one example of a lurid Hearst story, featuring a large full-color illustration in the artistic style of the era's pulp paperbacks, see Arthur V. Allen, M.D., "Animal Torture Worthless to Science: A Veteran Doctor Explains Why the Heart-Breaking, Barbaric Sufferings Inflicted upon Dogs in the Vivisection Laboratories Have Contributed Practically Nothing to Medicine in 300 Years," *American Weekly,* July 1, 1945, 6–7. This supplement was nationally syndicated; my copy was delivered by the *Syracuse Herald-American.*

51. For more on the efforts of Castle, Davies, and Hearst, see Susan E. Lederer, "Political Animals: The Shaping of Biomedical Research Literature in Twentieth-Century America," *Isis* 83:1 (March 1992), 63–64. Davies's popularity is confirmed by a full-cover painted image of her on *Movie Classic* magazine for March 1936, the same issue that, by an ironic coincidence, ran an article about a film filled with animal experiments, *The Story of Louis Pasteur.*

52. "*Life*'s Pictures," *Life,* October 24, 1938, 10.

53. "Animal Experimentation," 48.

54. Ibid., 50. The sources of the historical images were not indicated, but Harvey's portrait was a detail from the 1848 painting by Robert Hannah ("William Harvey Demonstrating His Experiments on Deer to King Charles I and the Boy Prince" at the Royal College of Physicians, London) and Pasteur's was a detail from Albert Edelfelt's 1885 painting discussed earlier. Lister's was taken from a photograph.

55. Ibid., 52–53.

56. Ibid., 53. The issue of November 7, 1938, carried several letters to the editor, both pro and con, including one from Irene Castle. The editors printed their own response to Castle's letter and to one claiming that anesthesia was not widely used in animal experiments. Among the more unusual support letters was one from a nun in Los Angeles, writing on behalf of the Franciscan Sisters of the Sacred Heart, "whose lives are devoted to the relief of suffering," to say "thank you for your contribution to the cause of medical science" (2–3).

57. *Life* was not alone among mass magazines in supporting vivisection in this era. Among the many sympathetic articles, I note a photoessay that appeared in *This Week* magazine, a syndicated newspaper supplement for October 26, 1947: James R. Miller, "Vivisection: Lifesaver or Fraud?" 4–5, 20–21. The copy in my collection was distributed with the *Sunday Bulletin,* Philadelphia. A boxed note, captioned "Profit and Loss on Vivisection," set the tone of this article. "Diabetes used to kill everyone it touched. Now insulin is keeping 1,000,000 Americans alive. The cost: 30 dogs. Until a few years ago, blue babies died by the hundreds. Now children . . . are being saved by an intricate new operation. The cost: 75 dogs." One photo of rabbits in a laboratory was captioned "Miracle drugs would be useless if not tested on rabbits first."

58. I suspect that people living on farms and in rural areas had so much exposure to the birth, death, and use of domestic animals (and probably to game animals and vermin as well) that medical experiments on animals were consonant with their experience and prompted no serious distress or indignation. Even in 1940 (fifty years after "the passing of the frontier"), about 44 percent of Americans lived outside cities (23 percent of these lived on farms and 21 percent in nonfarm rural residences). Additionally, a fair share of adult urban dwellers had grown up on farms. See "Population, by Sex, Residence, and Color: 1790 to 1950," U.S. Bureau of the Census, *Historical Statistics of the United States, Colonial Times to 1957* (Washington, D.C., 1960), 9.

59. *Life,* January 4, 1943, 42–43.

60. *Life,* January 3, 1944, 33–34, 37–38.

61. *Life,* March 14, 1949, 105–109. The following year, *Life*'s story about research on an artificial heart device that could temporarily substitute for a living organ opened with pictures of doctors doing surgery and diagrams of the machine and closed with a photograph of three happy dogs that had lived for various intervals of time on a mechanical heart. See "Artificial Heart: Mechanical Device Substitutes for Living Organ," *Life,* May 8, 1950, 90–92.

62. In 1946, the Friends of Medical Research inaugurated a prize named for Nobelist George Hoyt Whipple to honor animals used in experiments. Photographs of two dalmatians, the first recipients, honored for blood-plasma research at a ceremony at the American Museum of Natural History, were printed in newspapers and magazines. For two such photographs, see *New York Times,* February 7, 1946, 30; and Lederer, "Political Animals," 74. From 1946 through 1964, according to Lederer (ibid., 73), the Research Dog Hero Award was given annually by the National Society of Medical Research and publicized with press releases and photographs.

63. "Life on the American Newsfront: 8,000 Doctors Convene at Atlantic City," *Life,* June 21, 1937, 28–29. The letters to the editor can be found in issues of November 7, 1938 (p. 18), and November 21, 1938 (p. 4).

64. *Look,* January 17, 1939, 6–11, and January 31, 1939, 18–21.

65. Fishbein had earlier appeared as the author of a photoessay in *Look* magazine, "A Medical Student Becomes a Doctor: The Life of an Intern," October 25, 1938, 8–11. *Life* had its own photoessay on interns two years later in "The Interne," January 20, 1941, 58–65.

66. *Life,* May 2, 1949, 40–41.

67. *Life,* March 14, 1938, 45–53.

68. Ibid., 45.

69. Ibid., 46.

70. "A Wounded Veteran," *Life,* November 6, 1944, 79–80, 82, 84; "Teaching the Crippled to Walk," *Life,* May 5, 1947, 105–106, 108–111. See also "Hospital Ship Is a Floating Haven for

Navy Wounded," *Life*, January 11, 1943, 71–77; "Flying Nurses Aid U.S. African Campaign," *Life*, April 19, 1943, 41–42; "Repair of the Wounded: Soldiers Help to Heal Themselves," *Life*, July 19, 1943, 36, 39–40, 42; and "Prosthetics: Artificial Arms and Legs Repair the Handicaps of Battle Wounds," *Life*, January 31, 1944, 69–70, 72, 75.

71. "Sister Kenny: Australian Nurse Demonstrates Her Treatment for Infantile Paralysis," *Life*, September 28, 1942, 73–75, 77.

72. For a review of Kenny's career and its significance in the context of late-1940s controversies, see Naomi Rogers, "Sister Kenny Goes to Washington: Polio, Populism, and Medical Politics in Postwar America," in *The Politics of Healing: Histories of Alternative Medicine in Twentieth-Century North America*, ed. Robert D. Johnston, 97–116 (New York: Routledge, 2003). On Kenny, see also John R. Paul, *History of Poliomyelitis* (New Haven, Conn.: Yale University Press, 1971), chap. 32.

73. In the 1940s, Kenny was featured frequently in the popular media. Besides the two magazine issues just mentioned, Kenny's story was told in three different comic books (in 1942, 1944, and 1947), in a radio drama (in 1942), in a popular memoir (1943), and in a Hollywood movie (in 1946).

74. "Healer from the Outback," *Saturday Evening Post*, January 17, 1942, 18–19, 68, 70.

75. More than sixty years later, the stylish upper photograph on the splash page was closely imitated on the cover of *U.S. News and World Report* for April 3, 2006, "The World's First Cancer Vaccines: A Breakthrough That Will Save Thousands of Lives."

76. On this photographer's career, see Fritz Goro, *On the Nature of Things: The Scientific Photography of Fritz Goro* (New York: Aperture, 1993), with introduction by Stephen Jay Gould, biographical essay by Thomas, Peter, and Stefan Goreau, and "commentary by Nobel Prize–winning scientists." The chemists credited for the quinine synthesis were William von Eggers Doering and R. B. Woodward. This report was probably the source for a comic-book story about the synthesis two years later, "Quinine," *Marvels of Science* 2 (April 1946), 28–31, since at least two panel drawings closely match photos in *Life*'s article.

77. *Life*, June 4, 1945, 43–44, 46.

78. Another experiment using human subjects was featured just a few weeks later: "Men Starve in Minnesota: Conscientious Objectors Volunteer for Strict Hunger Tests to Study Europe's Food Problem," *Life*, July 30, 1945, 43–46.

79. *Life*, November 5, 1945, 65–70.

80. "Arthritis: Mayo Clinic Finds a Treatment for Man's Most Crippling Disease," *Life*, June 6, 1949, 106–113.

81. Ibid., 111.

82. *Life*, October 31, 1949, 54–56.

83. *Life*, December 21, 1953, 20–21.

84. Two years later, *Life* ran an article announced with this teaser on the cover: "Surgeon Deplores Blind Fear of Cancer." The surgeon was Dr. George Crile Jr. of the Cleveland Clinic. *Life* gave him this forum for "a broad public hearing" because of "the importance of the subject and the basic disagreement within the medical profession itself." The editors also included an opposing statement by several prominent physicians and eight further views about Crile's argument by individual medical authorities. See "A Plea against Blind Fear of Cancer: An Experienced Surgeon Says That Excessive Worry Leads to Costly Tests, Undue Suffering, and Unnecessary Operations," *Life*, October 31, 1955, 128–130, 132, 134, 139–140, 142.

85. *Life*, June 11, 1956, 151–152, 155–156, 158, 160, 163, 165–166.

86. John Hill of Hill and Knowlton wrote privately, "I think we are [now] on a better footing there." See Hill and Knowlton: Carl Thompson, "Meeting with Representatives of TIRC Members, Thursday, June 7, 1956," June 12, 1956, available online at http://tobaccodocuments. org/ness/4637.html; and Hill and Knowlton: John W. Hill, "re: Campbell-Johnson and British Tobacco People," June 25, 1956, Bates: MWC003510-MWC003511, available online at http://tobaccodocuments.org/ness/28035.html (both accessed June 3, 2008). The TIRC was the Tobacco Industry Research Council. I appreciate Allan Brandt's help in locating these documents.

87. "Clue in the Studies of Smoking Dangers," *Life*, April 22, 1957, 123–124. On the science of cancer etiology in the 1950s, see Colin Talley, Howard I. Kushner, and Claire E. Sterk, "Lung Cancer, Chronic Disease Epidemiology, and Medicine, 1948–1964," *Journal of the History of Medicine and Allied Sciences* 59:3 (July 2004), 329–374. Also relevant are four articles by Allan M. Brandt: "The Cigarette, Risk, and American Culture," *Daedalus* 119 (Fall 1990), 155–176; "'Just Say No': Risk, Behavior, and Disease in Twentieth Century America," in *Scientific Authority and Twentieth Century America,* ed. Ronald G. Walters, 82–98 (Baltimore: Johns Hopkins University Press, 1997); "Blow Some My Way: Passive Smoking, Risk and American Culture," in *Ashes to Ashes: The History of Smoking and Health,* ed. Steven Lock, Lois Reynolds, and E. M. Tansey, 164–191 (Amsterdam and Atlanta, Ga.: Rodopi, 1998); and "The First Surgeon General's Report on Tobacco: Science and the State in the New Age of Chronic Disease," in *Silent Victories: The History and Practice of Public Health in Twentieth-Century America,* ed. John W. Ward and Christian Warren, 437–456 (New York: Oxford University Press, 2007).

88. *Life,* January 24, 1964, 56a–62, 64.

89. "Project Needle-Lollipop: Utah Children Help Test Serum Which May Reduce Effects of Polio," *Life,* September 24, 1951, 71–72 (quotation on 71).

90. *Life,* July 13, 1953, 32–33.

91. *Life,* October 19, 1953, 127–128.

92. *Life,* October 27, 1952, 115–116, 118, 121 (quotation on 115).

93. William L. Laurence, "Vaccine for Polio Successful; Use in 1 to 3 Years Is Likely," *New York Times,* March 27, 1953, 1, 21.

94. "Tracking the Killer," *Life,* February 22, 1954, 120–122, 124, 126, 129–130, 132, 135.

95. "U.S. Gets Set for Polio Vaccine," *Life,* April 11, 1955, 35–39.

96. *Baltimore Sun,* April 12, 1955, 1.

97. "Polio Vaccine a Success," *People's World* (Los Angeles), April 13, 1955, 1.

98. *Life,* April 25, 1955, 36–37.

99. Medicine and science are largely ignored in the (otherwise strong) collection of essays edited by Erika Doss, *Looking at "Life" Magazine.* Bruce Lewenstein's unpublished Ph.D. dissertation and two articles derived from it do call attention to the science stories in *Life*'s first decade, but largely to connect those stories to the careers of Gerard Piel and Dennis Flanagan, who had been science editors at the magazine for a time. See Bruce V. Lewenstein, "Public Understanding of Science in America, 1945–1965" (Ph.D. diss., University of Pennsylvania, 1987); idem, "Magazine Publishing and Popular Science after World War II," *American Journalism* 6:4 (Fall 1989), 218–234; and idem, "The Meaning of 'Public Understanding of Science' in the United States after World War II," *Public Understanding of Science* 1:1 (January 1992), 45–68. Marcel C. LaFollette discusses *Life* in *Making Science Our Own: Public Images of Science, 1910–1955* (Chicago: University of Chicago Press, 1990), but it is not included among the magazines for which she did a thorough content analysis. *Life* is also discussed briefly in John C. Burnham, *How Superstition Won and Science Lost: Popularizing Science and Health in the United States* (New Brunswick, N.J.: Rutgers University Press, 1987), 191–192.

100. For easy comparison, a few examples are noted: Waldemar Kaempffert, "Medical Miracles: Newest Discoveries about Influenza, Cancer, Syphilis, Infantile Paralysis, *Look,* January 28, 1941, 36–41 (a cover story); Robert M. Yoder, "Healer from the Outback: Nurse Kenny, Enemy of Paralysis, Answered Critics with Cures," *Saturday Evening Post,* January 17, 1942, 18–19, 68, 70; Miller, "Vivisection: Lifesaver or Fraud?"; Richard Thruelsen, "Men at Work: Public Health Doctor," *Saturday Evening Post,* May 13, 1950, 36–37, 170; and William Manchester, "The Great Vivisection Dog Fight," *Look,* June 6, 1950, 22–27.

101. For a general exposition, see Stephen P. Weldon, "Secular Humanism," in *The History of Science and Religion in the Western Tradition: An Encyclopedia,* ed. Gary B. Ferngren, 208–213 (New York: Garland, 2000).

102. Alfred C. Kinsey, *Methods in Biology* (Chicago: Lippincott, 1937), 6; I was led to this book by Philip J. Pauly, "The Development of High School Biology, New York City, 1900–1925," *Isis* 82:314 (December 1991), 688.

103. Pauly, "Development of High School Biology," 676.

104. Ibid., 683.

105. For examples, see "These Are 'Angle Shots,'" *Life,* August 30, 1937, 12–13, 15, a feature about press photographers, showing them at work and illustrating the effects of their techniques (angle, lighting, etc.); and "Speaking of Pictures: What's Happening to These Men?" *Life,* November 5, 1951, 22–24, a story about techniques of posing football players for photographs.

106. Piel, "Reminiscences," 45–49.

107. Ibid., supplemented by a personal letter from Mr. Piel, September 7, 2003. See also Lewenstein, "Magazine Publishing," "Meaning of 'Public Understanding of Science'" (especially p. 50), and "Public Understanding of Science."

CHAPTER 10. THE MEANING OF AN ERA

1. "You and Your Doctor," cover story, *Life,* October 12, 1959, 26–27, 144–160.

2. "Big Pill Bill to Swallow," *Life,* February 15, 1960, 97–103.

3. "Doctors and the Rx Scandal: How Some M.D.s Short-Cut Ethics and Profit from Their Own Prescriptions," cover story, *Life,* June 24, 1966, 86–88, 92, 94–96, 98, 100, 102.

4. "Drug That Left a Trail of Heartbreak," *Life,* August 10, 1962, 24–36.

5. Renée C. Fox and Judith Swazey, *Spare Parts: Organ Replacement in American Society* (New York: Oxford University Press, 1992); and Bruce Lewenstein, "Science and the Media," in *Handbook of Science and Technology Studies,* ed. Sheila Jasanoff, Gerald E. Markle, James C. Petersen, and Trevor Pinch, 343–360 (Thousand Oaks, Calif.: Sage, 1995).

6. "Gift of a Human Heart: A Dying Man Lives with a Dead Girl's Heart," cover story, *Life,* December 15, 1967, 23–27.

7. "Houston's Two Master Heart Surgeons Are Locked in a Feud: The Texas Tornado vs. Dr. Wonderful," *Life,* April 10, 1970, 62B–74, with cover caption, "A Bitter Feud: Two Great Surgeons at War over the Human Heart."

8. *Life,* September 17, 1971, 56, 56A–56B, 58, 61–62, 64, 66, 68–70.

9. The filming of *Arrowsmith* was completed before *The Sin of Madelon Claudet,* but *Madelon Claudet* was rushed into an earlier release so that Mayer (and not Goldwyn) would get credit for bringing this famous stage actress to the screen. The popular success of these two films gave Hayes a new reputation, far beyond the circles of legitimate theater.

10. Radio versions of "Arrowsmith" starring Helen Hayes included these broadcasts: *Campbell Playhouse,* dramatized by Orson Welles on February 3, 1939; *Helen Hayes Theater of the Air* on CBS in 1940 and 1941; and *Electric Theater* on CBS in 1948 and 1949. For information about the *Campbell Playhouse* performance, see the RadioGOLDINdex database of old-time radio programs, http://www.radiogoldindex.com/cgi-local/p2.cgi?ProgramName= The+Campbell+Playhouse (accessed June 3, 2008). The two later productions are listed in Donn B. Murphy and Stephen Moore, *Helen Hayes: A Bio-Bibliography* (Westport, Conn.: Greenwood, 1993), 194, 198.

11. See, for example, "Polio: Summer Season Brings Epidemics of This Uncontrollable Disease," *Life,* August 15, 1949, 46–48, 51.

12. Helen Hayes with Katherine Hatch, *My Life in Three Acts* (San Diego: Harcourt Brace Jovanovich, 1990), 175.

13. Jane S. Smith, *Patenting the Sun: Polio and the Salk Vaccine* (New York: William Morrow, 1990), 271; and David M. Oshinsky, *Polio: An American Story* (New York: Oxford University Press, 2005), 86.

14. "Breath of Life" was broadcast on January 17, 1955, and "Hayes Talks" on August 29, 1954; both were on NBC. See Murphy and Moore, *Helen Hayes,* 200–201.

15. Kenneth Barrow, *Helen Hayes, First Lady of the American Theater* (Garden City, N.Y.: Doubleday, 1985), 157. In Hayes's last memoir, we find a slightly different account: "Jonas Salk later told me that press coverage of Mary's death helped him gain financing for his research" (*My Life in Three Acts,* 175).

16. Murphy and Moore, *Helen Hayes,* 200. From the title, one assumes the subject of the drama was the discovery of ether anesthesia in 1846.

17. "Dr. Rebecca Dorsey," with Helen Hayes, in *Hallmark Hall of Fame,* thirty minutes, broadcast on CBS, November 14, 1954, audiotape in author's collection. Other installments in this series during 1954 included stories of Madame Curie, Nurse Edith Cavell (also starring Helen Hayes), Dr. William Mayo, Albert Schweitzer, and William Harvey.

18. This scene resembles one in the 1937 film *The Green Light,* in which locals fear injections for Rocky Mountain spotted fever.

19. *New York Times,* March 30, 1954, 27; the article's spelling errors (Villroth and Koposi) have been silently corrected. See also a shorter obituary in the *Chicago Daily Tribune,* March 30, 1954, A6, which omits any mention of her teachers and credits her primarily with attending the birth of Earl Warren, former governor of California and then chief justice of the U.S. Supreme Court.

20. "Dr. Rebecca Lee Dorsey, Noted Obstetrician, Dies," *Los Angeles Times,* March 30, 1954, 20. This long article is clearly based on a series of three articles that this paper had published a few weeks earlier, based on one or more interviews with Dorsey; see Leonard Wibberley, "Story of Rebecca Lee Dorsey, M.D.," *Los Angeles Times,* February 3 (p. 5), February 4 (p. 5), and February 5, 1954 (p. 5). Dorsey's story was later recovered by reporter Cecilia Rasmussen, who generously shared with me an incomplete copy of Dorsey's unpublished memoir; for this, I extend my thanks to her and to the anonymous owner of that typescript and associated documents from Dorsey's early career. See Cecilia Rasmussen, "L.A. Scene: The City Then and Now; Medical Pioneer's Many Firsts," *Los Angeles Times,* February 3, 1997, B3; and idem, *L.A. Unconventional: The Men and Women Who Did LA Their Way* (Los Angeles: Los Angeles Times, 1998), 2–3.

21. "Anti-toxine in Town," *Los Angles Times,* January 16, 1895, 16.

22. "Helping Pasteur Fight Rabies," *Los Angeles Times,* January 25, 1954, A4.

23. Another example of Dorsey's placing herself into the most direct connection with the greats of medical history is that Dorsey claimed that only two people were injected with tuberculin by Robert Koch himself, Paul Ehrlich and herself (reported in the Wibberley article in the *Los Angeles Times,* February 4, 1954, 5). Needless to say, Koch did not develop his tuberculin until several years after Dorsey had already returned to the United States.

24. Pasteur Foundation Gala, April 19, 2005. Other photographs of the award ceremony may be seen at the Pasteur Foundation website, http://www.pasteurfoundation.org/pictures_gala 2005.html (accessed June 3, 2008).

Armed Forces Institute of Pathology, viii, 33,
  293n11
Army Medical Museum, 32
Arrowsmith (Lewis), 131, 151–152
Arrowsmith (film), 138, 151–153, 262
"Arrowsmith" (radio plays), 157, 262, 269, 327n10
Arrowsmith, Martin (character), 152, 158
arsenic, 143, 145; arsenicals, 240
arthritis, 242–243
artificial hearts, 202, 323n61
artificial limbs, 198. *See also* rehabilitation
  medicine
Asian American health hero, 198
aspirin, discovery of, 166
Atlanta Pasteur Institute, 293n12
"Attempted Assassination of the President"
  (*Frank Leslie's Illustrated Newspaper*), 39
Audit Bureau of Circulation, 311n24
Auenbrugger, Leopold, 307n39
Australia, 149, 196
autoexperimentation. *See* self-experimentation
autojector device, 201
autopsy, 277n61
Avery, Oswald, 296n2

bacterial and viral strains, typing of, 126, 130, 136,
  142, 194, 219, 247, 296n2
bacteriology, medical profession's hesitation
  about, 76–77
"Bad Case of Consumption—Reciprocity
  Lymph, A" (*Puck*), 89, Color Plate 8
Bailey, William C., 86
Bailey, Leslie, vii, 114
Baker, S. Josephine, 116, 158, 270, 307n33
Baltimore Pasteur Institute, 293n12
Balto, the sled dog, 190–191; scrapbook of
  clippings about, 315n76
Banting, Frederick G., 226, 307n33, 307n39
Barnard, Christiaan, 257–258
Barnum, P. T., 286n9
Barnum's American Museum, 65
Barrymore, Lionel, 264
Barton, Clara, 158, 193, 307n33
Baruch, Bernard, 198
Basalla, George, 202, 309n2
Bayer Aspirin, 166
beard as a symbol of a physician, 14, 24, 135
Beaumont, William, 26, 32, 136, 166, 283n47
beer and wine, preservation of, 45
Beerbohm, Robert, 310n4
Behring, Emil von, 94, 185, 264, 305n18, 307n39
Bell, Alexander Graham, 38–39

Bell, Charlie, 251
Bell, Clark, 17
Bellevue Hospital (New York), 22–24
Bell Syndicate, 313n41
Bennett, James Gordon, Jr., 48, 72
Bergh, Henry, 78, 285n9
Bergmann, Ernest von, 87
beri-beri, 185
Berliner Illustrirte Zeitung, 212
Bernard, Claude, 160, 168
Bernhardt, Sarah, 105
Bernstein, Roslyn, viii
Best, Charles, 307n33
Bethune, Norman, 159, 270
bichloride of gold, 91
Biggs, Hermann M., 77, 92, 279n8, 285n6,
  291n49
Billings, Frank Seaver, 55, 58, 62, 66, 76, 161
Billroth, Theodor, 264
biographical films. *See* biopics
biography as a form of medical history, 150–153
biologics, 106, 107, 109–110, 241, 305n18; produc-
  tion by health departments, 110; production
  by pharmaceutical companies, 110
biopics, 137, 143; historical inaccuracies in,
  302n55. *See also individual film titles*
biopsy, 215–217
birth defects, 257
Birth of a Baby, The (documentary film), 223
Bitterroot Valley, 141–142
Black Star magazine, 251
Blackwell, Elizabeth, 26, 158, 193, 270, 307n33
Blackwell, Emily, 26
Blackwell's Island institutions (New York), 21,
  86, 274n31
Blaine, James G. (in cartoon), 56, 89, 281n28
Blainiac rabies, 56, Color Plate 5
Blake, professor at Yale, 90
Blake, William E., 311n21
blindness, 116
blind patient in *Dr. Ehrlich's Magic Bullet*, 145
Bliss, D. Willard, 14
blood. *See* horses used in production of serum;
  transfusion of blood
blood plasma, 308n39
blue-baby breakthrough, 3, 80, 227–228
"Blue Baby Research" (*Life*), 228
Blustein, Bonnie Ellen, 288n25
Boaz, Franz, 183
Bodas, Carol, viii
Book of Marvels, The (Williams), 128–129
Boston Evening Transcript, 134–135

ABOUT THE AUTHOR

BERT HANSEN teaches American history and the history of medicine at Baruch College of the City University of New York. He holds degrees from Columbia College and Princeton University. His publications include *Nicole Oresme and the Marvels of Nature* (on scholasticism and science in the fourteenth century) and articles on various subjects in the nineteenth and twentieth centuries, such as public-health cartoons, medical education, physicians' views on homosexuality, popular images of laboratory science, and the careers of gay and lesbian physicians. His research has appeared in the *American Historical Review,* the *American Journal of Public Health,* the *Bulletin of the History of Medicine, History Now,* and other journals and books. One of his articles received an award for excellence in medical writing, and three others were reprinted in undergraduate textbooks: *Good Writing, Major Problems in the History of American Medicine and Public Health,* and *Sickness and Health in America.* He has taught at SUNY-Binghamton, the University of Toronto, and New York University.